Theoretical Basis of
OCCUPATIONAL
THERAPY

Third Edition

Theoretical Basis of OCCUPATIONAL THERAPY Third Edition

Mary Ann McColl, PhD, MTS
Associate Director, Centre for Health Services and Policy Research
Professor, Rehabilitation Therapy/Public Health Science
Queen's University
Kingston, Ontario, Canada

Mary Law, PhD, FCAOT
Professor Emeritus
School of Rehabilitation Science
McMaster University
Hamilton, Ontario, Canada

Debra Stewart, MSc
Associate Professor
School of Rehabilitation Science
McMaster University
Hamilton, Ontario, Canada

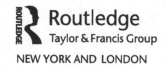
Routledge
Taylor & Francis Group

NEW YORK AND LONDON

First published 2015 by SLACK Incorporated

Published 2024 by Routledge
605 Third Avenue, New York, NY 10158

and by Routledge
4 Park Square, Milton Park, Abingdon, Oxon OX14 4RN

Routledge is an imprint of the Taylor & Francis Group, an informa business

Copyright © 2015 Taylor & Francis Group.

Library of Congress Cataloging-in-Publication Data
McColl, Mary Ann, 1956- , author.
  The theoretical basis of occupational therapy / Mary Ann McColl, Mary Law, Debra Stewart. -- 3rd edition.
      p. ; cm.
  Preceded by Theoretical basis of occupational therapy / Mary Ann McColl ... [et al.]. 2nd ed. c2003.
  Includes bibliographical references and index.
   ISBN 978-1-61711-602-5 (paperback : alk. paper)
  I. Law, Mary C., author. II. Stewart, Debra, 1954- , author. III. Title.
  [DNLM: 1. Occupational Therapy. WB 555]
  Z6665.O2
  615.8'515--dc23

                        2014042144

  ISBN: 9781617116025 (pbk)
  ISBN: 9781003526742 (ebk)

  DOI: 10.4324/9781003526742

CONTENTS

Acknowledgments

On behalf of the authors, I would like to thank several individuals who contributed very significantly to the completion of this book. We were fortunate to have the assistance of two student research assistants who painstakingly assembled the dataset that served as the basis for this book: Christine Gallah and Ishanee Jahagirdar.

We thank the contributing authors for their thoughtful chapters, and their assistance in developing the themes in this book. We appreciate those who have been with us from the beginning and have adapted their chapters for each successive edition. We also appreciate those who have come to this project with fresh eyes and a new perspective. We acknowledge the contributions of authors in previous editions, such as Lorna Doubt and Penny Bryden, whose efforts continue to be reflected in this version.

As in all my undertakings, I owe a huge debt of gratitude to my administrative research assistant, Lynn Roberts. She made countless contributions to this book, some obvious, such as the references and appendices, and some subtle, such as tactful correspondence, daily support, and astute observations.

On a personal note, I extend my sincere thanks to the students of Queen's University Occupational Therapy Class of 2015. We were together in an introductory theory course throughout the writing of this book. Their passion for their new careers, their earnest and probing questions, and their generous attention have contributed in innumerable ways to this third edition.

Mary Ann McColl, PhD, MTS

ABOUT THE AUTHORS

Mary Ann McColl, PhD, MTS is a Professor in Rehabilitation Therapy and Associate Director of the Centre for Health Services and Policy Research at Queen's University, Kingston, Ontario. She is also the Academic Lead of the Canadian Disability Policy Alliance.

Mary Law, PhD, FCAOT is a Professor Emeritus in the School of Rehabilitation Science, Occupational Therapy Program and co-founder of the *CanChild* Centre for Childhood Disability Research at McMaster University, Hamilton, Ontario.

Debra Stewart, MSc is an Associate Professor in the School of Rehabilitation Science, Occupational Therapy Program and an a investigator with the *CanChild* Centre for Childhood Disability Research at McMaster University, Hamilton, Ontario.

Contributing Authors

Briano Di Rezze, PhD, OT Reg. (Ont.) (Chapter 11) is an Assistant Professor in the School of Rehabilitation Science and Scientist at the *CanChild* Centre for Childhood Disability Research at McMaster University, Hamilton, Ontario.

Terry Krupa, PhD, OT Reg. (Ont.), FCAOT (Chapter 10) is a Professor in the School of Rehabilitation Therapy at Queen's University, Kingston, Ontario. She holds cross-appointments in both the Department of Psychiatry and the School of Nursing at Queen's University.

Nancy Pollock, MSc, OT Reg. (Ont.) (Chapter 5) is an Associate Clinical Professor in the School of Rehabilitation Science and a Scientist with the *CanChild* Centre for Childhood Disability Research, both at McMaster University, Hamilton, Ontario. She practices clinically with REACH Therapy Services.

Michelle Villeneuve, PhD, MSc, BSc OT (Chapter 12) is an academic and researcher in the Faculty of Health Sciences and an Associate of the Center for Disability Research and Policy at the University of Sydney, New South Wales, Australia. She is also cross-appointed to the School of Rehabilitation Therapy at Queen's University, Kingston, Ontario.

Preface

"He who loves practice without theory
is like a sailor who boards ship
without a rudder and compass,
and never knows where he may cast."

Leonardo da Vinci

Who would have thought that in the 8 years since the publication of the second edition of this book, the world would have changed so dramatically for students of occupational therapy? When we prepared the annotated bibliography that was a major part of the second edition, it still seemed like a significant contribution to making life easier for scholars and researchers. Now, not even a decade later, the concept of an annotated bibliography in hard copy is an anachronism. Why would anyone buy a book that does for them what they can do with a few keystrokes at their desktop computer, sitting in their pajamas at home with a cup of tea? We could not even imagine 10 years ago the ease with which students and other researchers access occupational therapy literature today.

So when the publishers told us they were sold out of the second edition and asked if we would consider a third, we realized that this meant considering a whole different type of book. Instead of an annotated bibliography, we had to offer something more than the casual searcher could readily find with a few quick search terms. We had to offer an analysis and synthesis that added value to this search process. Furthermore, with searching made so easy and democratic, we had to offer a search that had very explicit parameters so that readers could have confidence in what was covered and what was not. Finally, we had to bring to the enterprise a clear and compelling organizational structure that would make it all make sense.

With that in mind, we offer a third edition of *Theoretical Basis of Occupational Therapy* that we hope maintains some of its more effective features from previous editions and adds new features that ensure its continued relevance. In addition to updating the database of articles to 2012, we have done the following:

- Preserved the overall organizational structure, looking both at determinants and consequences of occupation
- Further developed the three metaphors—the filing cabinet, the toolbox, and the telescope—that helped us to organize and retrieve occupational therapy theory
- Invited contributing authors from previous editions to update their chapters and added new authors to supplement content
- Added sections about the major named occupational therapy models that are increasingly part of our dialogue

Instead of an annotated bibliography, we offer an appendix that catalogues the literature we have included. In each of the "determinants" chapters, we have asked invited authors to extract key themes, follow threads of theoretical development, reflect on external influences on occupational therapy theory, and comment particularly on developments since 2000. We hope that this edition contributes to the ongoing debates and developments in occupational therapy theory and raises at least as many questions as it answers!

Mary Ann McColl, PhD, MTS

Section I

Introduction

Determinants of Occupation

- Physical
- Psychological-Emotional
- Sociocultural
- Cognitive-Neurological
- Environmental

Occupation

- Self-care
- Productivity
- Leisure

Consequences of Occupation

- Health
- Well-Being
- Participation
- Community integration

1

Introduction

Mary Ann McColl, PhD, MTS

This is an introductory textbook to help occupational therapy (OT) students to understand how to think about occupation, the many factors that affect occupation, and how to use occupation therapeutically to promote health and well-being.

This is the third edition of this book. The aim of all three editions has been to help OT students, researchers, and clinicians by collecting together advances in theory published in the peer-reviewed literature. The first and second editions accomplished this task by providing annotated bibliographies of selected theoretical articles—from 1900 to 1990 for the first edition and from 1975 to 2000 for the second edition. In the third edition, we have taken account of the fact that the world has changed dramatically in terms of access to peer-reviewed literature. No longer is it necessary to go to the "stacks" of the library to consult bound editions of old journals or hard copies of current journals; neither is it necessary to order through inter-library loan copies of articles contained in journals not housed in the local library. Now we can each literally sit at our desktops and call up copies of articles of interest. What then is the relevant contribution of a book like this when the peer-reviewed literature is so readily available?

Like the two previous editions, this book offers "students" of OT, whether they be new recruits to the profession or lifelong learners, the results of an exhaustive review of international peer-reviewed literature in OT. We have searched 13 journals over 13 years (2000-2012) to provide a synthesis of current theoretical developments in OT and occupational science. According to Lee (2010), theory is typically presented in OT in the form of books, often by the authors of the theory itself. Peer-reviewed literature, on the other hand, offers a more democratic and critical perspective on theory:

- It invites a broader spectrum of participants into the debate on theory. One need not necessarily be able to write a whole book to participate in the debate on theory; one need only be able to prepare a journal article, typically some 3000 to 5000 words.

- Journal articles as a source for theory have the advantage of quality control; they undergo a degree of scrutiny in order to be published that is more rigorous than that done for books. The peer-review standards used by the 13 journals included in this book were sufficiently high to qualify them to be included in the Cumulative Index to Nursing and Allied Health Literature (CINAHL), one of the premier library databases in the health and social sciences. Peer review is the industry standard for quality and credibility and is usually interpreted as a proxy for the quality of the evidence and the absence of an editorial bias. Although books do undergo some degree of peer review at the publisher, there is more tolerance for an individual perspective or approach to be expressed in a book than in a journal article.

- Journal articles also tend to be more current and topical. It is considerably more timely to publish findings in a journal than in a book. Even with a journal there is some delay to allow for the peer-review process and administrative handling; however, especially with electronic journals, the time from submission to publication is always decreasing, to an average of about 3 months currently.

McColl MA, Law M, Stewart D.
Theoretical Basis of Occupational Therapy, Third Edition (pp. 3-6).
© 2015 Taylor & Francis Group.

This book also offers a classification system for theory, a digest of new developments in each area of the classification system, and a commentary on theoretical developments across theory areas that advance the knowledge and expertise of the profession as a whole.

Five Types of Knowledge Needed to Be an Occupational Therapist

In order to be an occupational therapist, five types of knowledge are required:

1. Knowledge about humans
2. Knowledge about our environments
3. Knowledge about disability
4. Knowledge about occupation
5. Knowledge about the therapeutic use of self

Knowledge About Humans

We need to understand human beings on all levels, from biological and psychological to sociological and anthropological. We need to understand how the human body and mind work; what keeps humans healthy and what makes them sick. We need to know the consequences of illness or injury and what can be done to help. We need to understand how humans relate to one another, how they behave in social circumstances, and how they participate in groups and societies.

Knowledge About Our Environments

Second, we need to understand the environments that humans participate in and the effects those environments have on them. Environments can be physical, such as buildings or landscapes; they can be social, such as families or peer groups; they can be institutional, such as workplaces or health care settings; or they can be societal, such as values systems or governments. Environments can be proximal to a person or distal; they can be hostile or friendly, reciprocal or authoritarian. We need to understand how different types and features of environments affect human beings and their health and well-being.

Knowledge About Disability

Third, we need to understand disability. *Disability* is broadly defined in terms of an activity or activities that individuals are unable to do, either because of impairment or because of an environment that does not adequately accommodate them (or both). Occupational therapists help others to "do," so people with disabilities are at the heart of OT, the primary clients of occupational therapists. Disability affects a person on many levels—physically, psychologically, socially, economically, vocationally, and spiritually. Occupational therapists need to understand all of these effects if they are to provide comprehensive, holistic care.

Knowledge About Occupation

Fourth, and not surprisingly, occupational therapists need to understand *occupation*—the things a person does that fill his or her time and give his or her life shape, context, and meaning. We typically classify occupations as self-care, productivity, and leisure, but occupation is much more than that. It includes both subjective and objective components; it strives for a balance that is compatible with health and wellness; it changes over the life course to meet the different needs of each life stage. The remainder of this book is devoted to understanding how occupational therapists think about the stunning complexity of occupation.

Knowledge About the Therapeutic Use of Self

Finally, we need a fifth and final area of knowledge in order to be effective occupational therapists. We need to know ourselves as *therapeutic agents*. We need to understand what it is about us that permits others to take chances, to make changes, to face challenges. It is not something someone else can tell us; we each have to figure it out for ourselves, and we spend the entirety of our professional careers doing so. It is, however, essential to being a good therapist—knowing whether it is your compassion, your sense of humor, your enthusiasm, your can-do attitude, or some other aspect of your personality that is your greatest asset as a therapist. This is often referred to as the "therapeutic use of self."

Occupational therapists use these five kinds of knowledge in every aspect of their professional lives, in every decision they make, in every observation they record.

- They use it to notice what is going on with patients, how they are functioning, and where their problems appear to originate.
- They use it to select the appropriate assessments to apply and to delve deeper into the scope, nature, and magnitude of the problems that clients bring.
- They use it to interpret the findings of their assessments and to synthesize an understanding of the factors affecting occupational performance and the potential for therapeutic effects.
- They use it to select possible intervention approaches, to estimate the prognosis for recovery, and to understand the impacts and consequences of particular therapeutic approaches.

This knowledge is acquired in a number of different ways throughout one's lifetime, such as during initial professional education; through experiences as occupational therapists; through our interactions with clients and their families; through our relationships with other professionals; through continuing education, workshops, journals, and books; and through life experiences, with maturity. In the absence of a way to file and organize all of this information, obtained at different times and in different ways, the result is a jumble of theoretical knowledge, somewhat akin to a big box of treasures acquired over a lifetime and stored in a cupboard or attic. The prospect of finding the thing you need in the box is daunting, requiring you to pull everything out and deal with the mess that you find. This prospect often puts one off from even looking, and instead we simply do without.

The parallel with OT theory goes like this: We know that we have learned something at some point in our education, continuing education, or other life experiences that will help with a particular situation, but we do not know where to find it or the details of it. The prospect of combing through our old notes, textbooks, and course handouts is akin to the prospect of going up to the attic and pawing through that big box of memorabilia. Instead, we come to simply do without theory. We operate intuitively based on what bubbles to the top of our memory, without attribution of ideas to their proper sources and without consideration of the corollaries and implications of those ideas. We justify this approach by calling it "eclectic."

What this book offers is not a new theory of OT but rather a way to gather, organize, and analyze the growing body of theory that each occupational therapist carries with him or her about humans, their occupations, and their environments. *Theory* refers to organized systems of ideas used to help explain or predict how things work. It has been defined in previous editions of this book as "tools for thinking" that offer us some degree of explanation for why things are the way they are. Theories are seldom "proven," but they are usually supported to a greater or lesser extent by research. Research provides evidence either for or against the claims a theory makes about why things are the way they are.

Theories are typically made up of concepts and principles. *Concepts* are important words that provide mental representations of the "things" the theory explains. *Principles* are statements about the relationships between concepts. Most people have heard of Einstein's theory of relativity. A small part of the full theory is this deceptively simple equation: $E=mc^2$. The theory represented by this equation is made up of three concepts: energy (E), mass (m), and the speed of light (c). The theory states the principle about the relationship between those three concepts; specifically,

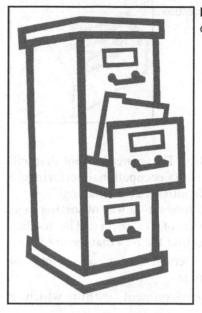

Figure 1-1. Filing cabinet.

that the energy produced by an object is related to the mass of the object multiplied by a constant factor—the speed of light, squared (c^2).

OT theory is also made up of concepts and principles. We do not usually express OT theory as equations, but we often show diagrams with arrows and lines connecting concepts and suggesting relationships among those concepts. Chapter 6 gives a number of examples of these types of diagrams. Theory helps occupational therapists to understand and to explain to others how we think about the relationships among important ideas, such as people, environments, and occupations; roles, habits, and skills; or sensation, tone, and movement.

Instead of carrying the five types of knowledge that occupational therapists need in an overwhelming jumble, we offer a virtual filing cabinet (Figure 1-1), wherein all of the knowledge that OTs acquire can be dutifully filed with related and compatible ideas so as to be readily available when needed. Each of the drawers of the filing cabinet corresponds to an important area of OT theory, and once we decide which drawer to open, all of the necessary information is there for our perusal. These drawers contain the ideas, assumptions, experiences, and learning that we acquire over the course of our education and our lifetime in practice. They help us make therapeutic decisions and understand our observations.

For that reason, we can think of them as tools for thinking and tools for acting therapeutically to improve occupation. Therefore, within each drawer, we need a toolbox that helps us to find the right theoretical tool for the job at hand. Do we need a tool that will help us observe the strengths and weaknesses of a person's occupational performance, or the stage and acuity of

Figure 1-2. Toolbox.

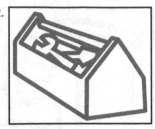

their illness or disability? Do we need a tool that will help us change the person's occupational performance or correct specific difficulties they are having?

We offer just such a toolbox—a way of sorting tools within a particular area of OT theory. The toolbox (Figure 1-2) helps us to find the tool that we need:

- To assess the person from a variety of different perspectives
- To assess the environment within which a person functions
- To assess the occupational performance of the person and any problems he or she may be experiencing
- To act therapeutically to correct dysfunction in the person
- To adapt or advocate for changes in the environment within which a person functions
- To intervene to improve occupation

Finally, in order to select the right theory and the right tools to be most helpful to a particular patient, we need a series of lenses that help sharpen our focus on the client and his or her needs (Figure 1-3). First and foremost, we need a lens that focuses on the client's occupation and occupational performance problems. Next we need to see the client in a lifespan perspective to understand his or her developmental stage and the particular issues and challenges that characterize it. The third focusing ring is a lens to help us consider the origins of the occupational performance problems. Do they originate in the person or in the environment? If they originate in the environment, which aspect of the environment is responsible—human or nonhuman, constructed or natural, proximal or distal? If they originate in the person, which component of the person seems most responsible—physical, psychological-emotional, sociocultural, or cognitive-neurological?

The fourth focusing lens relates to the tools and aptitudes available on the therapist's part to render assistance. For a person with a particular occupational performance problem, at a particular stage in life, with

problems originating from difficulties in a particular system or area of the environment, what types of assessments and treatments do we have at our disposal to assist? Finally, what outcome do we expect when we apply these tools under these circumstances? Where do we expect to get to, and in what interval of time, with what frequency and intensity of therapy?

Summary

This chapter introduced three metaphors that help occupational therapists know how to think and what to do for clients coming to them with occupational performance problems. It offers the filing cabinet as a way of storing, sorting, and retrieving all the important knowledge that occupational therapists carry with them. It offers the toolbox as a way of sorting the tools that are contained within each drawer of the filing cabinet—tools for thinking and tools for acting. Third, it offers the telescope (see Figure 1-3) as a way of sharpening our focus on the clients to help us select and coordinate the use of this knowledge and these tools.

As a final note about this book, we talk about formal theories that are published and known to us by a particular name, and we also talk about ideas, assumptions, experiences, and learning that we have acquired over the course of our educations and our lifetimes in practice. Both of these help us make therapeutic decisions and understand our observations. We refer to these two classes of theory as "big-T theory" and "small-t theory":

- "Big-T theory"—Theories that are formalized and widely known by a particular name, such as the Model of Human Occupation or the cognitive-behavioral approach
- "Small-t theory"—Fragments of important knowledge that have not been collected and formalized but are no less influential and informative in our daily functioning as occupational therapists.

Figure 1-3. Telescope.

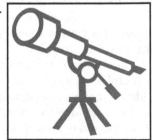

2

Development of This Book

Mary Ann McColl, PhD, MTS

What we have tried to do in this book is provide an introductory resource that builds on the previous two editions and categorizes and classifies theoretical literature published in the 20th and 21st centuries to date. This book, like the previous two, operates on a unique classification system that focuses on the determinants of occupation: physical, psychological-emotional, sociocultural, cognitive-neurological, and environmental. We use that classification system to offer ready access to new theoretical developments about the factors that affect occupation.

At the root of the organizational structure of this book is a set of beliefs about occupation that is derived from the literature in occupational therapy (OT) since the beginning of the 20th century. These ideas will be further developed in subsequent chapters, but for introductory purposes, let us simply say that occupational therapists believe the following:

- That occupation affects health
- That person and environment factors affect occupation
- That the person can be understood in terms of his or her physical, psychological-emotional, cognitive-neurological, and sociocultural components
- That the environment consists of physical, social, and societal influences
- That OT can affect the relationship of determinants to occupation and thereby ultimately affect health and well-being (Figure 2-1)

Chapters 3 and 4 introduce the two metaphors that are central to the organization of this book and to the way of thinking about OT theory that we propose: the toolbox and the filing cabinet. Their utility in studying and using OT theory throughout one's career is described in detail. Chapters 5 and 6 focus on the consequences of occupation: its relationship to health, well-being, participation, and community integration. Chapter 5 discusses the concept of occupation itself and historic developments through the 20th and 21st centuries. Chapter 6 deals with models that attempt to explain the relationship of occupation to health. These are referred to in other texts as "occupation-focused models." The chapter reviews a number of models most commonly seen in the literature and in practice. They are named theories that are widely recognized within the profession and typically associated with a cadre of authors. For each of these theories we provide a basic description of its historical development, its key concepts, and its fundamental principles. Consistent with the purpose of this book, we also provide a detailed analysis of theoretical developments published in the peer-reviewed OT literature since 2000.

Chapters 7 through 11 focus on the determinants of occupation—that is, those factors that affect occupation. These five chapters explore contemporary developments in theory within the professional OT literature about the determinants of occupation. This theory helps us understand possible factors responsible for things that may go wrong with a person's occupation or occupational performance. These determinants help us generate hypotheses about *why* a person might be experiencing a problem in occupational performance. Furthermore, they give us a starting place to begin considering how we might intervene to help overcome the problem.

McColl MA, Law M, Stewart D.
Theoretical Basis of Occupational Therapy, Third Edition (pp. 7-11).
© 2015 Taylor & Francis Group.

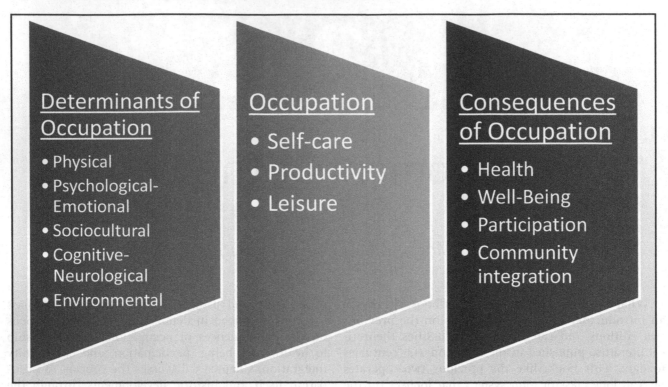

Figure 2-1. The determinants and consequences of occupation.

Each of these chapters explores one of the five determinants and the current state of knowledge about how it affects occupation. Each chapter was motivated by the following questions:

- What do we know about the physical, psychological-emotional, sociocultural, cognitive-neurological, environmental determinants of occupation?
- What physical, psychological-emotional, sociocultural, cognitive-neurological, environmental factors affect occupation, and what do we know about how they affect it?

It is important to stipulate that we are focusing on theory rather than "evidence" here—looking at models of the determinants of occupation rather than research evidence in support of individual factors.

Chapters 12 through 14 address models of practice and of service in OT. The bulk of the book to this point talks about how occupational therapists *think*, but these three chapters talk about what occupational therapists *do* and how theory helps them know *what* to do. In Chapter 12, we examine the third metaphor, the telescope, that helps us focus all this knowledge when addressing the problems of a particular client. In Chapter 13, we consider common modes of intervention used by occupational therapists, and in Chapter 14, we look at how occupational therapists interact with their clients and the organizations and systems within which they work.

Search Strategy

For Chapters 5 through 11, current information about OT theory was derived from an exhaustive search of the peer-reviewed literature in OT. The key database used for this search was the Cumulative Index of Nursing and Allied Health Literature (better known as CINAHL). Searches were limited to the English language and humans. The search focused on 13 years, from January 2000 to December 2012, and the 13 major OT journals listed in Table 2-1.

The articles that constitute the basis for this book were searched for initially using the keywords *occupation* and *occupational performance*. This preliminary cut at the published literature aimed to identify articles that attempted to explain or describe the key concepts of occupation and occupational performance. In other words, an article had to mention *occupation* or *occupational performance* in the title, the abstract, or the keywords in order to be eligible for further consideration in this book. I think the reader will agree that this is a basic condition for OT theory and would not prove too exclusionary when applied to the literature.

The search produced the following results: 889 articles were found that were considered to pertain directly to either occupation or occupational performance (see Table 2-1). The term *occupation* produced more results (673) than *occupational performance* (295).

Table 2-1
Results of the Literature Search by Journal

	Occupation	OP*	Either
British Journal of Occupational Therapy	110	45	140
American Journal of Occupational Therapy	89	54	134
Journal of Occupational Science	108	5	110
OTJR: Occupation, Participation and Health	80	31	100
Scandinavian Journal of Occupational Therapy	58	37	83
Canadian Journal of Occupational Therapy	50	36	76
Average	**51.8**	**22.7**	**68.4**
Australian Occupational Therapy Journal	43	21	62
Occupational Therapy in Health Care	35	14	42
Occupational Therapy International	22	20	41
Occupational Therapy in Mental Health	32	8	37
Physical and Occupational Therapy in Geriatrics	23	13	33
Physical and Occupational Therapy in Pediatrics	14	9	20
New Zealand Journal of Occupational Therapy	9	2	11
Total	**673**	**295**	**889**

*OP: occupational performance.

Four journals produced at least 100 articles each: *British Journal of Occupational Therapy, American Journal of Occupational Therapy, Journal of Occupational Science,* and *OTJR: Occupation, Participation and Health.* The average number of articles per journal was 68.4. Similarly, the average number of articles per year for the 13 years of the search was also 68.4.

For Chapter 6, on occupation-focused models, the titles of the models discussed were entered as keywords into the database for the period and journals specified. For Chapters 7 through 11, on the determinants of occupation, keywords were identified in collaboration with the chapters' authors and searched from the total set of 889 (Table 2-2). Based on these searches, the authors were provided with lists of annotated references pertaining to their theory areas (as well as copies of the first and second editions of this book).

On the basis of titles, abstracts, and keywords (sorted by relevance), authors indicated which articles they considered to represent a new contribution to theory in their area. Articles were included in the chapter if they did the following:

- Expressly mentioned a specific theory or a key concept of the pertinent theory area in the title, abstract, or keywords

- Developed, elaborated, or explained an idea that guides or underpins the practice of OT

Articles excluded from consideration were those designed as follows:

- Measurement studies or evaluations of psychometric properties of assessments related to a particular model or theory area

- Applications of a model or theoretical idea to a special population or setting

- Research studies testing the tenets of a theory

In most instances, it was possible to tell from the conclusion of the abstract if the article was aimed at advancing theory or providing a specific piece of evidence for a single theoretical principle.

Language

A final word about the language used in this book. We have chosen the language for this book in a very purposeful fashion. First, with regard to theory, we have attempted to avoid a proliferation of terminology. We do not use the terms *paradigm* or *frame of reference.* Instead, we use only two terms to talk about theory:

- Conceptual models—referring to models that help us to THINK

		Table 2-2
		Search Terms Used in Literature Search
Chapter	**Topic**	**Keywords: Occupation OR Occupational Performance AND...**
8	Occupation-focused models	Occupational Behavior, Model of Human Occupation, Canadian Model of Occupational Performance, Occupational Adaptation, occupational science, occupational justice, occupational identity, Ecology of Human Performance, Person-Environment-Occupation, Person-Environment-Occupational Performance
9	Sociocultural	Balance, belief, culture, family, group, habit, meaning, role, routine, social, society, spirituality, time, temporal, value
10	Psychological-emotional	Affect, agency, behavior, cognition, coping, emotion, interpersonal, identity, locus of control, mood, motivation, self-perceptions, self-awareness, self-esteem, self-efficacy, social, thoughts
11	Physical	Assistive devices, biomechanical, cardiovascular, compensation, endurance, energy conservation, fatigue, hand function, musculoskeletal, rehabilitation, remediation, range of motion, respiratory, skin, strength
12	Cognitive-neurological	Arousal, awareness, attention, central nervous system, cognition, coordination, executive, function, integration, memory, pain, plasticity, perception, spasticity, tone
13	Environmental	Access, accommodations, attitudes, barriers, built environment, disability supports, ecology, environmental adaptation, expectations, micro-, meso-, macro-environment, policy, services, systems, stigma, social support, tools, technology

- **Models of practice**—referring to models that tell us what to DO

Conceptual models are made up of *concepts* and *principles* (or statements about the relationships between concepts), and models of practice are made up of *assessments* and *interventions*. In this way, we have sought to use language that is descriptive and meaningful, to use terms that are already in our lexicon and avoid coining new terms, and to be consistent and predictable in our use of language. We do this to ease the burden on readers, but we also encourage readers to determine the terminology that fits best with their practice setting and regulatory requirements.

We also talk about theory that helps us understand the determinants and consequences of occupation:

- **Determinants of occupation**—These refer to the five factors that affect occupation: four aspects of the person (physical, psychological-emotional, cognitive-neurological, and sociocultural) and the environment. Each theory area contains all that we know about each of these determinants: How does the *physical* aspect of the person affect occupation? How does the *psychological-emotional* aspect,

sociocultural aspect, or *cognitive-neurological* aspect of the person affect his or her occupation? How does the *environment* affect occupation?

- **Consequences of occupation**—We have also observed through our literature searches that occupational therapists seek to help their clients achieve a finite but broad-reaching set of overall goals. They seek to restore their clients' health, promote their sense of well-being, enable their full participation and citizenship, and enhance their integration in the community. We refer to these broad outcomes as the consequences of occupation, because occupational therapists believe that these positive states are the result of a balanced and meaningful portfolio of occupations.

We are aware that there is considerable sensitivity regarding language that refers to *disability*. Some individuals and groups prefer what has come to be known as "people-first" language (that is, "people with disabilities"), whereas others state a strong preference to be referred to as disabled people. We use both forms interchangeably. Our guiding principle is "inclusivity." We seek to use language that invites others into the dialogue and welcomes a variety of perspectives. We refer to federal guidelines for nondiscriminatory language. We seek neutrality and clarity of communication in language and defer to the language preferences of the disability groups with whom we interact.

With regard to the recipients of OT services, again there is no consensus about the correct terminology for all settings. The term *client* appears to be most common in the OT literature; however, strictly speaking, it is inaccurate in many instances. Throughout the book, we attempt to use the following terminology:

- *Patient*, when referring to someone who is admitted to a health care facility
- *Resident*, when referring to someone in a long-term care or community residential facility
- *Client*, when referring to someone living in the community who engages the services of an occupational therapist
- *Consumer*, when referring to someone who is a member of a rights movement or group or a recipient of services from a community group embracing an independent living philosophy

With regard to cultural considerations, we acknowledge the presence of a Western cultural bias. This coincides with the largely North American and European origins of the profession of OT. It further reflects the sources of peer-reviewed OT literature in journals from Western nations. We strive for cultural sensitivity and cultural competence in all of our discussions.

Finally, with regard to the tone of the discourse in this book, we have sought above all to make it accessible and explanatory. It has been referred to as conversational in tone and has been critiqued both for being too complex and too simplistic! This leads us to believe that we have found just the right tone. This book is primarily an introductory textbook for OT students, whether they are undergraduate or graduate students. We do not wish to detract from the complexity of ideas by making the discussion too simple, nor do we wish to complicate ideas that are elegant and straightforward. We have tried to be direct and accurate. It is our contention that if one truly understands something, then one can communicate it simply and effectively. We seek to provide discussions that help occupational therapists communicate the ideas that guide them not only to other occupational therapists but also to clients and their families, to other professionals, and to administrators and payers.

3

The Occupational Therapy Toolbox

Mary Ann McColl, PhD, MTS

In the previous chapter, we referred to an occupational therapy (OT) toolbox (Figure 3-1). The toolbox is a metaphor for a system to sort the various types of tools that occupational therapists have at their disposal. Like the toolbox of a carpenter, our toolbox helps us to find the tool that we need to be able to think about the client, the problem, and its context. Just like in carpentry, tools do not do the job by themselves, but they assist us to do it. It is possible to use a number of different tools to do the same job; however, the correct tool does the job best and makes it easiest. Conversely, one tool may have applications in a variety of different situations. Different workers will have preferences for particular tools, with which they are most comfortable and familiar. Some people try to use the same tool for every application. I am sure you have seen people use a screwdriver to take the lid off a paint tin, to pry two surfaces apart, or to scrape off old paint. On the other hand, I am sure you have seen people use a knife or a dime to do the job of a screwdriver. If the only tool you have is a hammer, it is amazing how every problem begins to look like a nail!

The carpentry metaphor demonstrates the flexibility of tools, but it also shows how tools become compromised when used in applications for which they were not intended. Occupational therapists have at their disposal a broad array of tools, some of which are more appropriate for specific occupational problems than others. Most occupational therapists have favorite tools, preferences usually based on the area in which therapists practice, the tools favored by their colleagues, the tools that were prevalent when they were educated, the accessibility of particular tools, and the opportunities available to learn more about the tools.

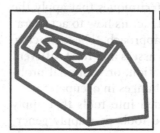

Figure 3-1. Toolbox.

OT tools may be separated into two main groups: tools to help us *understand occupation* and tools to help us *change occupation*. The former offer us ways to think about occupation, and the latter offer us ways to act therapeutically in relation to occupation. We call these two types of tools *conceptual models* and *models of practice*. Conceptual models help us think about occupation, what it is, what factors affect it, and what healthy and unhealthy occupation looks like. Conceptual models are made up of concepts, definitions, and principles about relationships between concepts. Models of practice help us act therapeutically to understand how occupation changes and how therapists may use this knowledge to help clients achieve their occupational goals.

Ideally, there should be relationships between conceptual models and models of practice; that is, we should be able to trace the link between the tools used for thinking about a client's problems (conceptual model) and the tools used for helping to overcome the problem (model of practice). A practice approach should reflect the conceptual ideas on which it is based. Assessments and interventions should mirror the understanding of occupation and human health on which they are based.

McColl MA, Law M, Stewart D.
Theoretical Basis of Occupational Therapy, Third Edition (pp. 13-15).
© 2015 Taylor & Francis Group.

Table 3-1 **The Occupational Therapy Toolbox**		
	About Occupation	**About Humans and Environments**
Tools for Thinking	Occupational conceptual models	Basic conceptual models
Tools for Acting Therapeutically	Occupational models of practice	Basic models of practice

The Model of Human Occupation is a good example of this. The conceptual model associated with the Model of Human Occupation gives us theory to explain the relationship among skills, habits, motivations, and human occupation. The model of practice associated with the Model of Human Occupation offers us assessment tools and intervention techniques that apply the conceptual model or that instruct us how to act therapeutically according to this approach. These practice tools are meant to allow us to assess and treat different types of performance, habituation, or volitional problems to produce predictable changes in occupation.

OT tools are further divided into tools that apply specifically to occupation and tools that apply generally to human beings and their environments. Tools focused on occupation are most often developed by occupational therapists and explain what occupation is, how it contributes to health, and how it relates to a variety of other factors. Tools borrowed from other disciplines help us understand human beings in context. They tell us more about the human organism, its component parts, its underlying processes, and its relationship to its environment. For example, anatomy, physiology, biology, pathology, kinesiology, and other basic biomedical sciences offer us tools that help us to understand the physical aspects of human beings.

The distinction between *occupational theory* and *basic theory* is important. Ideas classified as *occupational theory* describe occupation, each from its own particular perspective. For example, Mosey developed a theory in the 1970s entitled "recapitulation of ontogenesis" (Mosey, 1974). This would be considered *occupational theory* because it explains the development of occupation and discusses specific occupational tasks (such as vocational choice and self-care) from a developmental perspective. On the other hand, developmental theories like those developed by Piaget (1928) and Erikson (1959) would be considered *basic theories* because they discuss the development of human beings and of specific human components such as cognition and social relationships. Basic theories, then, describe the components necessary for the development of occupation, such as cognitive development, physical development, social development, and so on but do not address occupation directly.

For all of these tools, we need a toolbox—a system of organizing the many tools at our disposal to allow us to find the right one for the job at hand. The toolbox is a repository from which occupational therapists can select ideas, concepts, principles, assessments, and interventions that help them to understand and influence the occupational performance of their clients. The preceding discussion suggests that this toolbox should be divided into four quadrants (Table 3-1), to accommodate the following:

- Tools for thinking about occupation
- Tools for thinking about humans and their environments
- Tools for acting therapeutically with regard to occupation
- Tools for acting therapeutically toward humans in the context of their environments

To that end, we offer four terms and their definitions that will be used throughout this book:

1. *Occupational conceptual models* are tools for thinking about and understanding occupation. Occupational conceptual models help us understand occupation and the things that interfere with occupation to produce problems. For example, theories about how occupation is acquired and how personal factors can affect the acquisition of occupation would be considered occupational conceptual models.

2. *Occupational models of practice* are tools for acting therapeutically to make a change in occupation. This is theory that helps us to know how to act to help clients improve their occupation. As an example, theory about how the environment may be modified to enhance occupation would be considered an occupational model of practice.

3. *Basic conceptual models* are tools for thinking about humans and their environments. These include conceptual models from other disciplines that help us understand human beings in general. They do not deal specifically with occupation but rather with the components of people and environments that admittedly influence occupation. For example, basic conceptual models about how

muscles receive messages from the central nervous system to produce human movement would be found in this section of the OT toolbox.

4. *Basic models of practice* are tools for acting therapeutically to make a change in humans and their environments. Basic models of practice relate to specific components of humans and their environments. For example, theory about how occupational therapists might intervene with physical modalities to promote activity tolerance and endurance would be considered a basic model of practice.

In this textbook, we focus on theory from the first quadrant of the toolbox—that is, occupational conceptual models. These are theories that over the past century have helped us understand what occupation is and what factors affect it. Wherever possible, we offer examples of theories that would be classified in one of the other three quadrants of the toolbox: occupational models of practice, basic conceptual models, or basic models of practice; however, the purpose of this book is to search out, identify, and classify theory that explains the phenomenon of occupation.

4

The Occupational Therapy Filing Cabinet

Mary Ann McColl, PhD, MTS

This chapter introduces the occupational therapy (OT) filing cabinet (Figure 4-1), the second of three metaphors that we offer to help students understand and use OT theory. In the same way that the tools in OT theory need a toolbox, OT theory needs a filing cabinet to organize and classify ideas to make it easier for therapists to find the one that helps in a given situation.

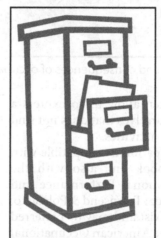

Figure 4-1. OT filing cabinet.

Occupation

In this book, occupation itself is typically thought to be made up of self-care, productivity, and leisure. *Self-care* refers to those activities that the individual performs for the purpose of maintaining the self in a condition that allows for function. Self-care occupations help one to be ready and prepared for other occupations. They include those referred to as activities of daily and community living. (Some definitions categorize sleep or rest in a separate area, but we include them under self-care.)

Productivity/Work refers to those activities that customarily fill the bulk of one's day and contribute to economic self-maintenance, home and family maintenance, service, or personal development. There is a component of obligation attached to productivity. In its most traditional form, productivity takes the form of salaried employment. However, it may also include work around one's home or voluntary work, if some commitment or obligation is implied in the performance of these duties. It may include child care

or other caregiving. Productivity may include those initiatives taken on by an individual in preparation for future productivity. These include developmental play in young children and education or training at older ages. Productive activities often represent our contribution to our home, family, community, workplace, or society. They validate our need to be useful and to feel that we accomplish something within our own sphere of influence.

Leisure includes those activities engaged in when one is free from the obligation to be productive. Leisure activities are defined by the personal preferences and interests of the individual. They may be either sedentary or active, social or individual, creative or technical. They are usually voluntary in nature and

McColl MA, Law M, Stewart D.
Theoretical Basis of Occupational Therapy, Third Edition (pp. 17-26).
© 2015 Taylor & Francis Group.

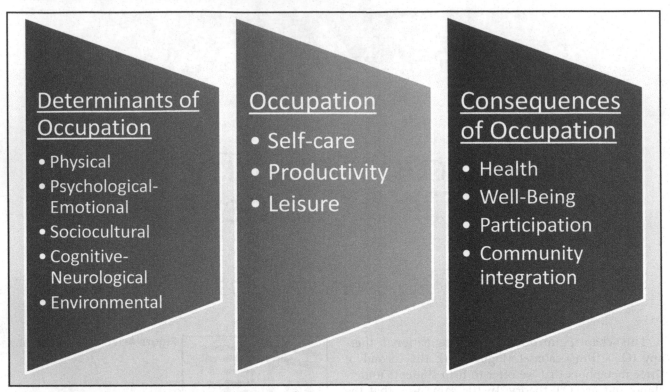

Figure 4-2. The determinants and consequences of occupation.

fully discretionary. They often allow us to express a creative or personal side of ourselves that does not find expression in our other daily activities.

This classification of occupation is compatible with previous editions of this book and also with the Canadian Model of Occupational Performance and Engagement (CAOT, 1997, 2002; Townsend & Polatajko, 2007). Other classifications exist and may be preferred by the reader. For example, the American Occupational Therapy Association's (2014) "Occupational Therapy Practice Framework, 3rd Edition" includes eight areas of occupation that can be mapped quite readily onto the three above: activities of daily living, instrumental activities of daily living, rest and sleep, education, work, play, leisure, and social participation. It is noteworthy that like the oldest classification on record (Meyer, 1922: "work, play, rest and sleep," p. 2), this classification includes sleep and rest.

Our understanding of occupation is further broken into both the *determinants* and the *consequences* of occupation (as well as, of course, understanding occupation itself) (Figure 4-2).

The *consequences of occupation* are the outcomes that occupational therapists typically seek: health, well-being, social participation, and community integration. The models that explain the relationship between occupation and these outcomes we call "occupation-focused models." They are found in the top drawer of the filing cabinet, and they are described in Chapter 6. Occupation-focused models tell us about

occupation and its relationship to health, well-being, participation, and integration.

In order to fully understand occupation, we also need to understand the *determinants of occupation*—that is, those factors that affect occupation. Determinants are those factors that affect, influence, or determine how occupation looks and feels. This book uses a classification of five determinants derived directly from the OT literature. Based on exhaustive literature searches conducted for the previous two editions as well as for this edition, we have discovered a high degree of consensus on the factors that occupational therapists believe affect occupation. These have been relatively consistent in the OT literature since the beginning of the 20th century (McColl, Law, & Stewart, 1993; McColl, Law, Doubt, Pollock, & Stewart, 2003). The literature showed that we typically think of occupation as being a function of either aspects of the *person* or aspects of the *environment*. The *person* is usually further broken down into four components: physical, psychological-emotional, cognitive-neurological, and sociocultural. The *environment* includes physical, social, cultural, economic, and political aspects. Figure 4-3 offers a depiction of the determinants of occupation.

You will find different labels for the determinants of occupation in other sources. For example, the "Occupational Therapy Practice Framework: Domain and Process, 3rd Edition" (American Occupational Therapy Association [AOTA], 2014) and the Canadian Model of Occupational Performance and Engagement

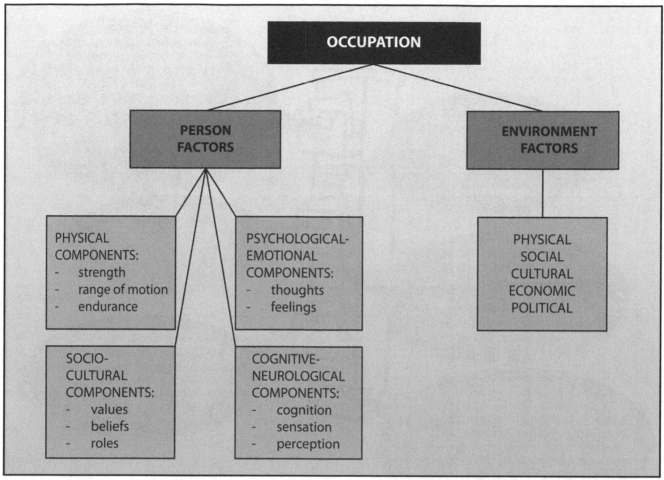

Figure 4-3. The determinants of occupation.

(Townsend & Polatajko, 2007) both use slightly different groupings of determinants; however, again, both systems can map easily onto these five simple determinants. We have found that this set of determinants has worked well over the past two editions of this book. It has effectively allowed us to classify OT theory according to determinants, and we therefore commend it to readers as a simple yet comprehensive way to think about the determinants of occupation, or the factors that can affect a person's occupation.

The Occupational Therapy Filing Cabinet

The OT filing cabinet contains six drawers that allow us to classify, store, and access OT theory readily when needed. You may prefer to think of them as six folders on the hard drive of your computer, but either way, they are six receptacles into which you may systematically file, sort, and preserve important documents. These six drawers/folders will help you go

directly to the area where the document you need is most likely to have been saved.

The top drawer contains OT theory that tells us about the relationship between occupation and outcomes that occupational therapists are ultimately interested in achieving. These outcomes include health, well-being, community integration, and social participation. These are referred to in Figure 4-4 as the *consequences of occupation*.

The next five drawers of the filing cabinet contain information about the *determinants of occupation*, or the factors that affect occupation. There are five determinants of occupation that correspond with the five factors most likely to influence occupation. A separate drawer in the filing cabinet is devoted to the knowledge of how five different types of factors *affect* occupation: physical factors, psychological and emotional factors, social and cultural factors, cognitive and neurological factors, and environmental factors. One drawer each of the filing cabinet is devoted to storing the knowledge associated with one each of these five determinants. The following discussion describes

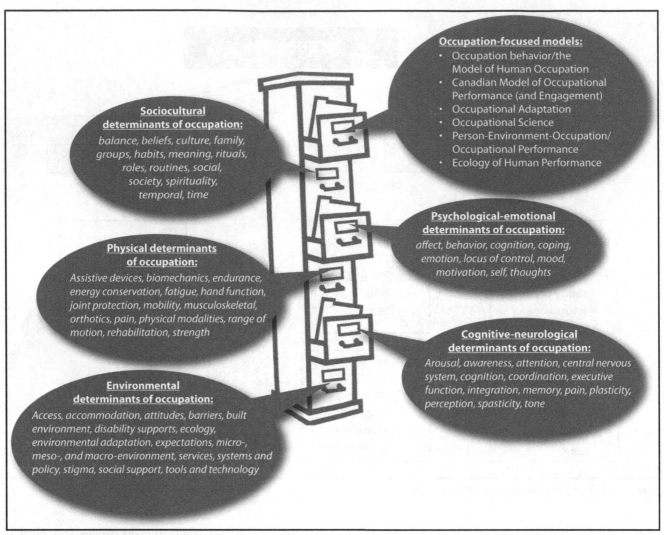

Figure 4-4. The OT filing cabinet.

more about what types of knowledge might be found in each of the "determinants" drawers.

The Physical Determinants of Occupation

The physical determinants of occupation refer to the physical factors that affect occupation. The physical determinants of occupation arise from the musculoskeletal system. To the extent that the musculoskeletal system operates effectively, it typically provides the needed resources for occupation—resources such as strength, range of motion, and endurance. However, if occupation is impaired, one cause of that impairment may be disorder or dysfunction of the musculoskeletal system or the physical aspect of the person. Therefore, the physical determinants of occupation are of interest to occupational therapists. For example, imagine a client who has a job such as a bank teller, where he or she stands all day. If this client lacks the endurance to stand for long periods, an occupational therapist might view the physical limitation of endurance as a determinant of the occupational performance problem.

The Psychological-Emotional Determinants of Occupation

Similarly, occupation may be affected by thoughts and feelings. Problems in occupational performance may arise from the *psychological-emotional* component of the person. Disordered or maladaptive thoughts and feelings can have a significant negative impact on occupation. For example, the persistent thought that one is unable to leave one's house for fear of contamination would have a significant negative impact on the ability to maintain relationships and roles. In this case, the occupational therapist might focus on those thoughts and feelings as psychological-emotional determinants of occupation. Therefore, another drawer of the filing cabinet contains everything we know about how thoughts and feelings affect occupation.

The Cognitive-Neurological Determinants of Occupation

The *cognitive-neurological* component refers to the central processing of internal and external stimuli. Another drawer contains all the information occupational therapists possess about how the central nervous system affects occupation. Cognitive-neurological determinants of occupation include the cognitive, sensory, perceptual, and neurological integration of input essential to one's ability to carry out daily activities with success and satisfaction. The cognitive-neurological component is distinguishable from the physical component in that it focuses on the central nervous system, whereas the physical component focuses on peripheral, musculoskeletal functioning. It also differs from the psychological-emotional component in that it emphasizes the ability to process incoming information rather than the psychological or emotional experience of it.

The Sociocultural Determinants of Occupation

The *sociocultural* component of the person includes learned beliefs, attitudes, roles, and behaviors that are a result of socialization or upbringing. Sociocultural determinants of occupation refer to the process of organizing one's occupation into social patterns or habits that conform to the social and cultural roles one fulfills. Occupational dysfunction occurs when performance and expectations diverge. Concepts are classified as sociocultural determinants that are socially defined, constructed, or mediated. Therefore, concepts such as time, roles, meaning, and spirituality may be considered parts of the sociocultural component, and knowledge about these is filed along with other social or cultural factors affecting occupation.

The Environmental Determinants of Occupation

Finally, the *environment* is defined broadly to include both the physical and the social environments. We also typically think of three levels of environment: the micro-environment, referring to the proximal environment, including one's home and those one lives with; the meso-environment, referring to one's community, workplace, neighborhood; and, the macro-environment, referring to the distal environment or the society in which one participates. The environmental determinants of occupation include any aspect of the environment that has the potential to either facilitate or impede occupation. In the AOTA practice framework (AOTA, 2014), contextual and environmental factors are organized into cultural, personal, physical, social, temporal, and virtual elements. In this book, environment is conceptualized as having physical, social, cultural, economic, and political elements. Occupational dysfunction arising from the environmental component would be the result of an inadequate, overly controlling, hostile, or perhaps simply indifferent environment.

It should be emphasized here that these five determinants need not be considered mutually exclusive of one another. A particular theoretical idea may be classified in more than one place depending on its context or the details associated with its application. We should also note that some well-known theories may not fit tidily into one theory area; elements of it may fit best in different theory areas. For example, the Model of Human Occupation contains ideas from a number of different theory areas. Concepts such as values, habits, and temporal adaptation fit well with the sociocultural theory area, whereas ideas such as personal causation, interests, and skill learning fit more comfortably in the psychological-emotional area. This should not be considered to detract from the credibility or effectiveness of either the taxonomy or the model. It is simply a product of the cross-section of two ways of looking at occupation. It is enormously beneficial in working with theory to be able to consider it from different perspectives and to be flexible in thinking about occupation.

What's in the Filing Cabinet?

What gets classified in each of these drawers and folders? Ideas about what occupation is all about, what things can interfere with occupation, what happens to people when components fail, and how occupational therapists can act to restore health and occupation. In fact, each drawer contains its own toolbox, with tools for thinking and tools for acting. Those tools are further sorted as tools specifically addressing occupation and tools that are more generally about humans and their environments. For example, the physical determinants drawer contains the following:

- *Basic conceptual models* that tell us about physical functioning in humans.
- *Occupational conceptual models* that tell us about the relationship of physical factors (such as strength, endurance, and range of motion) to occupation.
- *Basic models of practice* that offer us assessments and interventions aimed at altering the physical component of the person.

- *Occupational models of practice* that provide assessments and interventions aimed at improving occupation through physical skills and activities.

Each drawer of the filing cabinet also contains what we referred to previously as "big-T theory" (or named theories), and "small-t theory" (or generic, unnamed theory) in OT. Since the 1980s, a number of named big-T theories have emerged (such as the Model of Human Occupation, the Cognitive Disabilities Model, and the Person-Environment-Occupation Model). Usually a theory that merits a name is one that offers a systematic view of a particular domain; it purports to be a comprehensive, internally consistent theoretical tool. Very often, named theories also have a body of empirical evidence associated with them. They are structured such that it is possible to generate hypotheses from their stated principles and to test those hypotheses to support and validate the theory. They are intended to render the world more predictable and permit generalization about relationships between concepts of interest. These theories are usually easily recognized as theory because they are labeled as such.

However, equally important are ideas that guide and govern practice but are not incorporated into formal theoretical systems. For example, occupational therapists depend heavily on ideas about grading activity to present an increasing challenge toward mastery. This idea has been a part of OT thinking and culture since the early part of the 20th century and yet has never been associated with a particular author or named theory. As such, we refer to it as a "small-t theory" and consider it essential to capture in a book of this type. Another example of unnamed theory is the "4 Ps" of energy conservation: posture, planning, pacing, and prioritizing. This is an enormously useful intellectual tool or piece of theory about energy conservation, whose origins have been lost—it has become a part of the folk wisdom of OT. It has neither an author's name associated with it nor a body of research to support it, but this does not diminish its importance or utility in the consciousness and processes of OT. Therefore, we include it as theory, or as a tool for thinking, for the purpose of this book.

The filing cabinet offers the opportunity to classify both types of theory and also offers the flexibility to use more than one theory area to cover all the important aspects of a particular theory. Now let us look more closely at each of the drawers of the filing cabinet and their contents.

Second Drawer: Sociocultural Determinants of Occupation

The second drawer is labeled "Sociocultural Determinants of Occupation." Ideas and theories located in this drawer explain problems interfering with occupation as arising from the social and cultural groups that we grew up in, identify with, and affiliate to. By virtue of membership in these groups, we each internalize social and cultural concepts that shape who we become and how we undertake our occupation.

Occupational Conceptual Models

Occupational conceptual models falling into this category analyze occupation in terms of socially constructed phenomena, such as roles, habits, time use, and beliefs. As a result of belonging to certain social and cultural groups (such as the family, the peer group, the age cohort, the social class, the ethnic group), we adopt ideas about who we should be and how we should relate to others and participate in society. These values and beliefs about virtually every aspect of life shape who we are and govern our feelings about many occupations. Some of those beliefs and values are adaptive, meaning that they help us participate successfully and satisfactorily in occupation; other beliefs are maladaptive, meaning that they interfere with occupational performance. Models classified in the sociocultural area explain occupational dysfunction in terms of a disconnect or disharmony between our internalized values, beliefs, and norms and the requirements of our occupations. This is one of the oldest types of OT theory. Its origins are found in the early 20th century, when occupational therapists were first engaged to help inmates of institutions to be healthier by participating in occupations that simulated normal cultural expectations for time use and role participation.

Occupational Models of Practice

Occupational models of practice in this area generally aim at reconciling our social and cultural beliefs with the expectations and demands of our occupations. Assessments would typically seek to uncover values, beliefs, ideas, and expectations related to specific occupations. Interventions often result in restructuring social roles and occupational activities to enhance success.

Basic Conceptual Models and Basic Models of Practice

Basic conceptual models in the sociocultural area come primarily from sociology and anthropology and help us understand how humans function in groups, communities, and societies. Basic models of practice come from social psychology and pertain to the treatment of individuals in the context of groups, communities, and relationships.

Third Drawer: Psychological-Emotional Determinants of Occupation

Theory that pertains to the psychological and emotional aspects of the person would be located in the filing drawer labeled "Psychological-Emotional Determinants of Occupation." The theory found in this drawer helps us understand the thoughts, feelings, and behaviors of human beings and how those affect occupation. These theoretical ideas locate problems with occupational performance within the person—more specifically, in the psychological or emotional aspect of the person.

Imagine, for example, receiving a referral for a client who is seeking assistance developing work-related skills and aptitudes. You notice on the referral that the client has had a number of jobs over the past 5 years, but in each instance, employment has been terminated as a result of vague references to interpersonal difficulties. You suspect that these difficulties may be explainable by knowledge and theory contained in the psychological-emotional theory area.

Occupational Conceptual Models

Occupational conceptual models in this drawer help explain occupational dysfunction in terms of an individual's feelings, attitudes, motivations, and coping resources for occupation. You find both formalized theories with proper names as well as equally important ideas that have either been substantiated by research or by a tradition of practice wisdom. Both help us understand the psychological-emotional aspect of the person and how it affects his or her occupation. For example, we have occupational conceptual models that describe how motivation, volition, and the sense of personal causation affect a person's ability to engage successfully in productive occupation.

Occupational Models of Practice

Occupational models of practice include assessments and interventions to address psychological or emotional obstacles to occupational function. Using the example above, we might decide to perform a detailed occupational history assessment to try to understand better the patterns and circumstances that have affected the work history presented by our client.

Basic Conceptual Models and Basic Models of Practice

Basic conceptual models found in this drawer help us to understand the psychological and emotional aspects of human beings, but they have no particular focus on occupation. They typically arise from the disciplines of psychology, psychiatry, and neuropsychology. Basic

models of practice instruct us about how to assess and treat underlying psychological problems, such as depression or anxiety.

Fourth Drawer: Physical Determinants of Occupation

Theory that focuses on the *physical aspect of the person* as the root of occupational performance problems would be filed in the drawer of the filing cabinet labeled "Physical Determinants of Occupation." This drawer would contain all those ideas and practice tools pertaining to problems that can be located in the person—more specifically, in the musculoskeletal system. For example, if a client referred to you for difficulties with activities of daily living came limping into your office, wincing with pain, and had difficulty lowering him- or herself down into the chair, you would be justified in posing a working hypothesis that his or her occupational performance problems stemmed from underlying physical problems—that is, problems with bones, joints, muscles, or tendons.

Occupational Conceptual Models

Occupational conceptual models found in this drawer would explain occupational performance in terms of physical functioning, particularly strength, range of motion, and endurance. Problems of self-care, productivity, or leisure would be explained as a function of inadequate physical abilities to fulfill the requirements of the occupation. An example of occupational conceptual models of the physical determinants of occupation includes activity analysis. There is a rich historical tradition within OT of analyzing activities to assess the physical demands (among other types of demands) that they place on clients and the extent to which clients' physical abilities and disabilities permit them to participate in particular occupations.

Occupational Models of Practice

Occupational models of practice filed in the physical determinants drawer would include assessments and intervention approaches that remediate occupation through the use of physical rehabilitation activities. Following the occupational conceptual model of activity analysis (i.e., assessing the physical demands of a task and comparing those with the abilities of the client to meet those demands), an example of an intervention in this area would be an adapted self-care technique that took account of the physical limitation, such as one of the many bathroom adaptations that occupational therapists use to help people with joint limitations use their toilets or their bathtubs safely and without pain or injury.

Basic Conceptual Models and Basic Models of Practice

Basic conceptual models filed in this drawer would be aimed at understanding humans from a physical perspective. They would include the basic physical sciences such as anatomy, musculoskeletal physiology, kinesiology, and biomechanics. Our knowledge in these areas helps us understand the physical aspect of human beings and be aware of how the physical self can be injured or impaired. Basic models of practice would involve the use of physical modalities to improve physical functioning—in particular, to remediate strength, endurance, and range of motion.

This book focuses on *occupational conceptual models* and *models of practice* and refers readers interested in more information on basic models to textbooks in the respective disciplines mentioned throughout this chapter.

Fifth Drawer: Cognitive-Neurological Determinants of Occupation

The fifth drawer of the filing cabinet contains ideas and concepts that explain how the central nervous system affects occupation. These models understand occupational performance problems as a product of the functioning (or dysfunction) of the brain, the nervous system, and the sensory and perceptual mechanisms. Ideas found in the filing cabinet drawer labeled "Cognitive-Neurological Determinants of Occupation" locate problems interfering with occupation in the person, particularly in the central nervous system.

This area of theory might be invoked to address the occupational performance problems of a person who had recently had a stroke or who had a known neurological condition. Imagine receiving a referral to see a client who had recently suffered an acquired brain injury and was having difficulties with memory and executive functions. You might begin thinking about what you could offer this client by taking a look in the third drawer of the filing cabinet to see how an injury to the central nervous system (specifically the brain) could affect occupation and what could be done about it.

Admittedly, much of this consultation of theory in a particular drawer happens in seconds, particularly among experienced therapists. There is an immediate association between characteristics of certain brain lesions and their possible effects on common human occupations. It is not nearly as laborious in practice as opening a filing drawer and flipping through it to find the information needed. That is simply a metaphor to illustrate the process the therapist's brain undergoes in applying his or her knowledge to clients' occupational performance problems, to the underlying impairments and dysfunctions that give rise to those problems, and to the options for OT.

Occupational Conceptual Models

In this drawer you will find occupational conceptual models that explain difficulties with daily occupation as a function of the individual's inability to experience, process, and apply incoming information and subsequently produce motor outputs. These models locate occupational performance problems in the person and, more specifically, in the person's central nervous system—the brain and spinal cord. These structures govern cognition, perception, sensation, execution, coordination, and integration.

Occupational Models of Practice

The occupational models of practice in this drawer include assessments and treatments that would help you act therapeutically to optimize occupation by overcoming cognitive, perceptual, and integrative difficulties. In the example earlier, these practice tools would help the therapist better understand the nature of the memory and organizational problems and the effect those have had on specific occupations. Furthermore, this drawer would offer intervention tools that suggest how therapists might remediate or overcome occupational performance problems, depending on how they viewed the mechanisms of injury and recovery.

Basic Conceptual Models and Basic Models of Practice

Deeper in this drawer, you would also find basic conceptual models in the cognitive-neurological area that help us understand the human brain and nervous system in all their complexity. These theoretical tools come from a number of basic science disciplines, such as neuroanatomy, neurophysiology, and neuropsychology. Although these models can be highly influential in OT with clients who have had a neurological illness or injury, we need to be clear about which models actually address occupation (occupational conceptual models and models of practice) and which explain the human nervous system without particular reference to its impact on particular occupations (basic conceptual models and models of practice).

Basic models of practice would include assessments and interventions that do not refer specifically to occupation but offer tools for assessing and promoting the recovery of the brain and nervous system. These tools focus specifically on the neurological mechanisms and processes. In this area in particular, occupational therapists need to be clear about the distinction between tools that address occupation and those that do not. Both are valuable and indeed essential to effective practice in this area, and both need to be brought to bear on occupational performance problems.

When attempting to use the filing cabinet, therapists will sometimes be confronted with the question of what drawer to file something in and, subsequently, what drawer to go looking for something in. We acknowledge that the drawers of the filing cabinet may not be perfectly sealed and impermeable and that, in fact, information from a particular theory may fit into more than one drawer; therefore, it is important to recognize distinctions that help us to maximize the efficiency of the filing system. Two such distinctions arise with regard to cognitive-neurological theory: that between cognitive-neurological and physical determinants, and that between cognitive-neurological and psychological-emotional determinants.

First, you might say that the musculoskeletal system also includes nerves, so how do we decide which drawer to open in the case of damage to nerves? In this instance, we suggest that physical theory would be used to understand problems associated with damage to the peripheral nervous system, and cognitive-neurological theory would be used to understand problems associated with the central nervous system.

Second, you might say that the brain is implicated in both the psychological-emotional and the cognitive-neurological area, and of course, you would be right. Therefore, which drawer do we consult when we encounter a situation where thoughts and thinking impede occupational performance? In this instance, it would be important to ascertain whether the source of the problem is in the inability to engage in abstract or complex thought, such as in the case of a brain injury, a dementia, or a developmental disability. Theory on the cognitive-neurological determinants of occupation would assist us if this were the case. On the other hand, if it were disordered, distorted, or counterproductive thoughts that interfered with occupational performance, the theory about the psychological-emotional determinants of occupation would be most instrumental. Psychological-emotional theory would be useful to understand thoughts and processes that are maladaptive, whereas cognitive-neurological theory would be used to understand the inability to engage in particular cognitive processes.

Sixth Drawer: Environmental Determinants of Occupation

The sixth determinants drawer of the filing cabinet is substantially different from the other four. This drawer contains theory that locates the problem interfering

with occupation *not* in the person but in the environment. It starts from an assumption that every person has abilities and disabilities and that the extent to which a person is able to be successful in his or her occupation is a function of the barriers and supports encountered in the environment. This approach is consistent with the social model of disability, a model that has gained prominence in recent decades in our way of thinking about disability. Occupational therapists have theory that is entirely compatible with this way of thinking about ability, disability, and occupation, and this theory is typically found in the drawer of the filing cabinet labeled "Environmental Determinants of Occupation."

While every theory of OT acknowledges the influence of the environment on occupation, theory found in this drawer goes a step further. It rejects the medical model, which governed how occupational therapists thought about dysfunction for many years as located within the person and remediable only by realizing a change in the person. Rehabilitation in general, and OT in particular, has historically focused primarily on the remediation of individuals. Instead, environmental theories in OT say that the source of the problem, and hence the source of its remedy, is not found in the person but is located entirely outside of the person, in the environment. If the environment were more accommodating, more supportive, or more accessible, then the person would be able to be more effective and satisfied in his or her ability to fulfill occupations.

Occupational Conceptual Models

Like each of the other drawers, this one contains occupational conceptual models and occupational models of practice. Occupational conceptual models in the environmental category understand occupation in terms of the environmental forces that act on it. Environmental factors such as physical structures, attitudes, rules and conventions, policies and services, knowledge, and awareness can all affect the manner and scope of occupations a person can attempt and succeed at. Occupational conceptual models in the environmental theory area help us to understand these external influences on occupation.

Occupational Models of Practice

Occupational models of practice found in the environmental drawer include assessments and interventions that help us to optimize occupation by removing obstacles and barriers and enhancing support in the environment. This theoretical approach suggests a structural analysis of problems rather than an intrapersonal or interpersonal approach; therefore, assessments include environmental audits for safety, accessibility, attitudes toward disability, and availability of support.

Interventions include therapeutic efforts directed at the environment rather than at the client.

Basic Conceptual Models and Basic Models of Practice

Basic conceptual models help us understand the nature of environments and their effects on humans. These models come from a variety of disciplines, including geography, art, architecture, economics, politics, anthropology, and sociology as well as physics and ergonomics. Basic models of practice aim to change the environment, either through urban and social planning, advocacy, organizational tactics, or other methods of structural change.

Similar to the questions we encountered about the best place to file theory about the nervous system or about thoughts and cognitive processes, another query often arises regarding theory pertaining to roles and relationships affecting occupation. The question that arises is whether this type of theory is better filed under sociocultural determinants of occupation or environmental determinants. The correct place to file such theoretical ideas depends on whether the values and beliefs about roles, relationships, duties, obligations, and privileges are external to the individual or internal. If they are external—that is, if we are talking about the ideas that others hold about who the client should be and the effect that those ideas have on occupation—then that theory is best filed as part of the social environment. If, on the other hand, we are talking about how internalized values and beliefs about who one should be, how one properly fulfills certain roles, and what behaviors duly constitute a particular role, then we are using theory from the sociocultural area. In the former case, the cause of the occupational performance problem lies outside of the individual, in expectations that are inconsistent with our client's own values, whereas in the latter case, the cause lies within the client, in his or her own expectations of occupational performance.

5

The Occupational Therapy Telescope

Mary Ann McColl, PhD, MTS and Nancy Pollock, MSc, OT Reg. (Ont.)

We began this book by suggesting that three things are required for occupational therapists to be successful in practice. These three requirements are illustrated by three metaphors—the filing cabinet, the toolbox, and the telescope (Figure 5-1):

- The occupational therapy (OT) filing cabinet contains and organizes the knowledge that occupational therapists need about the relationship between occupation and health and about the five determinants of occupation, or the five types of factors that can affect occupation.
- The toolbox contains specific tools that occupational therapists use for thinking and for acting therapeutically.
- The telescope offers a way of focusing on a client and using the knowledge and tools (from the filing cabinet and the toolbox) to make a specific plan with each patient or client.

So far in this book, we have talked about theory in a general sense, without referring to a specific client. In order to be able to use theory, however, we have to apply it to the situation of the client in front of us. That is where the telescope comes in (based on the *McMaster Lens for Occupational Therapists*, Salvatori, Jung, Missiuna, Stewart, Law, & Wilkins, 2006). The telescope helps us to match the needs and the context of a particular client with the knowledge and tools that might be able to help him or her. The telescope uses five lenses to sequentially sharpen our focus on a

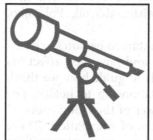

Figure 5-1. OT telescope.

client's issues, the nature and origins of the problem, the tools we have at our disposal, and the expectations we have of what we should be able to achieve. It allows us to use the knowledge we have accumulated and stored in order to serve our clients. In the remainder of this chapter, we assemble what we know about the five lenses that make up the telescope. These five lenses help us focus on the following:

1. The occupational performance problems experienced by the client
2. The lifespan or developmental perspective of the client
3. The probable origins of the problem and the factors underlying occupational performance problems
4. The practice tools available for therapy
5. The outcomes we expect to see at the conclusion of a course of therapy

McColl MA, Law M, Stewart D.
Theoretical Basis of Occupational Therapy, Third Edition (pp. 27-32).
© 2015 Taylor & Francis Group.

First Lens:
What Occupations Is the Client Involved With? What Is He or She Having Trouble With?

The first lens of the telescope focuses on the specific occupational performance problems the client is having. As occupational therapists, if we are going to be able to assist a client, then we need to begin by isolating the specific occupational performance problems that are affecting that person's health. We begin by asking what the individual has trouble *doing*—particularly in the areas of self-care, productivity, or leisure. A problem is typically something that the person wants to do, needs to do, or is expected to do but cannot do, does not do, or is not satisfied with how he or she does it (Law, Baptiste, McColl, Polatajko, Carswell, & Pollock, 2014).

In order to be able to understand a person's occupational performance problems and how they affect his or her health, we need models to guide how we think about occupation and its relationship to health. For this, we look in the "top drawer of the filing cabinet" at models of the consequences of occupation. These models help us understand how occupation affects health and how occupational performance problems cause problems in health, well-being, participation, and community integration. Here we find six big-T theories that give us a number of options for how occupational therapists think about the relationship between occupation and health, or the consequences of occupation. These six occupation-focused models provide the basis for how we think broadly about what we do as occupational therapists.

The choice of an occupation-focused model begins to populate our therapeutic landscape with a number of key concepts. These key concepts are things to which we pay particular attention in our initial observations of the client. For example, if we chose Occupational Adaptation, we would view occupational performance problems as inadequate adaptive responses to occupational challenges. In our initial assessment we would be attentive to the challenges in the environment and where the press for mastery comes from. We would be aware of the current repertoire of adaptive responses and the potential for using them to address new occupational challenges.

On the other hand, if we chose the Model of Human Occupation, we might consider occupational performance problems as problems of volition, habituation, and performance. Our attention would focus on the interests, values, and motivations for particular occupations; the roles, routines, and patterns of occupation;

and the skills available to accomplish them. Although we might not delve deeply into all these areas in our first meeting, it is worthwhile to make explicit how we think about occupation right from the outset. Thus our first focus on the client is on what his or her occupational performance problems are and how they appear to be affecting his or her health. In each case, we would consult the appropriate conceptual model from the top drawer of the filing cabinet to understand the relationship between occupation and health.

Associated with each occupation-focused conceptual model are models of practice that furnish us with ways of observing or assessing occupational performance problems. If, for example, we had chosen the Canadian Model of Occupational Performance and Engagement (see Chapter 7 for more information on all six of these models), we might use a tool such as the Canadian Occupational Performance Measure to initially identify occupational performance problems. This measure allows the client to identify, weigh, and rate three to five problems that we might reasonably work on together in therapy. Similarly, other occupation-focused models also furnish tools to help us with our initial assessment of the types of occupational performance problems the client is experiencing.

Second Lens:
What Is the Age and Stage of the Client in His or Her Development? What Are the Challenges and Skills That Go Along With That Stage?

The second lens of the telescope focuses on age and stage. Occupation changes across the lifespan. Not only do the things we are *able* to do change, but also the things we *prefer* to do, the things we *expect* to do, and the things that *others expect* us to do. We would consider it absolutely normal to see a 5-year-old sitting on the floor playing with a toy fire engine, but we would react differently to seeing a grown man doing the same occupation. We would expect a teenager to make his or her bed in the morning, but we would understand if an elderly person chose not to spend his or her limited energy making the bed or if a busy parent closed the bedroom door on an unmade bed in order to get everyone onto the school bus on time. These are simple examples of how age and life stage affect our occupation.

Cells and systems within the organism are programmed to respond in predictable ways to a variety of internal and external signals over time. For example, babies go from an unfocused stare to focusing on eyes and faces at a predictable interval after birth. Children share their toys with others at a certain stage. Young people choose careers and develop a worker identity. Families seek living quarters that are stable and safe. Older people give up regular work in exchange for the freedom to pursue other interests. Very elderly people reminisce about their lives—what was important to them, what they want to be remembered for. These are all examples of more or less predictable changes that humans go through at certain stages in the life cycle. At the root of the developmental perspective is the idea that development proceeds along predictable lines, and an appropriately designed challenge from a therapist may be the catalyst that stimulates development that has become stalled.

This developmental or lifespan perspective is important when trying to understand the occupational desires and difficulties of our clients. Therefore, the second lens of the telescope helps us focus in on the age and stage of a client and reconcile developmental expectations with occupational issues. After identifying the occupational performance problems he or she is experiencing (lens #1), it is essential that we put these occupations in perspective relative to the developmental continuum (lens #2).

Development refers to a predictable series of changes that an organism undergoes as it moves toward maturity. Development typically consists of two processes, maturation and adaptation. *Maturation* is a biologically determined change that happens to the organism even in the absence of outside influences (Mosey, 1986). For hypothetical purposes only, we imagine what would happen to a baby if it were isolated from all external influences. It would still change in some predictable and unavoidable ways; it would not remain a newborn perpetually. This process we call maturation, and we acknowledge that it is intrinsic, passive, sequential, and predictable. The organism is "hard-wired" to undergo these changes.

The other process that makes up development is *adaptation*. We do not raise babies in bell jars, sequestered from outside influences, so we also need to be able to talk about the changes that result from being exposed to influences from the environment. We use the term *adaptation* to refer to this more active process of change that accumulates in the organism as it responds to stimuli from within itself, such as hunger, curiosity, and attachment, and outside itself, such as sensory experiences, behavioral reinforcements, and expressed expectations.

Much has been written about the cumulative effect of biology and environment on human beings—on the effects of nature and nurture. Throughout the first part of the 20th century, it was assumed that development

was natural, preprogrammed, fixed, and hierarchical. More recent research in the area of motor development, for example, has suggested that change in the human organism may not be as predictable as previously believed (Thelen, 1995). Rather, it is more likely to be a response to changes in physical characteristics (e.g., weight, limb length) coupled with the innate drive to find the optimal movement solution.

The emergence of dynamic system models moved our thinking about development away from hierarchical models toward models that account for the influence of the interaction of multiple systems on behavior, including body systems, environmental demands, and the nature of the task. Thus it came to be understood that development occurred not only longitudinally, or vertically, over time, but also occurred horizontally, meaning across systems of the human being. It was a complex interaction of many factors both in- and outside the individual.

These newer theories of development raise serious questions about some models of practice, particularly those that became most prevalent in neurological rehabilitation, that are based on a hierarchical view of development. These theories also shift the balance between nature and nurture or between maturation and adaptation. They place more weight on skill acquisition as a function of the drive to adapt, with maturation being only one of the ingredients to be considered in the interaction between humans and environments.

There may also be some value in thinking about the predominance of the maturation factor at different stages throughout the lifespan. Biological maturation is very rapid during the first few years of life and often comes to the fore again late in life, when functional losses may occur as a result of aging. During the extended middle period of the lifespan, adaptation is most likely the main route through which occupation changes. Although maturational change is arguably still present among adults, it is likely to be very subtle.

The OT literature began to offer some intelligence on these issues in the 1950s and 1960s, about the same time that developmental psychologies were becoming popular. Occupational therapists mined the work of Gesell (Ilg & Ames, 1962) and other experts in physical development for clues to help us understand the impact of physical disability. Other influential schools of thought included Freud on psychosexual development (1905), Erikson on social development (1959), Piaget on cognitive development (1928), and Kohlberg on moral development (1981).

In 1949, Alessandrini recognized play as a child's central occupation and began to notice developmental similarities in the types of play that children engaged in. Throughout the 1950s and 1960s developmental schedules proliferated. Several notable contributions include Ayres's studies of perceptual motor development (1974);

Mosey's recapitulation of ontogenesis approach (1970), consisting of seven adaptive skills and the sequential patterns of their development; Fiorentino's work on the integration of primitive reflexes for motor development (1975); and Llorens's attempts to reconcile the many different developmental approaches and take a more holistic approach (1977).

The second lens of the telescope requires that we ask a number of questions about the contribution of age and stage to the problems that the individual is experiencing. What would we expect of an individual of a comparable age and life circumstance with regard to the occupation under consideration? Is the occupation one that is central to the developmental challenge of the client's age and stage?

Third Lens:
What Is at the Root of the Occupational Performance Problems the Client Is Experiencing? What Do You Hypothesize Is Causing the Problems? How Do Our Conceptual Models of the Determinants of Occupation Help Us Understand These Problems?

The third lens of the telescope focuses our attention further on what may be going on under the surface of the occupational performance problems. What underlying factors may be causing the problems? Literally, what are the determinants of the occupational performance problems we are seeing? What drawer(s) of the filing cabinet do we need to open to retrieve more information to help us understand the nature and origins of the client's occupational performance problems?

At this stage, we are generating hypotheses about where the problem lies. First we ask, "Is the problem in the person or in the environment?" If the response is the former, the person, then we ask whether the problem appears to be primarily physical, psychological/emotional, social/cultural, or cognitive/neurological. The responses to these two questions instruct us as to which drawer of the filing cabinet to open in order to access what we know about problems of this type.

You will remember that each drawer of the filing cabinet contains the assembled knowledge on one of the five determinants of occupation (physical, psychological-emotional, sociocultural, cognitive-neurological, and environmental). In other words, each drawer contains all that we know about one category of factors that might affect occupation or cause an occupational performance problem. Within each drawer of the filing cabinet lies a toolbox. As we have discussed previously, that toolbox contains tools for understanding (conceptual models) and tools for acting (models of practice). The knowledge pertaining to each determinant is organized within the drawer into tools that deal with occupation (occupational models) and tools that deal with an aspect of the person or the environment (basic models). Furthermore, it is organized into tools for *knowing* and tools for *acting*.

The next stage in using theory to assist clients is to figure out what we know about the kinds of problems the person is experiencing and what might cause those problems. For this we need occupational conceptual models and basic conceptual models. These help us delve deeper into the probable causes of the problems we are seeing. They help us understand what may be going on within the person or the environment to cause the occupational performance problems we are seeing. For example, if we judge that the reason for an occupational performance problem lies in the physical aspect of the person, then we will need access to our knowledge about bones and joints, muscles and ligaments, endurance and fatigue, and pain and pressure to discover what might be going on with the client. By opening the fourth drawer of the filing cabinet, we can flip through our accumulated knowledge of the physical factors affecting occupation to gain a deeper understanding of how the physical self contributes to occupational performance problems and, conversely, how the problem we are seeing in a particular client might have its origins in physical factors about the person. Perhaps his problem is that he does not have enough strength to do the occupation. Perhaps it is that he cannot move his limbs through the range of movement needed to complete the occupation, or perhaps he simply does not have the stamina to get through the occupation. The third lens of the telescope helps us identify probable causes for the problems we are seeing.

Fourth Lens:
What Assessments and Interventions Do We Have at Our Disposal to Address Problems of This Kind? What Additional Information Do We Need to Confirm Our Initial Impressions of the Problem?

The fourth lens of the telescope helps us focus on what we are going to do for the client. So far, we have identified occupational performance problems (lens #1). We have situated those problems in a lifespan perspective that allows us to understand how the client's age and stage of life affects the problems (lens #2). We have hypothesized about where the problems live—what factors are responsible for them, person factors or environment factors? Physical, psychological-emotional, sociocultural, or cognitive-neurological? We have consulted our theory base to discover what we know about problems with those types of origins or determinants (lens #3).

Now we must plan and execute a therapeutic approach. For this we turn again to the OT toolbox, and this time, to the side of the toolbox that contains models of practice. Models of practice tell us how to act therapeutically in order to help clients with their occupational performance problems. Models of practice can either address occupation directly (occupational models of practice) or they can address specific determinants (basic models of practice). In either case, models of practice are made up of two components: assessments and interventions. Models of practice typically correspond to the conceptual models chosen to explain the problem. In other words, lenses #3 and #4 are closely linked. Conceptual models and models of practice go together.

For example, if we have chosen the Model of Human Occupation as our overarching occupation-focused model (filing cabinet top drawer), then we may have identified problems related to roles and habits as potentially responsible for the occupational performance problems we are seeing (lens #1). With lens #2, we assemble what we know about the age and stage of the client and assess the extent to which these problems are typical or atypical for our client. Using lens #3, we focus further on the reasons for the problems our client is experiencing. Now we open the second drawer of the filing cabinet, in which lies all our theoretical tools that help us to understand roles and habits—theory about the sociocultural determinants of occupation.

Consistent with the Model of Human Occupation, our overall occupation-focused conceptual model, we seek to better understand roles, perhaps using a tool such as the Role Checklist (Oakley, Kielhofner, Barris, & Reichler, 1986). This measure provides a deeper, more informative perspective on roles—one of the sociocultural determinants of occupation. If a more detailed exploration of roles reveals that, in fact, the client is experiencing considerable role conflict by virtue of incompatible expectations around role performance, then we have the basis for planning interventions to mitigate role conflict. These interventions will also be found in our filing system under sociocultural determinants of occupation, on the side of the toolbox containing models of practice.

Fifth Lens:
How Long Should it Take to Make a Difference in the Problem We Are Addressing? What Should the Client Experience at the Conclusion of Therapy?

The final lens (lens #5) of the telescope focuses on the desired future we are seeking. Where should we realistically be able to get by the end of an interval of therapy? How will we know when we have reached the end of the therapeutic process? This stage requires clinical judgment and experience to identify what would be an achievable endpoint, what sort of frequency and intensity of therapy is required to reach that endpoint, and how long it should take us to get there. This endpoint is typically a function of health, well-being, community integration, or social participation. It is a direct result of the successful and satisfying performance of occupations that were previously problematic or troublesome.

Summary

This chapter presents the third of three metaphors for the tools used by occupational therapists. After assembling what we know about occupation (the filing cabinet) and choosing tools for thinking about occupation and for acting therapeutically (the toolbox), occupational therapists need to sharpen their focus on the particular patient or client in front of them (the telescope) in order to bring their knowledge and skill into practice. Whereas the filing cabinet and the toolbox refer generically to all OT knowledge and expertise, the telescope helps to apply that knowledge to the particular problems of a given client.

The telescope takes us through a five-step process that brings us closer with each step to knowing exactly what to do for a specific client. It considers his or her specific occupational performance problems (lens #1), his or her life stage and developmental challenges (lens #2), the possible reasons for the presenting occupational performance problems (lens #3), the tools available to address those problems (lens #4), and the expected outcomes (lens #5). Although this may seem like a long and tedious process to undergo for each client, experienced occupational therapists do all this focusing, opening, flipping, and hypothesizing in a split second. Knowledge about occupation, development, determinants, practice tools, and outcomes all interweaves seamlessly to create a cohesive picture of what is going on and what we as occupational therapists can offer.

6

How to Use the Toolbox, the Filing Cabinet, and the Telescope

Mary Ann McColl, PhD, MTS

When faced with a new client, how do we put our theoretical tools (the filing cabinet, the toolbox and the telescope) to work to mobilize our theory and optimize our effectiveness as an occupational therapist? We suggest a process that involves repeated consultations back and forth among the three tools (Figure 6-1). We outline here the typical process and then follow this outline with two examples.

1. Your new client has been referred to you on the basis of a presenting problem. Your first task as an occupational therapist is to pull out your **telescope** and try to see this person in terms of his or her presenting problems and stage of life (lenses #1 and #2).

2. In order to focus specifically on occupational performance problems, you go to the top drawer of your **filing cabinet** and select an overall *occupation-focused conceptual model* to explain the relationship between the presenting problems you are seeing (the client's health and well-being) and a set of occupational performance problems.

3. Within that top drawer, you find a **toolbox** containing occupational conceptual models and occupational models of practice. (Note that the toolbox in this top drawer does not contain any basic conceptual models and models of practice, because all of the models in the top drawer are explicitly related to occupation.) Once you have selected a conceptual model, then the *model of practice* typically follows. Choose an assessment from the model of practice to find out more specific information about the occupational performance problems the individual experiences and how they affect his or her health.

4. From the information assembled so far—the client's presenting health problems, his or her life stage, and his or her stated occupational performance problems—you almost automatically begin generating hypotheses about *why* the individual is experiencing these problems. These hypotheses involve one (or more) of the five determinants of occupation.

A. The presenting occupational performance problems may be a result of underlying sociocultural issues, such as role conflict, unbalanced time use, value dissonance, or nonadaptive habits.

B. They may be the result of psychological-emotional factors, such as inadequate coping skills, mood disorder, negative self-perceptions, or extremes of locus of control.

C. They may be related to physical determinants of occupation, such as impaired strength, range of motion, endurance, or pain.

D. They may be a function of underlying cognitive-neurological problems, such as disordered sensory processing, impaired executive functioning, lack of coordination, or excess muscle tone.

E. Alternatively, the presenting occupational performance problems may have less to do with the person and his or her abilities and disabilities and more to do with the environment that provides inadequate supports or that erects barriers, both physical and social.

This is also consistent with the third lens (lens #3) of the telescope, which we used to focus

McColl MA, Law M, Stewart D.
Theoretical Basis of Occupational Therapy, Third Edition (pp. 33-37).
© 2015 Taylor & Francis Group.

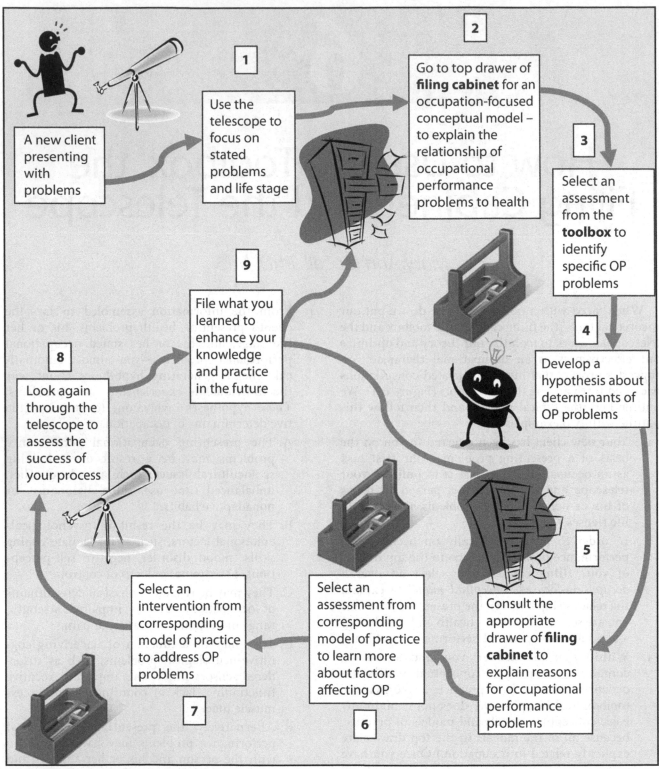

Figure 6-1. Using the toolbox, the filing cabinet, and the telescope.

in on the reasons for particular occupational performance problems.

5. Whichever of these hypotheses you feel does the best job of explaining the client's occupational performance problems leads you to the

drawer of the **filing cabinet** that contains this type of information. Within this drawer, you will find *conceptual models*—both big-T and small-t theory—that you have studiously filed there throughout your education, your career experience, and your continuing professional education. You have filed that information in anticipation of a moment like this, when you seek to explain the relationship of a particular group of determinants to a particular client's occupation.

6. That drawer of the filing cabinet sorts that information into four types of tools using a **toolbox**. Within each drawer of the filing cabinet, we find a toolbox that contains the following:

    - Tools that help us think about the factors that might be responsible for occupational performance problems (occupational conceptual models)

    - Tools that draw from our basic sciences and humanities knowledge to help us know more about those factors or determinants (basic conceptual models)

    - Tools that help us know how to assess and treat occupational performance problems affected by those factors (occupational models of practice). (This would constitute what has been called elsewhere a "top-down" approach to occupational therapy [OT], focusing first on occupational performance problems.)

    - Tools that guide us in directly treating deficits in the person or the environment, on the assumption that by doing so, these improvements will resolve occupational performance problems (basic models of practice). (This approach is consistent with what others have called a "bottom-up" approach to therapy, focusing on the determinants themselves rather than explicitly on occupation.)

    We have selected a *conceptual model* that affords us a deeper understanding of the possible reasons for the occupational performance problems we are seeing. Now we select a corresponding *model of practice*, including an assessment of specific determinants. Thus the assessment process in OT typically has two levels. The first level tells us *what* occupational performance problems the client experiences, and the second level gives us a deeper understanding of *why* the person is experiencing these problems—what physical and environmental factors are associated with or responsible for the occupational performance problems we are seeing.

7. Within the same drawer of the filing cabinet and associated with the conceptual model chosen from the **toolbox**, we also find intervention approaches that are consistent with that approach. Intervention approaches are methods for achieving change in the person, the environment (basic models of practice), or his or her occupation (occupational model of practice). This step is consistent with lenses #4 and #5 of the telescope, which sharpen our focus on the therapeutic tools we have at our disposal and our expectations of the outcomes of therapy.

8. The final step in using OT theory in practice is to reflect on the relative success of the process by taking another look through the **telescope** at the client and his or her occupational performance problems and health or well-being (lenses #1 and #2). This feedback loop allows us not only to evaluate the effectiveness of our treatment with that client, but also to evaluate the validity of our reasoning process, our identification of occupational performance priorities, our hypothesis about the reasons for occupational performance problems, and our choice of conceptual and practice tools.

9. This evaluation also contributes to our body of knowledge in the form of practical experience. It too is filed and stored in the filing cabinet for future use, thus constantly adding to the store of tools we have at our disposal for thinking about and enhancing occupational performance. As we acquire knowledge throughout our careers, we file it thus:

    - The top drawer of the filing cabinet if it pertains to the relationship between occupation and health

    - The remaining five drawers of the filing cabinet if it pertains to the factors affecting occupation, specifically to the four person factors (physical, psychological-emotional, sociocultural, or cognitive-neurological) or to environmental factors affecting occupation

    Within each drawer is a toolbox that helps us sort this knowledge further:

    - Tools that help us to understand the relationship between the specific person factor or environment and occupation (occupational conceptual models)

    - Tools that help us to better understand the specific person factor or environment itself (basic conceptual models)

    - Tools that help us know what to do to help someone improve occupational performance problems stemming from a particular cause (occupational models of practice)

    - Tools that help us know what to do to overcome that cause itself, whether it is an impairment that lies in the person or an obstacle that lies in the environment (basic models of practice)

Now let us examine the process in action, using the example of a particular client. Maria has been referred to a community occupational therapist upon discharge from an inpatient mental health facility. The referral states that she is seeking to return to her previous job as a paralegal in a large downtown law firm.

1. Using the **telescope**, we observe initially that Maria is a well-groomed, attractive woman in her mid-30s. She lives in a small condominium that is sparsely furnished and tidily kept. Maria states that she wants to return to work as soon as possible but cannot anticipate when the appropriate time might be and cannot imagine that she will be able to keep up with the demands of her former job.

2. Looking in the top drawer of the **filing cabinet**, we select Occupational Adaptation as the basis for our understanding of the issues Maria is facing. This model understands Maria's problems with return to work as a function of inadequate or insufficient adaptive responses.

3. This model further directs us to the **toolbox** for an assessment. We therefore look at Maria's desire for mastery and the demands from the environment to identify occupational challenges and occupational role conflicts. On this basis, Maria identifies three specific occupational challenges. She needs to be better able to organize her time to get things done; she needs to be able to explain her recent absence to colleagues at work; and she needs to manage stress and ask for help from coworkers when necessary. The Occupational Adaptation approach suggests that the way to health is through the development of a more effective repertoire of adaptive skills. Maria sets three goals associated with these challenges and agrees to work with the therapist on those for 1 month and then reassess her ability to return to work.

4. Maria's occupational performance problems, along with the other things we know about her, suggest that the main reason for her problems lies in the psychological-emotional area. It appears most likely that psychological or emotional factors underlie the occupational challenges she is experiencing.

5. This hypothesis leads us to the third drawer of the **filing cabinet**, where we find our accumulated knowledge about how factors like coping, stress, locus of control, and self-perceptions affect occupation.

6. From the **toolbox** within this drawer, we select specific assessments to correspond to these factors, such as a stress self-evaluation, a coping inventory, and an assessment of locus of control.

7. Armed with more detailed information about the psychological and emotional factors affecting Maria's occupation, we proceed to identify intervention approaches from the model of practice that might be effective in this situation. According to the Occupational Adaptation approach, intervention typically consists of evaluating existing adaptive strategies for their applicability to the current situation and, where necessary, adapting those strategies or learning new ones to respond to the occupational challenges at hand.

8. Having agreed with Maria at the outset that we would set ourselves a period of 4 weeks to work together toward the stated goals, the time comes to assess our progress and make a decision about terminating therapy and permitting Maria to get on with her life or identifying new goals and cycling around again toward further improvements.

9. The final stage in the process involves self-reflection on the part of the therapist to assess the effectiveness of his or her process in enhancing occupation for this client. The new knowledge gained from this case is then dutifully filed for future use in the ongoing process of learning about occupation, about people and their environments, and about the therapeutic use of self.

Here's another example using a different model and tool. The client is Matt, an inpatient in a rehabilitation facility. He has recently experienced a spinal cord injury and now that his fracture is stabilized, he has been referred to OT to begin preparing for return home.

1. Your first look through the **telescope** (lenses #1 and #2) shows a young man in his early 20s paralyzed from mid-chest down and still restricted to bed. He is overwhelmed and depressed by the changes to his life and cannot imagine what the next steps are.

2. Looking in the top drawer of the **filing cabinet**, we choose the Canadian Model of Occupational Performance and Engagement as our preferred way of understanding the relationship between Matt's occupation and his health or well-being. This model situates occupation as the medium through which humans and environments interact and specifies a client-centered approach.

3. This model offers the Canadian Occupational Performance Measure (COPM) as part of its model of practice. The COPM provides an opportunity for the therapist to hear from the client about his perceived occupational performance problems and how important these are in the context of his life. The COPM asks the client about the things he wants, needs, or is expected to do

but cannot or does not do or is not satisfied with the way he does them. On the basis of an initial COPM interview, Matt expresses his most pressing occupational performance problems as maintaining his relationship with his fiancée, figuring out how he is going to go back to working as a landscaper, and finding a place to live.

4. Based on what we have learned about Matt, it seems that the primary source of his problems lies in the supports available (or not available) to him in his home, workplace, and community.

5. We open the bottom drawer of the filing cabinet to understand better how accessibility and adaptive equipment, disability supports, and social supports affect occupation for someone like Matt.

6. From the model of practice section of the environment toolbox, we select a number of tools for more detailed assessment, such as a home accessibility checklist, a social support inventory, and a job analysis.

7. Also from the model of practice associated with the Canadian Model of Occupational Performance and Engagement, we select from the 10 enabling skills the ones that directly address the environment, specifically advocacy and support. With his permission, we begin making preliminary investigations with Matt's landlord, his employer, and his fiancée to assess the barriers and supports needed to achieve his goals.

8. This rehabilitation admission was planned to be 6 weeks in duration; therefore, we agree to reassess at 3 weeks.

9. As always, the cycle concludes with reflection on new learning and filing the experience in the appropriate place for future use.

Section II

The Consequences of Occupation: Health, Well-Being, Participation, and Community Integration

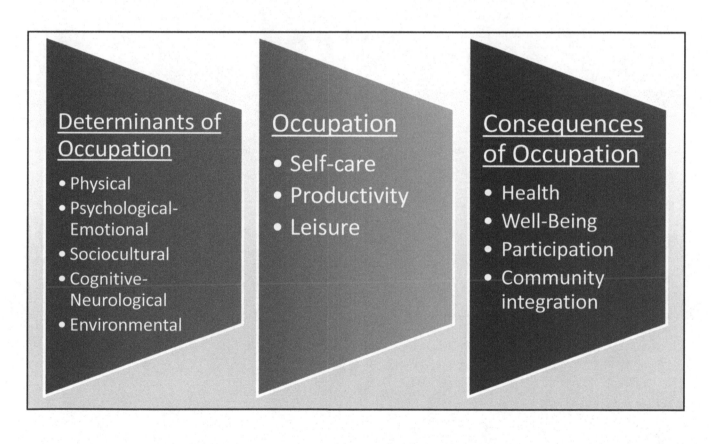

Determinants of Occupation

- Physical
- Psychological-Emotional
- Sociocultural
- Cognitive-Neurological
- Environmental

Occupation

- Self-care
- Productivity
- Leisure

Consequences of Occupation

- Health
- Well-Being
- Participation
- Community integration

7

Occupation in the 20th Century and Beyond

Mary Ann McColl, PhD, MTS*

Long before the profession of occupational therapy (OT) was conceived, the word *occupation* was used colloquially in much the same way that occupational therapists now use it—to refer to a meaningful way to use time. Jane Austen gave us an example of this in the novel *Sense and Sensibility*, when a distraught Colonel Brandon says to Eleanor, "Give me some occupation, or I shall run mad!" This, along with popular maxims such as "Idle hands are the devil's playground," tells us that not only the concept of occupation, but also its health-promoting effects were common knowledge at the beginning of the 20th century, when OT came into being. It is therefore only a short step to the definition of occupation advanced by the founders such as Adolph Meyer (1922): "a freer conception of work, including recreation and any form of helpful enjoyment."

This holistic view of occupation was soon challenged as the Cartesian mind-body dichotomy pervaded popular culture. It became important for health professionals to locate problems in either the mind or the body and to differentiate between interventions that were aimed at mind problems from those aimed at body problems. This was coupled with the intellectual pressure of the scientific revolution in the 1950s and 1960s, and soon the concept of occupation disappeared almost completely from the collective professional consciousness.

In 1962, Reilly refocused the attention of occupational therapists on the health-giving potential of occupation in her Eleanor Clark-Slagle lecture entitled, "Occupational Therapy Can Be One of the Great Ideas of 20th Century Medicine." Gender-specific language notwithstanding, the following quote stands out as a pivotal point in the history of the concept of occupation in OT: "Man, through the use of his hands, as they are energized by his mind and will, can influence the state of his own health" (Reilly, 1962, p. 1). This moment in time represents the beginning of a movement *away* from the tendency to reduce occupation to component parts and to focus treatment on smaller and smaller pieces of human beings. At the same time, it represents a movement *toward* a rediscovery of the therapeutic power of occupation for individuals, families, communities, and even society.

This chapter offers an overview of OT theory development over the period from 1900 to the present, decade by decade. In addition to encapsulating significant events in the theoretical development of OT, the chapter attempts to place these developments in the context of medical and societal developments.

*With thanks to Dr. Penny Bryden for contributions to the first edition of this book (1993).

McColl MA, Law M, Stewart D.
Theoretical Basis of Occupational Therapy, Third Edition (pp. 41-51).
© 2015 Taylor & Francis Group.

1900-1909

> *"How does occupation effect a cure?... One thing is certain, that the coated tongue, the obstinate constipation, the diminished secretions, the sallow complexion and the other symptoms of ill health that very stubbornly resist other methods of treatment gradually disappear when patients are engaged in suitable occupation, and we can nearly always look forward with confidence for a marked improvement in mental condition."*
>
> Moher, T. J. (1907). Occupation in treatment of the insane. *Journal of the American Medical Association, 158,* 1666.

> *"In these cases in which the tired mind tortures itself with doubts and fears and spends the long days in useless self-analysis, and in appreciation of mental and physical suffering, it is probable that progress toward health is often indefinitely delayed because no occupation is found or ever attempted.... A division of the twenty-four hours into changeable periods of work, rest and recreation, plenty of air, wholesome food, wise suggestions and such medical treatment as may be indicated—these simple elements, together with a pretty complete detachment from all other obligations in life, represent in brief the industrial system of treatment."*
>
> Hall, H. J. (1910). Work-cure: a report of five years' experience at an institution devoted to the therapeutic application of manual work. *Journal of the American Medical Association, 54,* 12-13.

North America embraced the 20th century with a sense of optimism, trusting that the New World had finally come of age. The ideal of a North American utopia gave purpose to a number of reform movements aimed at the development of social welfare services and industrial standards. Humanism was the dominant ideology, and women played an important role in social reform in addition to struggling for political equality for themselves. In the interest of women's rights, the first day care centers were established, women sought representation in industrial unions, and a balanced routine including physical activity came to be increasingly valued.

The advent of X-ray technology, blood transfusions, and early anesthetics allowed dramatic advances in surgical techniques and procedures. These changes in knowledge and technology brought about a positive shift in the valuing of health care professionals. Medicine began to be associated with science and technology in place of its historical association with charity. The reform impulse in the health care field aimed toward more effective and efficient treatment of the ill, thus ensuring the continuation of a progressive march toward the future. The predominant diagnoses that figure in the literature of the first decade of the 20th century are a variety of mental and nervous disorders as well as tuberculosis.

The humanitarian movement of this period contrasted sharply with the intolerance of weakness and abnormality seen in the late 19th century, associated with Darwinism and the notion of survival of the fittest. The early 20th century saw a renaissance of the moral treatment ideals of respect, kindness, religious attendance, daily routines, and diversion from morbid thoughts through labor. Physicians began to express the idea that people were healthier if they were meaningfully occupied. In fact, physicians took a sponsorship role in encouraging nurses and other health attendants to be aware of this idea and to put it into practice. They felt that the presence of occupation, or something to meaningfully occupy one's time, was the key to being healthy. Furthermore they suggested that one who was busy had no time to dwell on unhealthy notions or practices. Whereas in years gone by, a rest-cure had been a common prescription for ailments of a variety of types, physicians were beginning to talk about a work-cure. They began to prescribe a balanced regimen of work supervised by a new breed of health workers called occupational therapists.

1910-1919

> *"The benefits (of occupational therapy) are: (1) The employment of a large number of patients... which causes them to be less introspective; (2) the breaking up of a day full of monotony from which all hope and ambition is removed, into one which for several hours at least the individual has some real reason for existence; (3) the reeducation of patients and the training of habits which will permit them to go out into the world and lead a more or less self-sustaining life."*
>
> Ricksher, C. (1913). Occupation in the treatment of the insane. *Illinois Medical Journal, 23,* 385.

> *"At first the benefit of occupation was supposed to be in its time-killing characteristics. In certain advanced and chronic cases, this is all it can be claimed for. In other cases, however, in which there is hope of partial, if not complete, recovery, occupation is found to have certain definite effects. It centres the patient's attention away from himself. Thus mental debris is cleared away, and the real physical symptoms remain, which form a reliable index to the physician in diagnosis and prognosis. The effect of manual work is to strengthen muscles and coordinate the body. Change of occupation stimulates the brain, while continued occupation concentrates it."*
>
> Upham, E. G. (1917). Some principles of occupational therapy. *Modern Hospital, 8,* 409.

The second decade of the 20th century was dominated by the First World War, and the idealism of earlier years was dealt a crushing blow. The reform impulse that had characterized the first decade gave way to the need for efficiency and productivity in a tight wartime economy. It came to be believed that any given process, including the treatment of the ill, could be more effectively conducted if different specialists were responsible for each individual task. Science, efficiency, and progress were seen as inextricably linked.

Health care practitioners saw their roles greatly enhanced as the public became increasingly enamored of all things scientific. Wartime casualties brought a focus and legitimacy to physical disability that was previously unknown. Automation, industrialization, and the automobile brought with them industrial and vehicular accidents that often resulted in injury and disability. The polio epidemic of 1916 was another significant feature of this decade that focused the attention of the medical community on individuals with residual physical incapacities and paved the way for the development of the field of rehabilitation. In OT, the literature of this decade was dominated by a concern for returning veterans of the war and for their continued productivity, participation, and dignity. Previously, occupation had been applied primarily to mental disorders, but now its application for disabled veterans was readily apparent.

At the same time, the fundamental idea of occupation continued to be developed. Articles were devoted to determining the parameters of occupation and the principles for choosing and prescribing occupation relative to a specific problem. For example, occupation was felt to be most therapeutic if it was suited to the individual and therefore motivating and interesting. Furthermore, the notion of productivity was explored both from the perspective of a tangible end product as well as from the perspective of economic viability.

The ideas were introduced of preparing individuals for future remunerative work and of matching the individual's capabilities and interests to therapeutic activities. The importance of graded activity, or activity that could be adapted so that it continuously provided a challenge, was examined. In 1920, the first mention is made of OT with a child.

> *"We know we are helping these misfit children to self-possession in the broadest sense of the word, to realize that they are responsible little folks with real things to do. We help them to form good habits, to be observant, attentive, cooperative, honest, well-behaved children. We know that their salvation lies in handwork, and so we are encouraged to try again and again . . . ."*
>
> Bryant, L. C. (1926). Manual work with the mentally defective child patient. *The Modern Hospital, 27,* 63

> *"But occupational therapy has a very definite place, and it may be as a leading American psychiatrist of international reputation has said, 'occupational therapy will some day rank with anaesthetics in taking the suffering out of sickness.'"*
>
> Walker, J. (1930). Occupational therapy. *Occupational Therapy and Rehabilitation, 9,* 201.

1920-1929

The decade known as the "Roaring Twenties" was characterized initially by two significant movements: women's suffrage and prohibition. Women's groups were able to use their contribution to the war effort to promote their right to vote. By the early 1920s, most North American women had gained the right to vote, and the prohibition lobby attempted to capitalize on the austerity of the war years. It was not until later in the 1920s that North Americans began to experience the seemingly limitless optimism that usually characterizes popular accounts of the time. Industries began to respond to developments in technology, and consumers responded to the abundance of goods on the market. The result was an artificially high level of prosperity. Automobiles, telephones, and radios freed up large amounts of time, and people began to look for ways to spend their newfound leisure time. The collapse of the stock market in 1929 was an almost predictable response to the euphoric climate of investment and to the overextension of credit.

In the medical arena, the most significant advance of this decade was the popular acceptance of the "germ theory" of disease etiology and the corresponding development of vaccines and public health measures.

Epidemics of communicable diseases, such as typhoid and small pox, were virtually eliminated, making way for a focus on illnesses of a more chronic nature. Women played a vital role in educating the poor on the importance of personal and public hygiene as well as serving as primary caregivers in the recuperative process. Public hospitals flourished, and medicine became increasingly associated with the sciences. The biomedical model emerged, with its roots in utilitarianism, science, and rationality. It emphasized the importance of accurate diagnosis, using the most advanced technologies, and the application of scientifically sound treatments to cure pathology in the body and mind. In the mental health field, two other major schools of thought were emerging. The work of Freud and the psychoanalytic theorists and Pavlov and the behaviorists led to a view of mental illness as psychologically determined rather than physiologically or structurally caused.

OT services in chronic institutions expanded greatly during the 1920s, to the point where few were without occupational therapists. In addition, the discipline undertook a number of maintenance tasks, such as the development of professional associations, a journal, and educational standards. OT was defined in this decade as "any activity, mental or physical, definitely prescribed and guided for the distinct purpose of contributing to and hastening recovery from disease or injury" (Pattison, 1922). The literature still emphasized the use of graded, goal-oriented activity to motivate the patient toward recovery, and the balance of work, rest, and play in a person's daily occupations was considered vital to recovery. Seminal publications by Adolph Meyer and Eleanor Clarke-Slagle advanced the basic ideas underlying OT for this period: the idea of a balance of work, rest, and play for health, and the importance of regular, purposeful activity to organize one's time and roles.

In the last 5 years of this decade, the increasing influence of the medical profession and the emerging biomedical model can be observed in the OT literature. Some examples of these trends include the reference to the body as a "physical machine"; the need for basic science in OT curricula; references to OT as a medical, not a social field; and the increasing emphasis on return to work rather than the holistic curative aspects of occupation. The first reference to physical rehabilitation and to matching the activity to the disease (as well as to the person) appeared in this decade.

A debate also began to emerge about the economic aspects of therapy. Was therapy primarily curative, or should the products of therapy be economically useful and marketable? The works of Karl Marx brought new sensitivity to the issues of exploitation of workers, which had implications for the field of industrial therapy. In an effort to ensure that patients were not abused, some institutions shifted from involving patients in the actual work of the institution to simulated work, particularly crafts.

1930-1939

> *"Modern society is organized on an occupational basis, it is the occupation of the individual which gives him a feeling of independence and at the same time binds him to society."*
> LeVesconte, H. P. (1934). The place of occupational therapy in social work planning. *Canadian Journal of Occupational Therapy, 2*, 13.
>
> *"…a dementia praecox can play baseball, while a dementia paralytica can bowl."*
> Losada, C. A. (1936). Some values in occupational therapy. *Occupational Therapy and Rehabilitation, 15*, 288.

The decade of the 1930s was dominated by the Great Depression. Although predictable in hindsight, it took North America almost entirely by surprise. Business collapse alone would have made life difficult enough for North Americans in this decade, but combined with drought, thousands were left destitute. Relief programs ranging from agricultural support to job creation in industry and public works did not end the Depression, but at least they offered new ways of surviving it. This era marked the beginning of a more active role for government in the lives of individuals. However, the enclave of medicine remained relatively impervious to government intervention, despite calls for national health insurance to care for the illness and poverty caused by the Depression.

The expansion of OT services was dramatically halted in the 1930s. Although OT often contributed positively to the economics of a hospital by hastening recovery and discharge, many OT departments were reduced or closed. An appeal was made to therapists to continue their good works on a voluntary basis, harkening back to a time when all female labor was considered philanthropic. OT, however, was striving to be recognized as a legitimate profession within the medical care system and spurned these entreaties toward voluntarism. It was during this period that the debate began over diversional versus therapeutic activity and one of the original tenets of OT—that diversional activity *was* therapeutic—was temporarily lost.

The literature in this decade shows little real ideological growth because OT, along with society in general, was preoccupied with survival. Articles continued to reflect OT's commitment to the use of purposeful, productive activity to promote social and economic adjustment, and the debate over the need to produce articles of economic value in OT continued. Evidence abounds for the increasing influence of the biomedical model. Concepts of activity analysis and graduated exercise were central to the literature of this decade. Whereas several decades earlier, OT had dealt almost exclusively with mental health, by 1937 the tables had turned to the point where Clark (1937) suggested that OT should expand beyond physical activities into the psychosocial field!

1940-1949

> *"Civilization itself may indeed be defined to some extent as the ability of mankind to adjust itself to its handicaps by the successful application of the various modalities of occupational therapy and its related specialties .... When psychotherapy is crossed with physical therapy, we have occupational therapy, with the best characteristics of both parent specialties."*
>
> Bluestone, E. M. (1942). The argument for occupational therapy. *Occupational Therapy and Rehabilitation, 21,* 222.

> *"When the choice of activity was removed from the whims of the patient to the considered thought of the therapist, occupational therapy gained scientific status."*
>
> Licht, S. & Reilly, M. (1943). The correlation of physical and occupational therapy. *Occupational Therapy and Rehabilitation, 22,* 171.

With the memories of the First World War still fresh in many minds, Europe embarked on another "war to end all wars." Men and women from Canada and the United States responded to the call to arms and also to financially support the Allied war effort. On the home front, the last vestiges of the Depression vanished as industries sprang to work putting out war supplies. Women played a dominant role in factories as well as on farms, filling in for men who were fighting overseas.

The experience of war served to revive interest in health insurance and social security to combat the contingencies of unemployment, old age, and ill health. Preliminary discussions took place about the development of health insurance, but no real policy action was to take place until long after the war had ended.

In the medical field, a number of crucial developments during this decade changed the face of medical practice and rehabilitation. First, the discovery of penicillin and antibiotics put a virtual end to many communicable disease epidemics by 1950, making way for an increase in the prevalence of chronic conditions.

Second, medical and surgical improvements during the war led to the survival of casualties who would formerly have died of infection or other traumatic complications. Both of these developments required a tangible response from the medical profession and the emerging rehabilitation professions because of the increased prevalence of disability in society. In the mental health field, the advent of neuroleptic drugs and electroconvulsive therapy during the 1940s dramatically altered the practice of psychiatry. Instead of physical restraints, drugs rendered formerly unmanageable patients docile and amenable to psychological therapies.

Occupational therapists responded to these developments with formal techniques and programs of activities of daily living and vocational and prevocational assessment and training. These domains of occupation (i.e., self-care and work) came to be regarded as separate domains rather than as elements of an integrated and balanced occupational whole. Developments of synthetic materials for industry crossed over to the medical field to permit advances in prosthetic and orthotic technology. Again, occupational therapists responded with techniques to promote skill and expertise in their patients with these new devices, in much the same way that they sought skill and expertise in their own professional domain.

1950-1959

> *"Occupational therapy, born as a war baby during World War I, has had many years to mature, yet the question arises whether she has come of age. She often serves as one of the handmaidens of medicine; at other times she works alone without any seeming relationship to the great family of medicine. Some workers in the medical field question whether she is indeed a true member of the family."*
>
> Gordon, E. E. (1954). Does occupational therapy meet the demands of total rehabilitation? *American Journal of Occupational Therapy, 8,* 238.

> *"... Integrated function is the keynote. For this reason, the use of simple, normal, life-like activities is a logical treatment to encourage response in paresis in muscles. This, of course, is a principle of occupational therapy. Then occupational therapy should inherently, by the nature of its approach, be helpful in these cases."*
>
> Ayres, A. J. (1955). Proprioceptive facilitation elicited through the upper extremities. Part 3. *American Journal of Occupational Therapy, 9,* 121.

> *"In occupational therapy, the activities which you are going to do need to be done over and over and over, and they have to be fun, and they have to be done properly. We haven't done what we need to do in occupational therapy. We need to study. We need an understanding just as we need our basic science."*
>
> Rood, M. (1956). Neurophysiological mechanisms utilized in the treatment of neuromuscular dysfunction. *American Journal of Occupational Therapy, 10*(4), 224.

The decade of the 1950s was marked by the Cold War on the international front and by a buoyant economy on the home front. Business and industry flourished in a climate of almost insatiable demand for products of every description, from homes to cars to appliances to clothes. This era of plenty not only encouraged a dramatic rise in domestic population (the "Baby Boom"), but also lured hundreds of thousands of immigrants from war-torn European and Asian countries.

The 1950s were also a time of technological and scientific innovations. The exigencies of war and the continued participation in the Cold War had ramifications for advances in both the areas of space technology and medicine. While aeronautical engineers discovered new ways to broaden the world's horizons, medical researchers opened new frontiers in the treatment of illness. Pharmacological advances brought about a mentality that virtually every disorder could be treated with drugs, and physicians lost no time in prescribing new medications for mental and physical illness. Penicillin, the wonder drug of the previous decade, became widely used in the 1950s, and the discovery of the polio vaccine in the middle of the decade meant that polio was virtually eliminated, although many survivors experienced residual disabilities. In the newly recognized field of rehabilitation, territorial disputes were underway as the team concept developed. Instead of promoting cooperation and integration, the team concept brought pressure to bear on young health disciplines to differentiate themselves, to become increasingly specialized, and to claim their area of expertise through research and technology.

Developments in neurological research put information at the disposal of occupational therapists. Consistent with the prevailing biomedical, reductionist philosophy, occupational therapists began to apply this information to address specific physical or skill-related problems, consistent with a general trend to emphasize technique, rather than theory.

In the mental health field, dramatic changes were taking place. Theory borrowed from sociology underlined the importance of groups for social interaction and mental health. The group became a focus for therapy and was seen to have therapeutic properties unattainable in individual therapy. Applications of theory from psychology, particularly psychoanalytic theory, increased the awareness of occupational therapists of the power of the unconscious and the therapeutic benefits of unlocking information held at an unconscious level. Projective techniques became part of the arsenal of the occupational therapist, and different approaches were advanced to explore psychodynamic processes. Finally, the increasing sophistication of psychotropic drugs led to more freedom not only for patients in institutions, but also those in the community. Former mental patients began to be discharged to the community in unprecedented numbers, to be absorbed by an ill-prepared society.

1960-1969

> *"The logic of occupational therapy rests upon the principle that man has a need to master his environment, to alter and improve it. When this need is blocked by disease or injury, severe dysfunction and unhappiness result. Man must develop and exercise the powers of his central nervous system through open encounter with life around him. Failure to spend and to use what he has in the performance of the tasks that belong to his role in life makes him less human than he could be."*
>
> Reilly, M. (1962). Occupational therapy can be one of the great ideas of 20th century medicine. *American Journal of Occupational Therapy, 16*, 6.

> *"The social problem which really exists has to do with the treatment of long-term patients.... If occupational therapy is to contribute to a reduction of this great social problems it will be necessary for therapists to consider the way they approach treatment. They must be concerned with all the activities of living—not techniques but the use of the self in motivating and leading patients towards effective living."*
>
> Roberts, C. A. (1962). Healing the sick—responsibility or privilege—for the patient or the professional therapist. *Canadian Journal of Occupational Therapy, 29*, 13.

The continued economic boom throughout the decade of the 1960s provided the necessary stability for a fundamental reevaluation of the relationships, responsibilities, and obligations that society had forged. The solutions proposed were often radical, but the realization of inequities was something that no one could ignore. Protest groups fought for civil rights for people of color, and feminists attacked the hierarchical structure of North American society. In the face of continued pressure, government increased its capacity to function as both mediator and provider.

With Canadian and American governments showing increased concern about social and political rights of citizens, scientific advancements in both countries continued at astonishing speed. Vast sums of money were spent to encourage research and development, particularly in areas that would have an immediate effect on the well-being of the population. The health field especially benefited from this new focus, with important advances being made in techniques for diagnosis and treatment.

In OT, the speed and extent of change brought about a feeling of collective insecurity about the "complexity of illness relative to the simplicity of our tools" (Reilly, 1962, p. 2). The pride of the developing profession seen in previous decades was replaced by a sense of doubt and conflict. The professional literature illustrates a response to this crisis through an increasing focus on science rather than occupation.

1970-1979

> *"Imagine we occupational therapists are like a child standing on the sidewalk holding a balloon on a string, and watching a big parade of medical and scientific progress go by. Every now and again, like a child, we attempt to join the parade; we try to put on the regalia of professional jargon, but it doesn't fit too well. Despite the paternal amusement of our more sophisticated colleagues in other professions, we have not let go of the string of the balloon—at least, I hope this is true, for in my story, it is a beautiful balloon representing an understanding of the value of human potential."*
>
> Schimeld, A. (1971). Youth of today and their influences on the practice of occupational therapy. *Canadian Journal of Occupational Therapy, 38*(1), 3-14.

> *"One of the problems of moving from the medical model to the biopsychosocial model has to do with change itself. Any change is uncomfortable. However it must be remembered that occupational therapists really did not use the medical model for ordering a theoretical base or practice.... A realistic problem concerns the professional self-concept: a therapist who uses the biopsychosocial model has a much heavier emphasis upon the teaching-learning process."*
>
> Mosey, A. C. (1974). An alternative: The biopsychosocial model. *American Journal of Occupational Therapy, 28*, 140.

The relatively stable economies of the 1950s and 1960s left North Americans unprepared for the recession of the 1970s. In response, politicians began to seriously question the social and public policy goals of the previous generation in an attempt to come to terms with new realities. Events such as the Vietnam War and the Watergate scandal brought about a new period of popular cynicism. Radical movements were replaced by more moderate forms of protest, and fewer gains were made both by women and people of color. The economic recession predisposed politicians to careful evaluation of resource implications rather than to action.

However, this spirit of questioning and accountability had notable effects on the health field in general and OT in particular. A new emphasis was placed on quality assurance, standards of care, and the development of audit tools and methods. Also connected with the need for accountability was a strong push in the 1970s toward professionalism. The process of professionalization was seen to be initially related to the acquisition of the characteristics of true professions, particularly an exclusive body of knowledge. Thus the literature of the early 1970s is characterized by a preliminary discussion in nearly every article of the need for theory, accountability, and professionalism. This was a period of dramatic developments in the neurosciences, when occupational therapists made the most of an enriched understanding of the neuromuscular system.

1980-1989

> *"Occupation is a central aspect of the human experience. It is Man's innate urge toward exploration and mastery and his consequent ability to symbolize that makes him unique among animals."*
>
> Keilhofner, G., & Burke, J. (1980). A Model of Human Occupation, part 1. Conceptual framework and content. *American Journal of Occupational Therapy, 34*(9), 573.

> *"The challenge of the future will be to preserve and enhance a climate of caring for our patients in the face of a society increasingly dominated by technique and objectivism, a culture of narcissism that depersonalizes worth and trivializes play, in which medical science views Man as an object and the disabled as forever chronically ill, in which disabled persons while increasing in number might be provided with less of society's resources, and in which individuals are alienated and without social conscience because they have lost hope in creating change."*
>
> Yerxa, E. J. (1980). Occupational therapy's role in creating a future climate of caring. *American Journal of Occupational Therapy, 34*(8), 532.

The 1980s saw a renaissance of the concept of occupation as central to OT. OT theorists sought to refine the definition of occupation, to distinguish it from other related terms, and to develop a knowledge base about occupation that was theoretically consistent and empirically supported. The period began with numerous historical reviews of the profession of OT, with emphasis on the concept of occupation. Each of these articles summarizes with the same conclusion—that OT must return to its roots and reestablish its professional territory in the area of occupation. By the early 1980s, momentum had been established for the development of a science of occupation.

The mid-1980s also saw a focus on the environment as a target for treatment. The impact of the independent living movement had begun to be felt in the profession. According to the independent living ideology, disability was historically ill construed as a function of the person, when it was at least as much a function of an environment created to conform to an able-bodied bias. Thus disability came to be seen not simply as an organic reality, but also as a socially constructed phenomenon. Coupled with broad societal concern for the impact of the industrialized world on the physical environment, this trend had a significant impact on the field. The environment was defined, characterized, and conceptualized, alongside the person, as a legitimate focus of OT intervention. Theory from other disciplines, such as systems theory and ecological theory, helped inform this new approach.

Another notable undertaking of the literature of the 1980s includes attempts to study and understand the nature and characteristics of occupation, both as a naturally occurring phenomenon and as a therapeutic medium. With the development of qualitative research methods, occupation came to be understood not simply as an objective, observable phenomenon, but also as an experienced, personal, subjective one. Qualitative methods drew occupational therapists into a closer understanding of the unique nature of each person's occupational experience and the extent to which it was embedded in context. Numerous articles examined the extent to which particular features of occupation, such as choice, meaning, intensity, and purpose, affected overall outcomes. The nature of engagement in occupation was studied, with a number of articles focusing on the phenomenon of flow, or the altered perceptions that occur when one is optimally engaged in occupation. There was also a renewed interest in crafts as therapeutic media and a reexamination of the purpose and applications of crafts as occupations.

1990-1999

"The built environment, societal production of space, classification of individuals based on norms, the perception of disability as deviance, the power of health disciplines and bureaucracy [contribute] to the creation of disabling environments."

Law, M. (1991). 1991 Muriel Driver lecture. The environment: A focus for occupational therapy. *Canadian Journal of Occupational Therapy, 58*(4), 173.

"Evidence-based practice is a process of looking for understanding,...associated with research, [and]...a potential threat to the therapist."

Dubouloz, C. J., Egan, M., von Zweck, C., & Vallerand, J. (1999). Occupational therapists' perceptions of evidence-based practice. *American Journal of Occupational Therapy, 53*, 446.

"Spirituality is...a very important dimension of the health and rehabilitation of clients; however, less than 40% of the respondents indicated that addressing clients' spiritual needs was within the scope of their professional practice."

Engquist, D. E., Short-DeGraff, M., Gliner, J., & Oltjenbruns, K. (1997). Occupational therapists' beliefs and practices with regard to spirituality and therapy. *American Journal of Occupational Therapy, 51*(3), 173.

Yerxa (1991) and colleagues from the University of Southern California kicked off the last decade of the 20th century by coining and defining the term *occupational science* to refer to the scientific discipline associated with the profession of OT. Considerable discussion ensued about the ability of the profession to support a separate scientific discipline; however, its necessity was understood by all if the field was to advance as required. In addition to guidelines for education and research in the area of occupational science, there were even several attempts at the development of animal models for the study of human occupation.

The 1990s saw the development of graduate education in OT across North America, Great Britain, and Australia-New Zealand. Masters' and doctoral programs emerged to prepare occupational therapists to contribute to the body of knowledge in the field and to fill roles as researchers and faculty in an increasingly viable academic discipline. Theoretical developments accompanied the growth of many of these academic programs, and textbooks and resource materials proliferated.

The latter part of the century was also marked by a focus on client-centered practice as a basic approach in OT. This approach is based on beliefs about the dignity and autonomy of human beings and about the nature of therapeutic change. A number of articles and books appeared during the decade attempting to put this challenging concept into practice. All of these developments in the field took place against a background of enormous technological change and growth. It is hard to imagine that as recently as the 1990s, it was not uncommon to find desks without computers on them and telephones and paper mail still the main forms of communication in business, including health care. The implications of technological developments were not immediately clear to occupational therapists, but slowly over the decade, electronic communications began to be incorporated in OT processes, such as assessment and reporting. Electronic and computer-based solutions began to be available for problems in self-care, productivity, and leisure for disabled individuals.

Finally, the last decade of the 20th century was marked by a degree of millennial anxiety: What had been accomplished in the preceding 100 years? Was war truly the most significant characteristic of the 20th century? What fate did the next century hold in store for humanity? Was it too late to solve some of the problems—economic, social, environmental—that threaten the human race? In previous centuries, many people might have turned to their faith communities for answers to questions of this magnitude. At the end of the 20th century, however, organized religion had lost much of its stature in developed societies. In its place was an almost universal quest for spiritual (as opposed to religious) answers to these questions as well as questions of a more personal nature—how to find inner peace, what adds meaning to life, and how humans are related to one another and to their world. This quest for spirituality was also expressed in OT. Occupational therapists were reminded of their original commitment to health of mind, body, and spirit and sought to explore further what it meant for OT to include the spiritual dimension of clients within its domain of concern.

2000-present

> *"Engaging in occupation can reveal, explain, manage and overcome on-going health conditions. The core concept, 'occupation empowers', integrates the different roles of occupation and reflects the meaning of occupation for people with on-going health conditions."*
>
> White, C., Lentin, P., & Farnworth, L. (2013). An investigation into the role and meaning of occupation for people living with on-going health conditions. *Australian Occupational Therapy Journal, 60*(1), 20.

> *"Occupational therapists have devoted their interest to balance in life ever since Meyer spoke about a balance between work, play, rest, and sleep."*
>
> Wagman, P., Håkansson, C., Jacobsson, C., Falkmer, T., & Björklund, A. (2012). What is considered important for life balance? Similarities and differences among some working adults. *Scandinavian Journal of Occupational Therapy, 19*(4), 377.

It is difficult to examine history from a proximal perspective, and so we restrict our discussion of the 21st century to noting a couple of clear trends. We pursue a fuller discussion of the theory and developments since the turn of the millennium in subsequent chapters.

The latter part of the 20th century saw ideas from postmodern thinking pervade OT—ideas such as skeptical or critical analyses of accepted truths, rejections of objectivity, reductionism and causality, and a wholesale belief in the interconnectedness of all phenomena. The 21st century so far has seen a reaction to these ideas that includes a yearning for universal truths balanced against an awareness of the relativity of existence and the importance of context. Issues such as climate change, financial crises, and geopolitical instability evoke the need for a balance between reason and passion, hope and caution. As we see in subsequent chapters, these sensibilities have been represented in the OT literature since the year 2000. We see critiques of fundamental ideas in OT alongside appeals to basic beliefs about occupation and health.

The 21st century finds occupational therapists still struggling with the concept of occupation. Pierce (2001) noted the need to create bridges that bring occupational science to OT. She developed the notion of therapeutic power to assess what makes an occupation useful as a therapeutic tool. The therapeutic power of an occupation is made up of the intrinsic appeal of the occupation, the extent to which the environment supports the occupation, and its fit with therapeutic goals.

Several other authors also have responded to the challenge of the growing body of knowledge in OT by noting the need for connection between how we think about occupation and what we do as occupational therapists. In this book, we talk about conceptual models and models of practice. Conceptual models help us to think about the relationship of occupation to other factors, and models of practice tell us how to change occupation or its determinants using assessments and interventions (see Chapter 2). Ikiugu (2008) made a similar distinction between organizing models (those that provide an overall perspective for understanding the patient's problems) and complementary models (those that offer tools for practice). Ashby and Chandler (2010) also talked about two types of models that needed to be compatible: conceptual knowledge and procedural knowledge. The former aims at understanding occupation, and the latter aims at acting to change occupation.

In 2004, Polatajko et al. responded to the need for clarity and consistency in language about occupation by offering the Taxonomic Code for Occupational Performance. This hierarchical taxonomy consisted of seven levels, from basic voluntary movements around a single joint to movement patterns, actions, tasks, activities, occupations, and occupational groups (e.g., self-care, productivity, and leisure). Paley, Eva, and Duncan (2006) acknowledged the 50-year history of attempts to classify occupation but severely criticized the taxonomy and concluded that occupation is just too complex and context dependent to be subject to a rigid hierarchy.

Hocking (2009) also took a stab at clarifying language and concepts. She offered nine parameters for describing and discussing occupation that are reminiscent of activity analysis frameworks from earlier decades:

1. Knowledge, skill, and attitudinal requirements of the occupation
2. Who usually does the occupation
3. Rules, norms, and processes associated with the occupation
4. Spatial requirements and resources
5. Temporal aspects, such as duration, season, time of day, sequence, pace
6. Outcomes or products (tangible or ephemeral)
7. Meanings (personal, social, cultural)
8. History (economic, political, cultural, geographic)
9. Impact on health

She advocated for the need to describe occupations independent of the experience of doing them—what Nelson (1988) referred to as *occupational forms*.

An interesting undercurrent arises in the theoretical literature of the 21st century. Are some occupations inherently good, valued, worthwhile, and health promoting, or is occupation entirely subjective and context dependent? Is there anything we can say with certainty about the value of specific occupations? For example, is it always good to make your bed, or are there situations in which a compelling argument can be made for leaving the bed just as one got out of it? Morgan (2010), in his discussion of occupational satisfaction, suggested that some occupations are more likely than others to contribute to human flourishing and occupational fulfillment. These occupations he described as having value, worth, weight, or purpose. They provide substance to the occupational life. He characterized his perspective as normative, meaning that it referred to a standard or a convention. He did not say that any particular occupation is universally right for everyone; rather, he said that persuasive arguments can be made, based on evidence, that some occupations are more likely than others to lead to occupational satisfaction and health. These occupations have been shown in research to be related to desired outcomes, such as health, satisfaction, and well-being, and thus can be considered to have value or worth.

On the other side of the argument, and by far the more popular side, are those who take a relativistic view of occupation and its relationship to health. They focus on the subjective aspect of occupation and its situation in context. Kantzarksis and Molineux (2011), for example, characterized occupation as entirely socially constructed, meaning that it has no objective reality, only the meaning that individuals create for it. They resisted Western notions about occupation because of their origins in power structures and patterns of domination and exploitation. In particular, they took exception to the ideas that occupation is *active, purposeful,* and *temporal*—meaning that it involves doing, is goal oriented, and occupies time. They equated the idea of good and bad occupations with religious strictures on behavior and strenuously resisted such judgments.

A related concept that continues to be highly prevalent in the OT theory literature is the concept of meaning. Keponen and Kielhofner (2006) studied the meanings ascribed to occupation and noted the importance of creating the narrative of occupation as a means of finding meaning. They emphasized the link between saying and doing and the necessity of interpreting occupation for finding meaning and satisfaction. Reed, Hocking, and Smythe (2011) also explored meaning and determined that meaning derives from the feeling of being called to a particular occupation, from the potential for being with others, and from the possibilities of future benefits associated with the occupation.

Another elusive concept in OT is the notion of occupational balance. Wagman and colleagues conducted a scoping review over 15 years and found 43 articles dealing with balance (Wagman, Håkansson, & Björklund, 2012). The only conclusions they could draw were that occupational balance is subjective and that it exists on a continuum from better to poorer. They noted that balance has variously been described in terms of the mix of occupational areas; the characteristics of various occupations (physical, mental, social); the challenge presented by occupations; the patterns, roles, and routines shaping occupations; the time spent on different occupations; and the environments engaged in.

Finally, several articles shed light on the relationship between occupation and well-being in the period between 2000 and 2013. Kaponen and Keihl (2006) explored occupational disruption and found that the ability to find satisfaction in occupations was related to the enjoyment they produced, the challenge they posed, their intensity or demand, and their opportunity for social interaction, particularly the opportunity to share something in common with another. Pierce (2001) suggested that the appeal of an occupation lay in the fact that it provided pleasure, produced something, and restored energy. Doble and Santha (2008) found five critical issues that affect occupational well-being, some of which we discussed earlier: meaning, balance, belonging, choice, and subjectivity. They further stated that occupational well-being was associated with meeting the seven occupational needs: accomplishment, affirmation, agency, coherence, companionship, pleasure, and renewal. McColl (2002) also produced a similar list of needs that could be met by occupation, especially when stressful times amplify the demands on individuals. Occupation was an integral part of meeting basic survival needs as well as the need or drive for mastery, diversion, support, identity, habit, and spirituality.

Summary

The second section of this book began with a brief excursion through more than 100 years of OT history. This review has shown the rise and fall of some ideas, the persistence of many, and the demise of a few. The next chapter looks in detail at six occupation-focused models that offer a view of the relationship between occupation and health or well-being.

8

Occupation-Focused Models

Mary Ann McColl, PhD, MTS

The first step in thinking like an occupational therapist is to focus on occupation—that is, to try to understand occupation and its proposed relationship to health (lens #1 of the telescope). In order to do that, we need ways of thinking about occupation that help us to elaborate the construct and identify and analyze its parts. This chapter deals with occupation-focused models—those models that define, describe, and explain occupation and its relationship to health and well-being.

Occupation

Occupation is the central construct that defines and unites occupational therapy (OT) theory. *Occupation* is used throughout this book to refer to *purposeful or meaningful activities in which humans engage as part of their normal daily lives.* We use this term not in the colloquial sense, to refer to one's vocation, job, or field of professional expertise. Instead, we use occupation in the historical sense within OT, to refer to all aspects of daily living that contribute to health and fulfillment for an individual (as we have in previous editions). Occupation is the touchstone that helps to focus the practice of OT, and it is the overarching idea that gives unity and meaning to the theory base of OT.

A number of other words are sometimes used synonymously with occupation, such as *activity*, *task*, or *function*. We suggest that within the technical lexicon of OT, *occupation* has no synonyms. It is the most important word in OT, and as such, it needs to be used with precision and intention. We may use other words colloquially and generally, but we must use occupation technically and specifically. As Pierce (2001) suggests,

occupation is individually constructed and context dependent. Thus when we use occupation in this book, we refer to purposeful and meaningful activities enacted in the context of daily life. At its simplest, occupation refers to the things we *do*. The concept of *doing* is central to understanding occupation. Occupations do not necessarily need to be overt actions. They also can be thoughts, intentions, or plans.

Another term we often encounter in OT theory is *occupational performance*, referring to the actual *doing* of occupation. Thus *occupations* are the things we *do*, and *occupational performance* is the *actual doing* of occupations. Can occupations exist in the absence of the doing of them? Why do we make this distinction between occupation and occupational performance? At their simplest levels, occupations are abstract concepts. They are ideas about the things we do; they are the names we give to the things we do and how we think about them. For example, it is possible to think about the occupation of horseback riding without actually getting onto a horse. We each carry an idea in our minds of what horseback riding is. That idea consists of a number of smaller activities and tasks that make up the occupation. It may have emotional overlay associated with it, and it may be associated with specific other people and things as well as the background against which that occupation typically occurs. All of these aspects of an occupation exist in our minds at the mention of the occupation. Plato referred to the form of an object as its ideal essence, existing on a plane above the reality of the actual object. Thus, horseback riding exists both in the abstract and in the concrete. In the abstract, we refer to it simply as an occupation (or perhaps an occupational form). When we actually go to a

McColl MA, Law M, Stewart D.
Theoretical Basis of Occupational Therapy, Third Edition (pp. 53-66).
© 2015 Taylor & Francis Group.

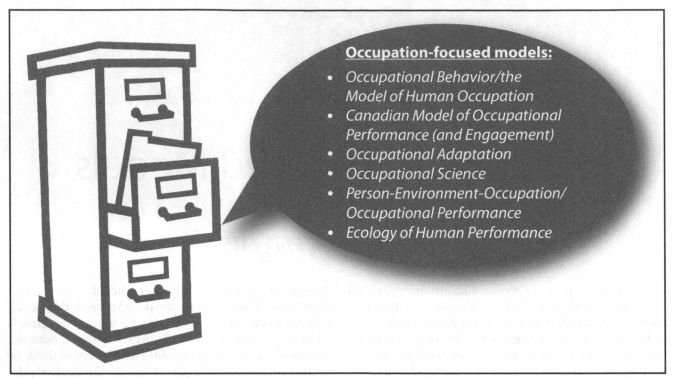

Occupation-focused models:

- *Occupational Behavior/the Model of Human Occupation*
- *Canadian Model of Occupational Performance (and Engagement)*
- *Occupational Adaptation*
- *Occupational Science*
- *Person-Environment-Occupation/ Occupational Performance*
- *Ecology of Human Performance*

Figure 8-1. The first drawer of the occupational therapy filing cabinet.

stable, get on a horse, and ride off into the sunset, this we call performing the occupation of horseback riding.

Nelson (1988) referred to this abstract notion of an occupation as the "occupational form," perhaps invoking Plato's notion of forms. According to Nelson (1988), to fully understand occupation, we have to separate the occupation itself from the context within which it exists and on which it is fully dependent for its final representation or performance. He coined the term *occupational form* to represent the decontextualized image of the occupation. He suggested that occupational form interacts with the individual's developmental level, resulting in meaning (perceptual, symbolic, and affective meaning), purpose, and ultimately occupational performance.

Why is this distinction important? Although it may seem unnecessarily abstract, it is important to recognize that we carry around with us these ideas of what occupations are. We make assumptions about how an occupation is performed, what it feels like, what is needed in order to do it, and what constitutes successful performance. Furthermore, these assumptions need not necessarily be shared; they may even differ between clients and therapists. Thus before an occupation can be discussed, it is essential that it be fully described, so that assumptions become explicit. If there are important differences in how different individuals understand an occupation, these then can be explored and reconciled.

For example, making the bed is a relatively simple occupation, and one that most readers will readily be able to think about in fairly concrete terms. What constitutes the occupational form of making the bed? Are we starting from a bare mattress, choosing the right-sized sheets, doing hospital corners, making sure the pillow cases are pointing the right way, pulling the covers to a taut finish that will bounce a coin? Are we simply pulling up the duvet and fluffing the pillows? Are we rolling up a sleeping roll on the floor of a shelter? All of these are versions of "making the bed" for different people in different settings. The occupational form of making the bed, however, is the generic activity that would be fairly consistent across contexts. When we analyze an occupation for its demands and requirements, we typically analyze the *occupational form*, whereas when we assess a client's ability to do something, we assess their *occupational performance*.

Occupation-Focused Models

OT theorists have proposed a number of conceptual models to help us think about occupation and its relationship to health outcomes (Figure 8-1). These models seek to define the basic parameters of occupation, its inherent nature, the relationships among its component parts, and ultimately its relationship to health and well-being.

In this chapter, we review the most commonly known and used theories describing occupation and its relationship to health. These theories share the following characteristics:

- They are all what we refer to as "big-T" theories"—that is, they have a formal title, and there are specific authors and researchers associated with each in the literature.
- They are typically attributed to OT authors and derive from the OT literature.
- They have occupation and health as key concepts.
- They do not focus on a particular determinant of occupation (e.g., physical, psychological-emotional, sociocultural, cognitive-neurological, or environmental); rather, they look at the effect of occupation (self-care, productivity, and leisure) on health and well-being.
- They are conceptual models that help therapists to know how to think about occupation and health. They exist to explain relationships between concepts rather than instruct therapists about how to assess and intervene (models of practice).

Consistent with the scope of this book, the intent is to focus on conceptual models (rather than models of practice) and to emphasize new theoretical developments found in the peer-reviewed literature since 2000. Most of these models were developed prior to that date and have been fully described in books or articles by their founding authors. They also have been reviewed and summarized in previous editions of this book and in other theory textbooks. Therefore, after a brief introduction to each model, the discussion emphasizes new findings in the professional literature.

1. Occupational Behavior and the Model of Human Occupation

Occupational Behavior and the Model of Human Occupation (MOHO) are regarded together in this book, because the latter derives directly from the former, and contemporary developments tend to refer exclusively to the MOHO.

The Occupational Behavior model was founded by Mary Reilly in the late 1950s-early 1960s. She asserted the need for a model that focused on the core concept of occupational behavior and brought together numerous themes in OT (Reilly, 1962). *Occupational behavior* was defined as the activities that occupy time, produce achievement, and sustain the individual. Drawing on a background in the social sciences, she moved away from the dominance of the medical and neurological sciences to reestablish occupation as the core concept in OT. The model brought together many historically familiar and relevant topics, such as the work-play continuum, roles and routines, temporal rhythms, mastery, and adaptation.

The Occupational Behavior approach focused on disruptions to occupational functioning, particularly work and work satisfaction. It brought together three bodies of knowledge from the social sciences to inform thinking about occupation:

1. Developmental theory contributed an understanding of the relationship between play and work, the development of social behavior, and the balance of activity and rest.
2. Achievement theory contributed the ideas of mastery and coping, the intrinsic drive to explore and understand the environment, and social learning models.
3. Role theory contributed knowledge about routines, habits, and roles; the behaviors that constitute these roles; and the rhythm of role performance over time.

In the early 1980s, three of Dr. Reilly's students (Kielhofner, Burke, and Heard) fulfilled the destiny of the Occupational Behavior approach by synthesizing and publishing key ideas in a series of papers and later books that introduced the MOHO (Kielhofner, 1980; Kielhofner & Burke, 1980).

The MOHO adds general systems theory to the Occupational Behavior approach. It represents the person as an open system with three hierarchical, interrelated parts:

1. The *volition* subsystem, including the interests, personal causation, and values. These provide enjoyment, meaning, and effectiveness to occupation
2. The *habituation* subsystem, composed of habits and roles—the routines and patterns of behavior that facilitate and streamline occupation
3. The *performance* subsystem, made up of the skills and abilities that are the building blocks of occupation

Health is achieved when these three subsystems operate in a coordinated fashion to meet the demands of the environment and adapt to challenges. The model is accompanied by a number of assessment and intervention tools available through an online clearinghouse, making it the most well-developed and widely known of all OT models (www.cade.uic.edu/moho/default.aspx).

The most recent edition of the model (Kielhofner, 2008) identified its outcomes as *occupational identity* and *occupational competence*, both contributing to *occupational adaptation*. Rather than viewing the three subsystems (performance, habituation, and volition) as hierarchical, the fourth edition of the model describes them as heterarchical. Rather than having higher-order values, interests, and volition dependent on lower-order habits, roles, and skills, the 2008 model saw the three subsystems as mutually influencing one another, with no expectation of an orderly or predetermined direction of the effects of one subsystem on another. Finally, the fourth edition described the individual as a dynamic system rather than an open system. This distinction invoked the idea that human occupation is not predictable according to a specified formula; rather, it is highly complex, constantly changing, and not subject to formulaic explanation.

The research since 2000 on the MOHO has been by far the most prolific of the models considered. A wealth of research has been published on the model by both the original authors and later adherents and critics. According to a scoping review conducted by Lee (2010), as of mid-2009, 433 books, chapters, and articles had been published focusing on the MOHO (compared with between 12 and 31 for other models over the same period). This can in part be accounted for by the fact that the MOHO has been around 10 to 15 years longer than other models.

On the strength of Lee's scoping review, the MOHO is the only occupation-based model that can be considered "evidence-based." The body of knowledge on the MOHO is made up primarily of articles exploring application of the model to particular areas of practice, patient populations, or geographic contexts. It is estimated that about 60% of the published research falls into this category. The literature provides examples of the use of the MOHO to promote wellness among Japanese elders (Yamada, Kawamata, Kobayashi, Kielhofner, & Taylor, 2010), to increase physical activity among people with mental illness (Cole, 2010), and to assess employment needs of people with intellectual disabilities in Bulgaria (Raber, Teitelman, Watts, & Keilhofner, 2010).

Another 30% of the literature is made up of psychometric and validation studies on the 20 assessments associated with the model. A surprisingly low 5% of articles are studies of the effectiveness of interventions based on the model. One example is another scoping review by Lee and Kielhofner (2010) of 45 studies looking at the MOHO as the basis for intervention aimed at employment. They showed that significant improvements in work performance could be achieved using structured intervention approaches based on the model.

Finally, the remaining 5% of articles associated with the MOHO are theoretical articles aimed at further exploring concepts or principles associated with the model and subsequently reflecting on or refining the theory. These latter few are the articles that are of particular interest in this book.

The MOHO research group conducted a survey of 1000 occupational therapists, leading to three publications about how the model is used in practice (Lee, Taylor, Kielhofner, & Fisher, 2008; Lee, Taylor, & Kielhofner, 2009, 2010). They concluded that therapists who use the MOHO do so because they find it client centered, occupation focused, and holistic (Lee, Taylor, Kielhofner, & Fisher, 2008). The availability of practice tools, such as assessments and structured interventions, also significantly affects uptake (Lee, 2010).

The main impediment to practicing using the MOHO concepts is lack of in-depth knowledge among therapists and the high degree of support needed to successfully implement it in a practice setting. Wimpenny and colleagues reported on a 2-year-long initiative to establish the MOHO as the basis for OT in their setting (Wimpenny, Forsyth, Jones, Matheson, & Colley, 2010). The process included monthly meetings and support provision for the first year, with additional expert consultation monthly for another year. This intensive process resulted in a community of practice that enhanced theory uptake. Melton, Forsyth, and Freeth (2010) also commented on the challenge of practice development and showed the need for institutional support and attention to individual differences in learning preferences and application styles. According to Lee (2010), evidence continues to be generated and interest sustained in the MOHO.

2. The Canadian Model of Occupational Performance

About the same time, the early 1980s, another occupation-focused model was developed through an entirely different mechanism. Rather than emerging from a strong academic tradition, like the Occupational Behavior model and the MOHO, the Canadian Model of Occupational Performance (CMOP) (Figure 8-2) arose out of a national consensus process initiated by government. In partnership with the Canadian Association of Occupational Therapists, the Department of National Health and Welfare in Canada established a national task force to see what therapists, educators, and researchers thought were the key ideas driving OT practice in Canada.

The model that emerged showed three concentric circles. At the center was the individual, with his or her physical, mental, social, and spiritual components. The individual interacted through the medium of occupation (self-care, productivity, and leisure) with the environment (including the physical, social, and institutional environment). Health was achieved when both performance and satisfaction with occupation were optimized. A key tenet of the model was a client-centered approach to practice. Practice tools were developed to accompany the model, including

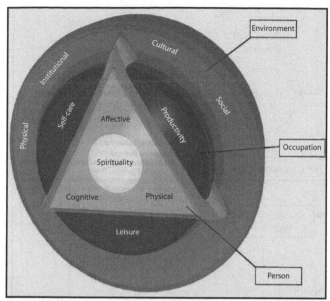

Figure 8-2. The Canadian Model of Occupational Performance. (Adapted with permission from [CMOP-E] Canadian Model of Occupational Performance in Polatajko, H., Townsend, E., & Craik, J. (2007). *Enabling occupation II: Advancing an occupational therapy vision for health, well-being & justice through occupation.* Ottawa, ON, CAOT Publications. p. 23.)

the Canadian Occupational Performance Measure (COPM) and intervention guidelines.

In 1997, the model was altered to feature the spiritual component of the individual at the center of everything, presumably elevated above the physical, mental, and social components of the person (CAOT, 1997, 2002). Subsequently, Townsend and Polatajko (2007) added the idea of engagement and renamed the model as the Canadian Model of Occupational Performance and Engagement (CMOP-E). The term *occupational engagement* was substituted for occupational performance to invoke the idea of *involvement* in occupation beyond the mere performance of it. The model itself remains unchanged; it still consists of three concentric shapes, with occupation as the medium through which individuals and environments interact.

The more recent publications (CAOT, 1997, 2002; Townsend & Polatajko, 2007) focus to a greater extent on the therapist and the skills and attitudes he or she must possess; thus, the latest version functions more as a model of practice than a theoretical model. The later versions feature the idea of *enabling* occupation, and the therapist's role is outlined as consisting of 10 skills: adapt, advocate, coach, collaborate, consult, coordinate, design and build, educate, engage, and specialize. Later editions also included the Canadian Practice Process Framework, an eight-step cycle from admission to discharge. This takes the place of Fearing and Clark's (2000) Occupational Performance Process

Model, featured in previous editions. Both of these "process models" show the steps engaged in by occupational therapists in collaborating with their patients, but they say little about the nature and extent of the relationships between elements of the person, the environment, occupation, and health.

Since 2000, four articles were found in the international peer-reviewed OT literature that focused on the CMOP or CMOP-E, and 110 articles were found on COPM (Law, Baptiste, Carswell, McColl, Polatajko, & Pollock, 1991, 2014). In two articles, the CMOP was used to give structure to clinical planning and service delivery—specifically, the model was used to classify occupations as self-care, productivity, or leisure or to identify the focus of intervention as person, occupation, or environment (Galvin, Randall, Hewish, Rice, & MacKay, 2010; Guay, Dubois, Desrosiers, & Robitaille, 2012). Another article cited the CMOP as the basis for exploring spirituality among elderly clients (Griffith, Caron, Desrosiers, & Thibeault, 2007). The fourth article focused on embedding the CMOP as the basis for practice for a whole department. Boniface and colleagues (2008) described the process of action and reflection associated with changing culture and practice to adopt a client-centered occupation-focused practice. The articles associated with the COPM focused on applicability in certain settings or populations, psychometric properties, or practice utility (for more information, see McColl et al., 2006).

In summary, it seems that the main contributions of the CMOP are as follows:

- Its simple yet pervasive characterization of occupation as self-care, productivity, and leisure
- Its emphasis on occupation as the medium through which person and environment interact
- Its consideration of spirituality as part of the domain of OT
- Its client-centered perspective on service delivery
- Its use as a means of initiating the model in practice

A critique of the model might point to the relative absence of a research base associated with any of these principles. Further, the treatment of key concepts can be considered somewhat superficial. Like many theories in OT, the CMOP points to the presence of a relationship between occupation and various concepts but offers relatively little in terms of empirical substance regarding the nature and extent of the proposed relationships. With regard to measurement, the COPM has been remarkably pervasive internationally as a generic measure of occupational performance, but it is only a first step in identifying occupational performance problems. It is not yet accompanied by a suite of measures of other key concepts in the model.

According to Ashby and Chandler (2010), the CMOP/CMOP-E and the MOHO are the two most

Figure 8-3. The Occupational Adaptation Model. (Reprinted with permission from Schkade, J., & Schultz, S. (1992). Occupational adaptation: Toward a holistic approach for contemporary practice, part 1. *American Journal of Occupational Therapy*, 46(10), 829-829.)

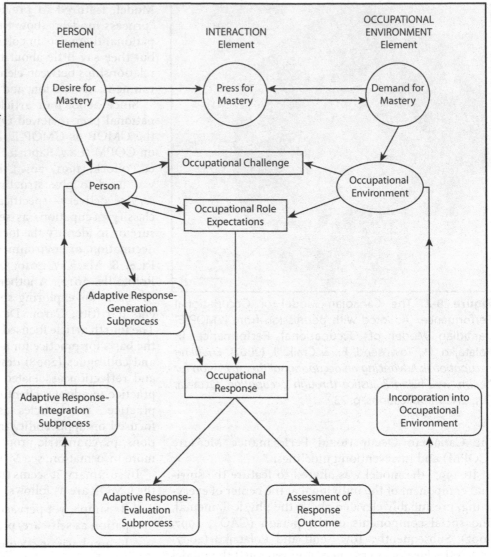

widely taught occupation-focused models in educational programs in Canada, the United States, the United Kingdom, and Australia. Virtually all programs in these four regions explicitly teach both of these models to their students as the basis for their understanding of what it means to be an occupational therapist. These two together then form a key basis for the practice of OT in the English-speaking world.

3. Occupational Adaptation

The ideas that humans adapt and that occupation is the mechanism that promotes human adaptation have been a part of OT since the earliest days. In 1984, Reed and Sanderson outlined three main ideas that have persisted throughout the history of OT: that the occupations of self-maintenance, productivity, and leisure persist across the lifespan; that they exist in a dynamic balance; and that they are the medium through which humans adapt to their environments.

In the early 1990s, adaptation became further formalized in a model published by Schkade and Schultz (1992) entitled *Occupational Adaptation* (Figure 8-3). This model arose in an academic environment (Texas Women's University) as the basis for the development of a graduate program in OT.

Unlike the two previous models (MOHO and CMOP), this model has at its center not the person but the process of adaptation. *Adaptation* is characterized as a normative, lifelong process that is a response to the internal and external pressures for mastery. These pressures, along with occupational role expectations, create occupational challenges. Over the lifespan, new challenges arise and new demands are made by the human and nonhuman environment. At any point in the life trajectory, illness or injury can impose new occupational demands, some of which may exceed the adaptive capacity of the individual.

In response to these challenges, the individual generates options. He or she can marshal existing adaptive behaviors, modify old responses, or generate entirely new ones. Depending on how effective the response is, it may either be integrated and stored for future use or discarded. The individual is endowed with a finite amount of adaptive energy that can be applied to adaptive challenges. The challenge of occupational adaptation is to use one's energy to produce occupational responses that are efficient, effective, and satisfying. Occupational therapists assist in that process by working toward occupational readiness (using skills and training) and occupational activity (performance of roles).

The Occupational Adaptation model includes a model of practice consisting of four main principles:

1. The focus of practice should be on "adaptiveness" rather than performance; on process rather than on outcome; on new adaptive skills rather than on new performance skills.

2. The adaptive capacity of the client is the key outcome rather than any particular occupation.

3. The client is the agent of change.

4. The therapist's main tool is the questions he or she asks rather than any particular technique or skill:

    What are you needing to do, and who says so?

    What would you customarily do when faced with a challenge like this?

    How will you know if that's not working and what might you do to modify it?

    Are there other, perhaps new, options for responding to this situation?

    What will happen the next time you are faced with a situation like this?

Only one practice tool, the Relative Mastery Measurement Scale (George, Schkade, & Ishee, 2004) has been developed for applying this relatively complex model.

In the literature of the 21st century to date, 27 articles were identified by the phrase "occupational adaptation." On closer examination, however, it became clear that this search term would not exclusively identify literature associated with the big-T theory called "Occupational Adaptation" as developed by Schkade and Schultz (1992). There were a number of other ways that the phrase was used:

- In several articles, it was used to refer to adaptations or modifications made to a particular occupation to promote independence (Lexell, Iwarsson, & Lund, 2011).

- In other articles, "occupational adaptation" referred to adjustments a person might make in response to inability (Lee et al., 2006).

- Adaptive strategies used to promote return to work were also called occupational adaptations (Soeker, 2011).

- Occupational adaptation is one of the key outcomes sought in the MOHO (Cahill, Connolly, & Stapleton, 2010).

- *Occupational adaptation* is a term also associated with *Occupational Science*. In one study, there was another theory attributed to Frank (1996) that was also entitled "occupational adaptation." Frank's theory is considered a part of occupational science, however, and is discussed later.

- Occupational adaptation was also used to refer to the generic outcome of successfully engaging in occupation in several studies (Klinger, 2005; Pepin, 2011).

- In one study, occupational adaptation was used to refer to an occupational therapist's adaptation to working conditions (Walker, 2001).

What is immediately evident is that we use both of the terms *occupational* and *adaptation* almost colloquially in OT. Not only that, but we use both words to refer to both processes and outcomes in OT. We talk about *adaptation* as both the process of adapting and also as the endpoint of successfully adapting. Similarly, we use the term *occupation* to refer to both the means through which occupational therapists operate and the end that they hope to achieve. With all this ambiguity in language, it can be readily understood how it might be challenging to pinpoint theoretical developments in the field of Occupational Adaptation.

For our purposes, we focused our search by eliminating articles that use the term occupational adaptation in any of these other senses and reported only on articles that referred to the proper name of the theory by Schkade and Schultz. We have also followed our usual decision rules and included only articles that developed or clarified the theoretical ideas. We excluded articles that merely applied the theory in a particular setting, that looked at measures or measurement properties, or that provided empirical evidence for a single principle of the model. That left us with seven articles that advanced ideas about Occupational Adaptation. These tended to appear at the beginning of the 13-year period studied (2000-2012), whereas the more colloquial uses of the term tended to appear in the more recent literature.

Jackson and Schkade (2001) contrasted the Occupational Adaptation approach to the biomechanical approach in the care of patients with hip fractures. They found that although functional outcomes were not significantly different between Occupational Adaptation and biomechanical approaches, the former achieved those outcomes more efficiently and afforded patients more satisfaction. They pointed to the importance of understanding the demand and press for mastery as motivating factors. These same factors were found to be important in the rehabilitation of people who had strokes (Gillot, Holder-Walls, Kurtz, & Varley, 2003). Johnson (2006) focused on the process of adaptation as a lifelong, normative, cumulative process. She differentiated it from coping, which is situational and episodic.

Bouteloup and Beltran (2007) emphasized the importance of understanding the underlying processes in adaptation. The Occupational Adaptation model refers to primary and secondary energy to denote the degree of cortical involvement in the effort associated with adaptation. To the extent that adaptation becomes subcortical, adaptive energy is freed for new learning, and higher cognitive processes are enabled. Finally, in several of the articles, it was emphasized that identification of occupational challenges and evaluation of outcomes in Occupational Adaptation are subjective assessments of effectiveness, efficiency, and satisfaction. In this way, the model acts as a stimulus for occupation-focused, client-centered practice.

Lee's (2010) scan of the theoretical literature in OT found similarly few articles in the peer-reviewed literature focusing on Occupational Adaptation. Ashby and Chandler (2010) found that of 64 OT training programs surveyed, only British and American schools covered this model, or a total of about one-fifth of programs. No Canadian schools reported explicitly addressing this model in their educational programs.

The Occupational Adaptation model is critiqued for focusing almost entirely on the internal processes in the person and ignoring the environment as a locus for intervention. Its strengths, however, are its focus on the complexity of the adaptive process and its emphasis not only on the "what" but also on the "how" of the OT process. Considerable scope still exists for development in this model.

4. Person-Environment-Occupation/ Occupational Performance

The Person-Environment-Occupation (PEO) model grew out of the work of Mary Law, focusing on the environment as an essential yet largely neglected aspect of OT (Law, 1991). The model asserts that person, occupation, and environment are in constant relationship with one another (Law et al., 1996). Unlike prior models that discussed the interaction of person and environment through the medium of occupation, Law and colleagues proposed that the relationship was "transactive." Rather than portraying person, occupation, and environment as three independent constructs acting on each other in predictable ways (interactive), they characterized them as dependent and mutually influential (transactive). This distinction resulted in

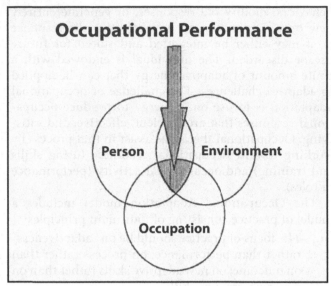

Figure 8-4. The Person-Environment-Occupation Model. (Reprinted with permission from Law, M., Cooper, B., Strong, S. C., Rigby, P., & Letts, L. (1996). The person-environment-occupational model: A transactive approach to occupational performance. *Canadian Journal of Occupational Therapy, 63*, 1-15.)

a model that is more organic than mechanistic, more complex and less predictable; thus intervention cannot be prescriptive but must be viewed as incremental. This is similar to the contention in later versions of the MOHO that the person is a dynamic system rather than an open system.

The principal tools associated with practice according to the PEO model (Figure 8-4) are the COPM and the Perceived Efficacy and Goal-Setting Measure. The PEO model includes a lifespan perspective, recognizing the potential for age-related changes in the needs and capabilities of the person, the demands and expectations of the environment, and the complexities and range of occupations.

According to the PEO model, optimal occupation performance may be achieved by altering any of the three components of the model: person, occupation, or environment. Change may be accomplished through adaptation of the individual, modification of the occupation, or adjustments to the environment. Intervention can be targeted at any of these three levels, and health is achieved when this dynamic relationship is effectively managed. The desired outcome of the model is to meet the intrinsic human needs for self-maintenance, expression, and fulfillment. Across the lifespan, it is understood that the three components of the model change in content and priority.

At approximately the same time, Christiansen and Baum (1991) produced a model to act as the basis for a comprehensive new textbook in OT. They called

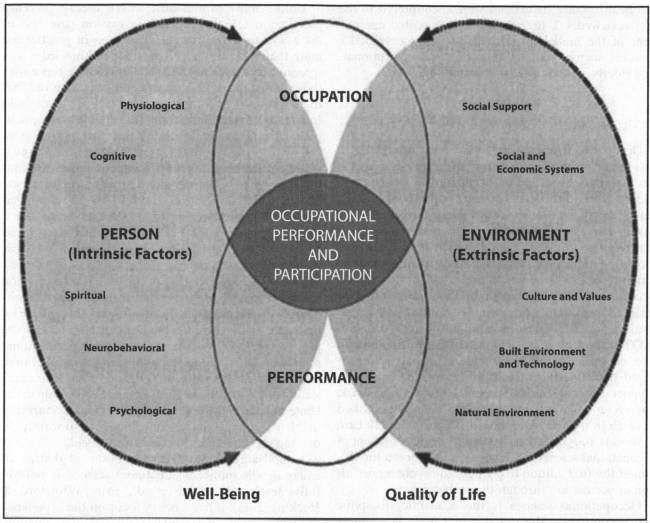

Figure 8-5. The Person-Environment-Occupational Performance model. (Reprinted with permission from Law, M., Cooper, B., Strong, S. C., Rigby, P., & Letts, L. (1996). The person-environment-occupational model: A transactive approach to occupational performance. *Canadian Journal of Occupational Therapy, 63*, 1-15.)

their model the Person-Environment-Occupational Performance (PEOP) model (Figure 8-5). The model builds up occupational performance in layers. At the first layer are intrinsic (person) and extrinsic (environment) factors. Once again, the person is made up of numerous component parts, and the environment contains physical, social, and societal factors. Person and environment are bridged at the second level by occupation and performance. Occupations are human pursuits that are goal directed, context dependent, recognizable, and meaningful. They are built up hierarchically from abilities, actions, and tasks, and they are organized into roles. Finally, at the third level, occupational performance and participation represent the ultimate outcome—the totality of occupations that constitute an individual's overall participation. As previously discussed, *occupation* is conceptualized as separate from performance in this model, suggesting that occupations exist in the abstract as well as in the

practical reality of their performance or doing. There is a broad array of occupations out there that an individual can potentially do, and these occupations become tangible and real when they are performed.

The model of practice associated with PEOP is client centered and occupation focused, or top down. The *top-down* approach refers to starting with occupation as the focus of therapy—that is, self-care, productivity, or leisure as the basis for the OT interaction. The alternative is to use a *bottom-up* approach, meaning starting with the deficits in skill components and working on those, assuming that improvements to occupational performance will follow from improved skills and abilities (Trombly, 1993). Assessment strategies include occupational history, role profile, perceptions of occupational disruption, and short- and long-term goals.

Research since 2000 is sparse substantiating both of these views of the relationship between occupation and health. Only six articles were encountered in the peer-reviewed OT literature. All represented applications of the model in particular settings or practice contexts, such as neonatal intensive care, institutionalized elderly, and knowledge translation.

5. Occupational Science and Occupational Justice

Occupational science is not so much a model as a movement promoting the body of knowledge associated with the concept of occupation. Occupational science arose in the late 1980s and early 1990s looking much like a new model—coining new terms and proposing principles about relationships between concepts that required further research. *Occupation* is defined according to occupational scientists as chunks of daily activity that can be named in the lexicon of the culture. *Occupational science* is an umbrella term covering all research leading to a better understanding of occupation. It was conceived to underpin the doctoral program in OT at the University of Southern California in 1989. The development of occupational science acknowledged that a sufficient body of knowledge existed to support doctoral studies. Kramer, Hinojosa, and Brasic Royeen (2003) pointed to the compilation of published research in the first edition of this book (McColl, Law, & Stewart 1993) as an early step in the development of occupational science. In particular, they noted the section of the first edition that tracks the evolving definition of occupation through the 20th century.

Occupational science is the academic discipline that accompanies the practice of OT. It is a movement for the legitimization of the practice of OT and a research enterprise with core concepts, methodologies, and dissemination vehicles. Conducted primarily by researchers, occupational science provides sound evidence on which to base our understanding of occupation and our profession. Its aim is to study the *form, function,* and *meaning* of occupation (Zemke & Clarke, 1996). According to Hocking (2009), occupational science consists of identifying the essential elements of occupation, describing occupation, and demonstrating its relationship to health.

What does it mean to be a science? Sciences are typically governed by assumptions about the nature of reality and the potential of humans to discover the principles that underlie that reality. Science literally means the application of the scientific method: to observe a problem, to generate a hypothesis, to gather data, and to interpret those data to reflect on the original problem. Science is by definition related to the gathering and interpretation of data. Those data may be qualitative or quantitative, inductive or deductive, context neutral or context dependent, rational or phenomenological.

Unlike most professions, where theory precedes practice, in OT the practice profession gave rise to the academic discipline. OT had been in practice for more than 60 years before the body of knowledge was recognized as a science. As such, there were those who thought that the profession was doing just fine and that there was no need for a separate enterprise to study it. In fact, there was concern that the emergence of occupational science would undermine the profession of OT by drawing resources away from it. Mosey (1997) made a distinction between occupational science and OT research. The former she defined as the basic science related to occupation, and the latter as the applied study of the effectiveness of OT. She advocated for a partition between the basic and applied sciences so that both can flourish and one does not overshadow the other.

While we may joke that occupational science is the science of qualifying every noun in the English language with the modifier "occupational," this enterprise has generated a considerable body of literature in the past 20 years. More than 250 articles on occupational science qualified for our dataset from the international peer-reviewed literature in OT since 2000. Honorary lectureships (such as the Ruth Zemke Lectureship in the United States and the Frances Rutherford Lectureship in New Zealand) have contributed significantly to moving the yardsticks forward in this field.

Several authors have recently observed that as an emerging discipline, occupational science is not yet fully developed (Pierce et al., 2010; Whiteford & Hocking, 2012). It has a heavy focus on the experience of occupation and personal narrative about occupation. By contrast, there is relatively little population-based or longitudinal research on occupation. The vast majority of articles dealing with occupational science employed qualitative methodologies. They tended to focus on describing occupational experiences through personal narratives. An extraordinarily high proportion of the occupational science literature is nonempirical—that is, it is theoretical, discussion-oriented, or commentary rather than data driven (Hocking, 2009; Pierce et al., 2010; Wright-St. Clair, 2012).

Some important ideas have emerged from the occupational science approach, including the concepts of *occupational justice* and *occupational identity*. Based on the assumption that humans need occupation in order to be healthy and well, *occupational justice* is a framework for examining the effects of inadequate engagement in occupation. The occupational justice approach began in the 21st century and is said by some to be a reaction to globalization and increased awareness of geopolitical forces shaping occupation and inequities in access to meaningful occupation. It adopts a social justice perspective, looking primarily at the environmental conditions that inhibit occupational choice and give rise to occupational deprivation, occupational alienation, and occupational imbalance. The role of the therapist is to enable occupation, thereby promoting occupational engagement or occupational participation.

Research on occupational justice since 2000 includes 38 articles found in the peer-reviewed literature. Many applied the occupational justice perspective to a particular disadvantaged or vulnerable group, such as victims of war or violence, refugees, immigrants or people with mental illness or disability. They involved both domestic and international settings and often invoked other theoretical or service perspectives, such as the human rights approach, the capabilities approach, or community-based rehabilitation. Methodologies used were often participatory action research or emancipatory research. The research tended to be overtly politicized, with no pretext of objectivity or neutrality, but rather with an explicit sociopolitical agenda aimed at removing barriers and alleviating inequities. The OT role is specified as advocacy and social action. Several authors noted that this approach hearkens back to some of the more politicized social justice campaigns of OT pioneers in the early 20th century.

Occupational identity is another important concept that arose out of the occupational science enterprise. Occupational identity is based on the belief that through occupation, we not only construct our world, but we also construct our selves. As Christiansen put it (1999; Christiansen & Townsend, 2004), we become who we are through what we do. Our identity is built from the way we interact with objects and humans and the social feedback we receive as a result of those interactions.

Since 2000, the research literature has offered a number of important ideas about occupation and identity. This literature was almost exclusively qualitative in its methodology, reflecting the social science origins of this area of inquiry (Phelan & Kinsella, 2009). Much of it reflected a lifespan perspective and the importance of continuity of identity throughout life (Howie, Coulter, & Feldman, 2004; Purves & Suto, 2004; Unruh, 2004; Wiseman & Whiteford, 2007). Through narrative approaches, several authors discussed the impact of disability or chronic illness on the life trajectory and the importance of occupation as a means of upholding identity and overcoming occupational disruptions (Jakobsen, 2001; Unruh & Elvin, 2004; Vrkljan & Miller-Polgar, 2007). Several authors situated the concept of occupational identity squarely within Western culture, with its emphasis on the individual and on achievement (Phillips, Kelk, & Fitzgerald, 2007; Rudman & Dennhardt, 2008).

6. Ecology of Human Performance

As its name suggests, the Ecology of Human Performance (EHP) model stresses the impact of context on occupation. It was designed for use not just by occupational therapists, but also by other health professions. As such, we do not find the word *occupation* featured as prominently here as we did in other models. Instead this model refers to *tasks*, meaning behaviors necessary for goal attainment. Tasks may be organized into role performance and occupational performance.

The EHP model (Figure 8-6) was developed by Dunn and colleagues at the University of Kansas Medical Center to guide their curriculum, research, and service. The model begins with the person but portrays him or her as entirely embedded in the "ball" of context or environment. So inseparable is the individual from his or her environment that it is only by artificially "cutting away" a part of the ball that we can see the person at all.

The ball is made up of four aspects of context: temporal (including age, developmental stage, life cycle, health status) and three types of environment: physical, social, and cultural. The entire universe of tasks is theoretically available to all people; however, most individuals engage in only a finite slice of these tasks. The spectrum of tasks available to a given individual is a function of the interaction of person and context. The person brings skills and abilities, and the environment supplies supports and resources.

A final interesting feature of this model is the designation of five therapeutic interventions used to promote task achievement. At this point, the conceptual model becomes a model of practice, telling therapists what they might DO to promote success with certain tasks: 1) establish or restore skills and abilities; 2) alter the context/environment; 3) adapt the task; 4) prevent, substitute for, compensate for, or work around dysfunction; or 5) create a perspective or view compatible with health.

Although the EHP is identified by Lee (2010) as the fourth most prevalent approach in occupation-focused practice, only two articles have appeared in the international peer-reviewed OT literature since 2000. One described the model as a basis for exploring service transitions in infancy and childhood (Myers, 2006), and one evaluated the effectiveness of a community program based on the task performance of adults with mental illness. It appears that the model has not widely penetrated the practice of OT.

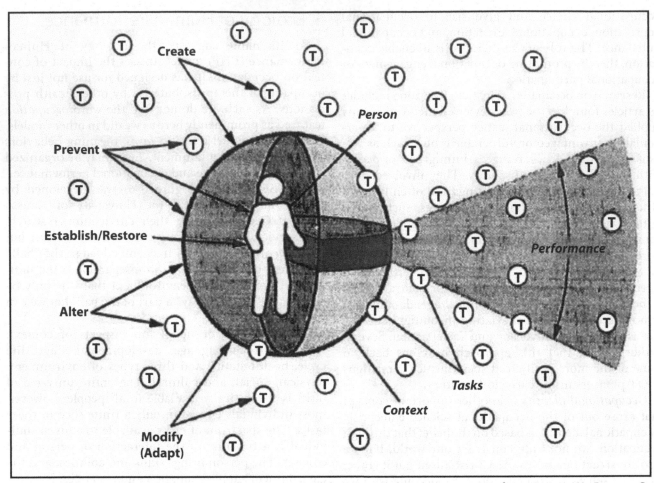

Figure 8-6. The Ecology of Human Performance model. (Reprinted with permission from Dunn, W., Brown, C., & Mcguigan, A. (1994). The ecology of human performance: A framework for considering the effect of context. *American Journal of Occupational Therapy, 48*, 595-607.)

Summary

This chapter contains the knowledge or information that we would find in the top drawer of the OT filing cabinet, knowledge about what occupation is and how it contributes to health and well-being. The six models discussed in this chapter provide us with definitions of occupation, key concepts associated with occupation, and a view of how occupation affects health. These six models were chosen for detailed consideration because they are most widely represented in the literature. Furthermore, other authors have agreed that these are the models most commonly used in practice and taught to students. We judge it to be a sign of the health of the profession of OT that there is both unity and diversity among the ideas expressed in these six models. In this summary, we discuss what they have in common and where they differ—what they all agree on and where each makes a unique contribution to the body of knowledge.

Common to all six of the models discussed is a consensus that we need to focus simultaneously on individuals, their occupations, and the environments within which occupations are undertaken. Although the models may differ in the relative emphasis they place on each of these constructs, all three constructs are present—in fact, prominent—in each of the models.

The models differ—sometimes meaningfully so, sometimes merely semantically—in what they call *occupation*. For example, the terms *occupational behavior, occupational performance, occupational adaptation,* and *task performance* are all used to represent the medium through which humans and environments interact. Furthermore, some models acknowledge a distinction between an abstract notion of occupation and its real-world performance, whereas others focus only on the latter.

Also common to all six models is the idea that occupation is basic to human existence, that to be human is to be occupied, and that to be healthy one needs to be meaningfully occupied. The models each suggest explanations for the relationship between occupation and health. For instance, Occupational Adaptation suggests that health and well-being exist when the adaptive capacity of the person corresponds to the demands from both internal and external sources. By contrast, the MOHO suggests that health is achieved when the individual's skills and abilities contribute to identity, competence, and adaptation.

There is plenty of evidence in the literature for a relationship between occupation and health; however, the nature and parameters of that relationship are not clear (Creek & Hughes, 2008; Yerxa, 1998). It is probably overly simplistic to assume that the relationship is direct or linear. Instead, it is more likely that it is affected by numerous factors in numerous ways. Hasselkus (2006) described the relationship as complex, with "delicate layerings of everyday occupation" (p. 627).

Intermediate in the relationship between occupation and health may be a concept referred to as occupational satisfaction, fulfillment, or well-being. This concept appears to be a subjective phenomenon whereby positive affect is associated with certain occupations. There has been a tendency to assume that all occupations have the potential to be healthful, depending on their meaning and value to the individual. However, recent research suggests that in fact some occupations are inherently more likely than others to be associated with positive health outcomes. Doble and Santha (2008) showed that occupational need fulfillment is the key to occupational well-being. Occupational needs include accomplishment, affirmation, agency, coherence, companionship, pleasure, and renewal. Thus the more an occupation meets one or more of these needs, the more likely it is to be associated with health and well-being. Morgan (2010) suggested that depth, focus, and commitment determine the value of an occupation and therefore its association with health. A decade apart, Yerxa (1998) and Hocking (2009) suggested that much more research is needed to understand the personal, occupational, and social context of occupations in relation to health.

Also common to most of the models in this chapter is the idea that occupation can be thought of in three main categories: self-care, productivity, and leisure. Although different words are used in different models or jurisdictions, these three components typically make up the totality of occupation. These three areas of occupation have guided the profession for more than a century, since its inception. Recently, however, there have been a number of critiques of this conceptualization of occupation. Various authors have found it limiting in one way or another. Reed and colleagues (2011) suggested that self-care, productivity, and leisure fail to adequately take account of the individualized meaning of occupations. Hammell

(2009) criticized them as biased toward Western culture, ableist and elitist. Polatajko and associates (2004) noted the potential for confusion and ambiguity when these words are used specifically by the profession and generally in the popular culture. Nevertheless, these words and ideas are pervasive in the theory of OT from the outset. Furthermore, they appear to have intuitive meaning in the discourse of OT. To date, nothing has been proposed that could be considered a reasonable substitute.

Another commonality is the idea that among the many terms used to describe what people do, there is an implicit hierarchy. In many of the models, occupations are thought of as divisible into smaller parts—typically activities, tasks, skills, and actions. Occupations can also be combined and built up to form larger concepts, such as roles or projects. Although there is no official consensus on the definitions of the many words used to describe what people do, there have been numerous attempts to define these words and a considerable degree of consistency in how they are used colloquially among occupational therapists.

Another similarity is the way humans are viewed by occupation-focused models. Human beings are typically divided into component parts representing different structural and functional aspects. Commonly, humans are thought of as physical, psychological, and social beings, with some taxonomies also including cognitive, sensory, neurological, or spiritual components. These differences may be somewhat confusing for those reading about OT for the first time, but it soon becomes apparent that they are somewhat arbitrary.

Perhaps more important than these similarities are the differences between the six types of occupation-focused models, because these differences are associated with preferences for particular models and suitability of certain models for particular applications. In the final section of this summary, we focus on what is unique and special about each of the models.

Beginning with the oldest model, the Occupational Behavior perspective and the MOHO have as their particular strength their roots in the social sciences. They focus to a greater extent than some others on roles, values, time use, and other socially constructed factors. As such, the MOHO has been more fully developed for use in mental health practice, and more evidence is available for it in that context. It also has the broadest range of associated practice tools and the fullest body of literature and evidence.

The CMOP, like the PEO model, has the advantage of wide recognition and simple concepts that are broadly applicable across settings and cultures. The three concentric circles/shapes of the CMOP or the three overlapping circles of the PEO are intuitively appealing to occupational therapists. This simple model helps to deal with the complex practice environment and organize it so that it is readily understandable and easily explainable to clients, families, teams, and agencies.

The occupational science perspective has as its primary advantage the emerging body of knowledge that is accruing to validate the process and the practice of OT. That body of knowledge has a number of acknowledged weaknesses, but it is nonetheless the seed of an empirical science associated with occupation. Furthermore, it has associated with it a unique social justice perspective on occupation and OT. Rather than the neutrality typically associated with a science, the occupational justice movement is a call to action that may serve as the basis for practice not only in the developed world but also in the developing world.

The EHP model is favored by some readers for its applicability to a wide variety of professions. The use of the word *task* instead of *occupation* broadens the appeal of the model to professions other than OT. Another interesting aspect of this model is its emphasis on the environment and the inextricable association between the person and his or her environment. Like the PEO model, the EHP model sees the relationship of the person to the environment as transactional rather than interactional, emphasizing the interdependence of person, task, and environment, mutually influencing one another at each stage. Also attractive about this model are the categories of intervention outlined in the model of practice.

Finally, the Occupational Adaptation model is unique in its emphasis on the generation, integration, and evaluation of adaptive responses. Whereas adaptation is a fundamental notion to many OT models, there is perhaps no other model that does such a detailed job of exploring the potential of *adaptation* to inform what occupational therapists do. Ultimately it is all about adapting—to one's abilities and limitations, to one's social and vocational circumstances, to one's physical environment, to one's thoughts and feelings. This model, however, is the only one that offers any specific intelligence on what adaptation means and how it is accomplished.

Summary

Despite OT's background in the health care system and the medical sciences, the six most popular models describing occupation and its relationship to health currently focus on the social sciences. They emphasize the social context in which occupation is embedded and the intrinsic and extrinsic social forces that act on the occupational being. Although therapists and therapeutic settings may demonstrate preferences for particular occupation-focused models, it remains the purview of every therapist to specify how he or she thinks about occupation and health. The models described in this chapter provide a starting place for discussions and deliberations about how we explain what we do and decide what to do next.

Section III

The Determinants of Occupation

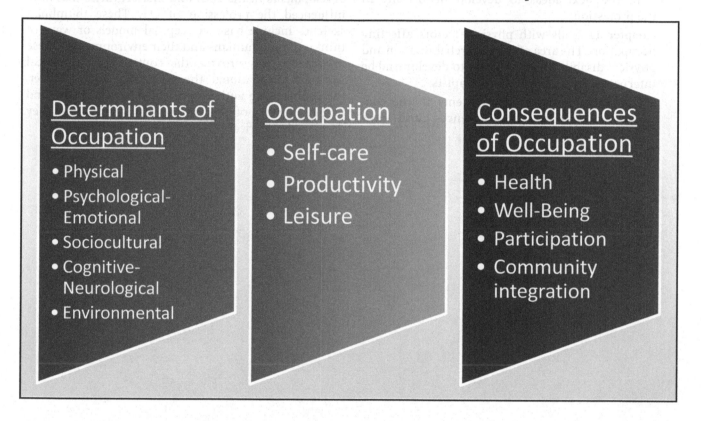

Determinants of Occupation
- Physical
- Psychological-Emotional
- Sociocultural
- Cognitive-Neurological
- Environmental

Occupation
- Self-care
- Productivity
- Leisure

Consequences of Occupation
- Health
- Well-Being
- Participation
- Community integration

The third section of this book elaborates on the relationship that occupational therapy (OT) theorists have postulated between occupation and its five identified determinants—four person characteristics and the environment.

- *What do we know about the [physical, psychological-emotional, sociocultural, cognitive-neurological, environmental] determinants of occupation?*
- *What [physical, psychological-emotional, sociocultural, cognitive-neurological, environmental] factors affect occupation, and what do we know about how they affect it?*

As explained in Chapter 2, each chapter builds on the work of the previous two editions of this book and adds to it the evidence from most recent peer-reviewed literature. Details of specific search strategies are specified at the beginning of each chapter. It is important to remember that these chapters do not represent

"theories" in themselves but rather categories of theory (or drawers in the OT filing cabinet). They contain all the theory that links a particular determinant (physical, sociocultural, psychological-emotional, cognitive-neurological, or environmental) to occupation. The chapters therefore include a summary of what is known about how each of these aspects of the person or the environment affects occupation.

In this book, our main aim is to catalogue and organize the body of knowledge that is used by occupational therapists. However, we also have another goal: to give a historical perspective on the body of knowledge used by occupational therapists and to situate OT theory in the context of other intellectual and cultural developments. We seek not only to understand where our ideas about occupation have come from, but also to honor the intellectual heritage of the profession. We show how the development of knowledge in OT marches alongside the development of knowledge in other disciplines. To that end, we offer five chapters dealing with the determinants of occupation in historical order, from the earliest ideas to the most recent.

- Chapter 9 discusses some of the founding ideas in OT about the relationship of social and cultural concepts to occupation, ideas such as habits, balance, roles, and groups.

- Chapter 10 covers the relationship of psychological and emotional factors to occupation. These were the next ideas to develop historically in the profession.

- Chapter 11 deals with physical factors affecting occupation. The area of physical rehabilitation and physical disability were the next to develop and be interpreted by occupational therapists.

- Chapter 12 discusses developments in the cognitive and neurological sciences and how central nervous system factors have been shown to affect occupation.

- Chapter 13 covers the most recently developed OT theory area. This chapter deals with the environment and how it affects occupation.

Not only is this section of the book organized chronologically, but each of the next five chapters is also organized chronologically. For each chapter, we offer a brief introduction to social and ideological developments in the 20th and 21st centuries that have influenced the profession of OT. These thumbnail sketches include basic conceptual models or ways of thinking about humans and their environments. These important ideas provide the context for theoretical work by occupational therapists. For each chapter, the contributing authors provide a more specific and targeted history of concepts within OT and how they developed historically.

9

The Sociocultural Determinants of Occupation

Mary Ann McColl, PhD, MTS

Introduction

Some of the most fundamental ideas in occupational therapy (OT) stem from the social-cultural area of theory—ideas about human beings that reflect their social nature and their membership in groups. Theory found in this category, the *sociocultural determinants*

of occupation, links occupation to a number of socially constructed concepts, such as values, beliefs, roles, habits, expectations, and norms. This theory area shows how these abstract concepts, if we internalize them and they become a part of who we are, affect our occupation (which in turn, of course, affects our health and well-being). This theory area includes some of the original ideas that led to the formation of the

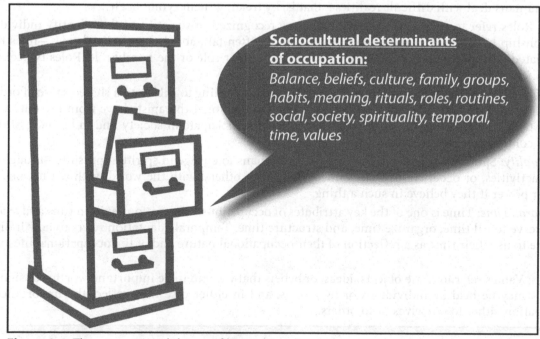

Sociocultural determinants of occupation:
Balance, beliefs, culture, family, groups, habits, meaning, rituals, roles, routines, social, society, spirituality, temporal, time, values

Figure 9-1. The occupational therapy filing cabinet.

McColl MA, Law M, Stewart D.
Theoretical Basis of Occupational Therapy, Third Edition (pp. 69-79).
© 2015 Taylor & Francis Group.

Concepts and Definitions

- *Balance*: The idea of a balance of human occupations has long intrigued occupational therapists. It suggests that one may have too much occupation, too little, or just the right amount. That right amount may be a function of time, variety, intensity, or some other quality.

- *Beliefs*: Beliefs are ideas that individuals hold deeply, even in the absence of evidence or the presence of evidence to the contrary. Beliefs are so much a part of the person that they are not subject to usual empirical standards.

- *Culture*: Culture refers to the ideas, customs, and social behaviors of a particular group of people. Culture may be a function of one's country, one's social groups, one's ethnic origins, or one's social circumstances.

- *Family*: Family refers to a group of people related by blood, marriage, or social convention. Families may be made up of many different combinations of adults and children of various ages. They may include parents, partners, siblings, offspring, or extended family such as grandparents, grandchildren, aunts, uncles, and cousins. Families are our primary source of socialization and typically fulfill unique roles in our lives.

- *Groups*: As social beings, individuals typically belong to a number of different groups, each of which may exert expectations and offer support to our occupations. These may include work groups, social groups, peer groups, religious or cultural groups, or recreational groups.

- *Habits* and *routines*: A habit refers to a regularly performed activity that is not entirely consciously mediated. Habits are behaviors that we perform commonly without thinking about them too much, thus they free up the conscious mind for engaging in other pursuits. Routines usually refer to more complex sequences of actions or behaviors.

- *Meaning*: Meaning is one of the most commonly invoked outcomes sought by occupational therapists. Meaning refers to the significance attributed to an object, event, or idea. Meaning may be either personal (i.e., an object or idea has meaning because of who the individual is), social (because of the groups he or she belongs to), or spiritual (because of symbolic significance or transpersonal attachment).

- *Rituals*: Ritual refers to a series of actions or behaviors that take on special meaning when performed to celebrate or commemorate. Occupational therapists acknowledge that rituals are an important part of how humans deal with difficult realities—that is, by treating them symbolically.

- *Roles*: Roles refer to patterns of behavior that are recognized in society and that identify individuals in relationship to others. Occupational therapists most often talk about occupational roles—roles that are associated with particular occupations, such as the worker role or the family role. Roles typically carry with them privileges, responsibilities, and expectations.

- *Social/Society*: Society refers to groups of people living according to rules and a shared sense of order. The adjective "social" refers to aspects of that society. Occupational therapists have from the outset understood their role as being one of helping individuals to participate in society and to be successful in the social context in which they operate.

- *Spirituality*: Spirituality refers to the capacity of humans to engage in spiritual pursuits—thoughts, feelings, activities, or occupations that connect them with others, with the world, with nature, and with a higher power if they believe in such a thing.

- *Temporal/Time*: Time is one of the key attributes of occupations. Occupations exist in time and space, and they serve to fill time, organize time, and structure time. Temporal adaptation refers to how individuals choose to use their time as a reflection of their occupational nature and of the occupational lifestyle they seek.

- *Values*: Values refer to those objects, ideas, or beliefs that we hold to be important, worthy, or significant. Values may be held by individuals or by groups, and in either case they reflect the importance of an occupation either to ourselves or to others.

profession of OT and that continue to play a vital role in theory and practice today.

The sociocultural determinants of occupation consist of social and cultural factors that affect occupation. Many of them are listed in the box at the beginning of this chapter. Theory classified in this "drawer" of the filing cabinet (see Figure 9-1) helps us understand how each of these concepts affects occupation. These socially or culturally constructed phenomena affect what we do and how we do it. Theory in the sociocultural area attempts to explain how the relationship works between abstract sociocultural concepts and occupation.

As occupational therapists, we use theory about the sociocultural determinants of occupation to understand how occupation is affected by internalized social and cultural factors (occupational conceptual models). Our literature helps us understand how concepts such as roles, beliefs, and values shape the occupations in which we choose to participate and how effective we are able to be at those occupations. For example, as a well-educated woman in Western society, what do I feel is expected of me? To what extent am I able to meet those expectations? Do my personal values collide with those of my social environment: my family, my friends, and neighbors, my colleagues and superiors at work, the broader society or culture? If so, which of my occupations are affected by that conflict, and how do I seek to resolve the tension? These are all issues that theory about the sociocultural determinants of occupation helps us to understand.

An occupational therapist might "open this drawer of the filing cabinet" in situations like the following:

- A young woman with a spinal cord injury wishes to live independently, but her family insists that she stay with them, because it is their duty to care for her (values, roles).
- A busy executive is admitted to the hospital and refuses to return to home or work. His only stated reason is that he cannot do it anymore (time, balance).
- An elderly client who was formerly active sits in a chair day in and day out after a stroke that leaves her unable to communicate. The only thing she can say is, "What's the point?" (meaning, spirituality).
- A middle-aged woman presents with depression. After the death of her husband, she has left the family farm to be nearer her children and moved to an apartment in the city (social participation, habits).

These are examples of situations in which a client presents for OT, and the occupational therapist determines that the origins of his or her problems lie in the social or cultural aspect of the person. After identifying occupational performance problems that the client wishes to work on, the occupational therapist speculates about the possible reasons for these problems. If those reasons relate to the sociocultural concepts described earlier, then the obvious place to look for guidance is the theory area associated with the sociocultural determinants of occupation—specifically, the occupational conceptual models and the occupational models of practice found in the second drawer of the filing cabinet.

The sociocultural area of OT theory contributes to our understanding of how internalized social and cultural factors shape our occupational performance. As a product of social processes, such as our upbringing, education, and acculturation, we develop and internalize messages about who we are and how we should behave in accordance with our social and cultural context. These socially and culturally mediated ideas play an important role in governing our occupational performance.

In examining the theory in this area, it is important to distinguish it from theory about the social environment and how it affects occupation. Theory in the sociocultural area is about beliefs and values that are internalized within the person. Sociocultural determinants of occupation include concepts that one has taken in and made one's own. For example, how a person thinks about his or her roles has important consequences for occupation; however, the ideas of others about the individual's roles also have the power to affect occupation, as we discuss later in the chapter on the Environmental Determinants of Occupation (Chapter 13).

Basic Conceptual Models Underpinning the Sociocultural Determinants

In order to understand how the social and cultural determinants affect occupation, we must first understand the person as a social and cultural being. For that, we rely on basic conceptual models from the social sciences, such as sociology, anthropology, and even theology. We use theory from the social sciences to help us to understand the social and cultural nature of human beings (basic conceptual models): how and why we affiliate with groups, how groups instill in members their norms and expectations, and how values are communicated, enforced, and altered. Social and cultural ideas become internalized and exert profound influences of who we think we are, what is expected of us, how we should behave, and how we should relate to others. Occupational therapists need an understanding of these basic sciences if they are to understand how the sociocultural aspect of the person affects his or her occupation. These basic conceptual models help us understand the social and cultural aspects of human beings and bring that understanding to our therapeutic efforts toward improving their occupational performance.

Theory about the sociocultural determinants of occupation was influenced by three social movements that were prevalent in the early part of the 20th century: the mental hygiene movement, the arts and crafts movement, and the settlement house movement. (For a fuller discussion of these, I refer the reader to *Restoring the Spirit* by Judith Friedland [2009]).

The mental hygiene movement was definitively described by Dr. Adolph Meyer in 1918 as follows (Meyer, 1918, p. 632):

> The problems of mental health…must be attacked beyond the walls of the hospitals which to-day deal with mental defect and mental disease…. They require more extensive training of the average physician in the timely understanding of mental difficulties; provision for the means and taste of the patient; and a more sympathetic and hopeful attitude on the part of the public.

The movement had its roots in moral treatment ideology, a psychiatric approach begun in the late 19th century that emphasized freedom from physical restraints, humane treatment, and normalization of routines and patterns in the patient's life. Among several pioneers of the movement was C. K. Clarke, a psychiatrist at the Rockwood Asylum in Kingston, Ontario, where treatment emphasized craftwork and sheltered work as diversions from pathological self-absorption and unhealthy thoughts.

A second social movement that provided a context for theoretical developments in OT was the arts and crafts movement. The arts and crafts movement was a sociopolitical response to the mass industrialization of the 19th century. Collectives of artisans responded to the alienation of workers, the mechanization of work, the segmentation of production, and the separation of workers from the outcomes of their labor. Instead, the arts and crafts movement focused on small-scale production, handmade works, and acknowledgment of individual achievement and creativity. It was a celebration of beauty and ingenuity and a return to valuing what humans create with their hands and minds.

The third social movement that gave rise to OT theory was the settlement house movement. Settlement houses were community centers, typically located in poor or immigrant communities, that provided life skills, literacy, and hygiene training. Growing out of the social gospel movement and focusing on social inequities associated primarily with ethnicity and poverty, the settlement house movement attracted primarily privileged women to volunteer their time and talents in poorer communities. Developments in public health and hygiene contributed to improvements in sanitation and food storage and preparation as well as child-rearing and housekeeping skills.

The reader will find these ideas reflected repeatedly in the developments throughout the 20th century in OT theory:

- Respect for the dignity of human beings, regardless of their infirmities
- Belief in the need to be occupied in order to resist unhealthy impulses
- Honoring of human work
- The capacity of humans for creativity and ingenuity
- The importance of life skills and literacy
- Women as lay purveyors of health education.

Occupational Conceptual Models Associated With the Sociocultural Determinants of Occupation

The field of OT began near the turn of the 20th century in response to social movements (described earlier) that called for more humane treatment of people who were disadvantaged in society. Since the latter part of the 19th century, the Moral Treatment and Mental Hygiene philosophies emphasized the value and potential inherent in all human beings, even those with severe disabilities and mental illnesses. One corollary of the approach was the idea that for individuals to be healthy, the patterns of their lives had to also be healthy, including patterns of activity and rest. This idea is memorably advanced for occupational therapists by the psychiatrist, Adolph Meyer:

> "There are many rhythms which must be attuned to: the larger rhythms of night and day, of sleep and waking hours, of hunger and its gratification, and finally, the big four—work and play and rest and sleep, which our organism must be able to balance even under difficulty. The only way to attain balance in all this is actual doing, actual practice, a program of wholesome living as the basis of wholesome feeling and thinking and fancy and interests."
>
> Adolph Meyer, *Archives of Occupational Therapy*, 1922, 2.

In this quote, Meyer introduces a number of the ideas that are prevalent in the early literature and form the foundation of modern OT:

- There are rhythms or patterns inherent in everyday activity (roles, habits, routines).
- Occupation is constituted of work (productivity), play (leisure), sleep, and rest (self-care).
- There is a balance among productivity, leisure, and self-care.
- Occupational dysfunction can be remediated by occupation, or doing.

What all the theoretical ideas associated with the sociocultural area of OT theory have in common is that they all involve abstract concepts that are socially mediated, socially constructed, or socially defined phenomena. They all have considerable potential to affect occupation. Theory about the sociocultural determinants of occupation shows how occupation is affected by relationships to primary (family) and secondary (friends, colleagues) groups in society. It also shows how individuals internalize their culture, how beliefs and values affect occupation, and how habits, rituals, and customs shape occupation. Finally, this area of theory includes spirituality and its effect on occupation, because religion, faith, and spiritual issues are all part of our internalized social and cultural ideology.

These ideas guided the emerging profession of OT through the first four decades of the 20th century. The 1950s and 1960s, however, brought about a trend toward objectivity and empiricism. Science was touted as the savior of the fledgling profession. The scientific revolution hit OT with all its reductionist fervor and nearly led to the demise of some of our most fundamental ideas. It threatened the validity of many sociocultural ideas such as the use of time, the patterns of occupational activity, and the importance of values and beliefs. Despite a few excellent articles published in this period, the literature on sociocultural theory is thin throughout the middle decades of the 20th century (Dodson, 1959; Dyer, 1963; Mielicke, 1967; Sanchez, 1964).

In the early 1970s, the literature in OT began to recover some of the ideas that had gone out of fashion, with a particular emphasis on the relationship between work and leisure (Matsutsuyu, 1971; Maurer, 1971). In 1971, Bockoven underlined the value of Moral Treatment principles for contemporary OT, and in 1977, Meyer's seminal article was reprinted for the benefit of future generations of occupational therapists.

Time

Time and its relationship to occupation is one of the most fundamental ideas that drive the thinking and the actions of occupational therapists. Adolph Meyer (1922, 1977), a founding "father" of OT, identified time as a key factor underlying "problems of living" and advocated the systematic engagement of interests to enhance a person's use of time and productive work. Seventy-five years later, Clark (1997) emphasized the importance of time use, suggesting that occupational science could produce a "blueprint for global health" by marshalling intelligence on occupation and time use.

It was not until 1977 that theory about occupation and time began to be developed in the OT literature. It was introduced by Kielhofner as part of his renaissance of occupational behavior (Kielhofner, 1977; Reilly, 1962) and the Model of Human Occupation (MOHO; Kielhofner, 1978). Temporal adaptation referred to two aspects of how time affects human occupation: first, time is used to organize occupations within a given day, and second, time over the lifespan affects how humans engage in occupation in a longitudinal perspective. Clark (1997) labeled these two ideas *tempo,* meaning the immediate use of time to pace and schedule occupations, and *temporality,* to refer to the past, present, and future of occupations.

Katz (1985) underlined the importance of time use as part of the legitimate domain of concern of OT and kicked off a flurry of theoretical development in this area over the next two decades. Several authors discussed the commodification of time and the assumptions in Western society that time is something over which humans have dominion. For example, Peloquin (1991) referred to the social construction of time and its representation as watches and clocks. She highlighted cultural messages received from media suggesting that if we construct time, then we can control time.

In the literature of the 21st century, Persson and Erlandsson (2002) challenged the postindustrial ethics of time use and the assumption that time serves the productive machinery of society. Larson and Zemke (2003) referred to *time sovereignty* to mean the sense that one has control over one's use of time and that time pressures (the tension between the time available and the time needed) can be managed. Green (2008) interpreted the elimination of sleep from most taxonomies of occupation as a reflection of the view that time can be budgeted and optimized, or wasted.

Larson and Zemke (2003), in a comprehensive examination of time use in OT, referred to three sets of factors that affect time use:

1. Biotemporal factors, such as survival needs, circadian rhythms, or lifespan changes

2. Sociotemporal factors, such as cultural norms and role expectations for time use and family needs

3. Occupation-temporal factors, such as the complexity, demands, coordination, and resource requirements of the activity itself

Larson (2004) referred to the task-scape or environment of an occupation, the cultural habitus or beliefs that surround the occupation, and the complexity of the occupation as key determinants of time use. She presented a very detailed model entitled the Dynamic Occupation in Time that aims to balance all those factors to optimize the use of time for occupation.

Several authors pointed to a reciprocal relationship between occupation and time (Pemberton & Cox, 2011). They noted not only that time does affect occupations, but also that occupations influence how we think and feel about the passage of time. Larson (2004) noted that time can be perceived as passing in six ways, depending of the occupations that fill that time: protracted, compressed, synchronized, ruptured, interstitial, or flowing. The idea of flow, or the unconscious passage of time, has been explored by a number of authors who sought to identify factors that could allow therapists to identify the "just-right challenge" for their patients (Jonsson & Persson, 2006). Flow (or

timelessness) occurs when the skill level of the person and the complexity of the occupation are balanced perfectly (Larson & von Eye, 2010).

In recent years, there has been considerable emphasis on the concept of balance in occupation and the desire of humans to avoid under- or over-occupation and instead to achieve a sense of homeostasis in the use of time to accomplish meaningful occupations (Bejerholm, 2010; Eklund, Leufstadius, & Bejerholm, 2009). Jackson and colleagues used the term *lifestyle redesign* to refer to a purposeful selection of occupations that promotes health and life satisfaction (Jackson, Carlson, Mandel, Zemke, & Clark 1998). Backman (2004; Anaby, Backman, & Jarus, 2010) traced the history of the idea of occupational balance and reminded us how elusive this notion is. At least four ways have been identified for conceptualizing balance: as the right number of occupations, as the appropriate occupations to fulfill roles, as value integrity (Pentland & McColl, 2008), and as compatibility of occupations (Matuska & Christiansen, 2008; Wada, Backman, & Forwell, 2010; Wagman, Håkansson, & Björklund, 2012).

Finally, there have been a number of articles that have looked at time use from the perspective of being vs. doing. Rowles (1991) referred to the spatiotemporal setting of an occupation as not only the locus of doing, but also the location of the life-world of the client. He emphasized the importance of understanding this spatiotemporal location as well as abilities and disabilities.

Habits, Routines, and Rituals

Another of the founding members of the profession of OT, Eleanor Clark Slagle, developed similar ideas to those of Meyer about the health-producing effect of activity taken in patterned and predictable ways. She became known for a therapeutic regimen called "habit-training" whose primary objective was to provide meaningful occupation for hospital patients, thereby preventing them from spending their time in morbid and unhealthy ways (Slagle, 1924). These habits were constituted to simulate the cultural ideal of a productive lifestyle. The notion of normality and the pursuit of integration pervaded the literature of the period and extended through to about 1950 (Nash, 1938; Pollack, 1938; Stanley, 1942).

In the 1980s the idea that habits affect occupation was reintroduced to the theoretical foundation of OT. With the introduction of the MOHO, a number of fundamental ideas, among them habits, found their way back into the consciousness of occupational therapists (Kielhofner, Barris, & Watts, 1982). Habits organize behavior into adaptive patterns that in turn integrate into higher levels of behavioral organization, such as roles and interests. Habituation was one of three hierarchical subsystems that govern human occupation: the performance subsystem, the habituation subsystem and the volitional subsystem.

In 1985, James offered a cognitive-neurological explanation for the power of habits to free the conscious mind. She conceptualized habits as pathways of electrical activity in the brain. Dunn (2000) also described the neuropsychological underpinnings of habit theory, based on the concepts of activation thresholds, habituation, and motivation. She defined four types of response to incoming stimuli, all of which seek the elusive state of homeostasis: low registration, sensitivity, sensation seeking, and sensation avoidance.

Ludwig (1997) suggested that habits and routines affect occupational performance in terms of nine adaptive outcomes: meeting obligations; remaining active; maintaining health; anticipating the future; asserting control; balancing work, rest, and play; achievement; continuity; and sense of self. In summary, habits reinforced both identity and relationships with others and thus had an indirect effect on well-being (Fearing & Clark, 2000).

A special issue of the *Occupational Therapy Journal of Research* in 2000 was devoted to habits and represented a consolidation of the importance of habits for occupational performance as well as a springboard for further research. A number of important ideas came out of the conference where these papers were first presented. Habits can be both healthy and unhealthy (Clark, 2000; Rogers, 2000). Habit domination, or an excess of routine, can lead to boredom and underperformance, whereas habit impoverishment can result in chaos and overstimulation (Clark, 2000; Dunn, 2000). Habits may be especially important for people with disabilities and chronic conditions as a means of promoting coping efficacy (Clark, 2000). Rogers (2000) emphasized the relationship between skill and habit and underlined the importance of consolidating skill training by habit training.

There are nine types of habits, and they exist on a continuum from micro-level behaviors, such as tics and conditioned responses, to macro-level patterns that govern a person's entire personality. Routines and rituals are types of habits; routines are more complex, multidimensional patterns of behavior, whereas rituals include affective and symbolic content (Clark, Sanders, Carlson, Blanche, & Jackson, 2007; Evans & Rodger, 2008; Segal, 2004).

Recent research on habits and routines has focused on the family as a system wherein habits and routines are reinforced. Family routines around standard daily occupations, such as bedtimes or mealtimes, have been shown to promote order and balance at the level of the whole family. They also appear to promote intimacy and interaction in relationships and to enhance identity in individuals (Evans & Rodger, 2008; Howell & Pierce, 2000; Koome, Hocking, & Sutton, 2012; Marquenie, Rodger, Mangohig, & Cronin, 2011; Segal, 2004; Schultz-Krohn, 2004). There have also been several negative side effects pointed out. Wallenbert and Jonsson (2005) observed that attachment to some habits and routines can be a deterrent to adaptation.

Roles

Role theory, originating in psychology, is an important part of understanding how the social and cultural nature of the person affects his or her occupational performance. Roles are patterns of behavior that are related to an individual's position in society (Toal-Sullivan & Henderson, 2004). Roles reflect both individual and internalized societal expectations and govern particular areas of life or particular relationships (Hughes, 2001).

Prior to the 1970s, the only role that was discussed in any detail in the OT literature was the worker role (LeVesconte, 1934, 1935). Despite the notion that a balance of work, rest, and leisure is ideal for health, the early OT literature was dominated by the need for recipients of OT to have work roles. Work roles result in a tangible product and produce an attendant sense of accomplishment. They contribute to the welfare of the institution or the community, thereby reinforcing the sense of belonging and responsibility. Work roles occupy the main part of the day and provide structure and normalcy to the waking hours.

The idea of roles became more prevalent in the OT literature in the 1970s and 1980s. Borrowing from sociology, roles came to be understood as a necessary shorthand for the organization of occupation across a person's day, week, and year. Roles were made up of skills, behaviors, and habits (Heard, 1977), and they were understood to change in relation to context and time. The notion of an occupational career was introduced (Black, 1976) to show that roles had meaning not only cross-sectionally, but also longitudinally. They were expected to change over the lifespan in predictable ways.

In the 1980s and 1990s, the idea of roles was further revitalized when it was included as a major concept in the MOHO. Roles were part of the habituation subsystem, and as such were shown to be associated with occupational performance and life satisfaction (Elliott & Barris, 1987). Age was shown to be a significant determinant of occupational role performance (Bränholm & Fugl-Meyer, 1992). While the middle decades of adulthood are relatively stable in terms of roles, the first decade (late 20s-early 30s) represents a period of role acquisition, and the fourth decade (the 50s-60s) sees retrenchment and forfeiture of roles. Disability is also typically associated with a loss of roles, particularly roles such as worker and caregiver, which have been shown to be considerably less common in disabled subsets of the population (Versluys, 1980). An important distinction was made between the "sick role" (Talcott-Parsons in Jones, 1974) and adaptive roles in rehabilitation.

Research on roles since 2000 has attempted to elaborate not only the fact of a relationship between roles and healthy occupation, but also the nature and parameters of that relationship (Erlandsson, Eklund, & Persson, 2011). Several researchers have also showed that some roles are valued more than others. The worker, family member, and friend roles tend to be the most highly valued in Western society. Furthermore, a higher number of roles are usually associated with higher quality of life (Eklund, 2001; Hachey et al., 2001).

Beagan and Saunders (2005) pointed out that there is often a reciprocal relationship between roles and factors such as gender, social status, and success. They use the example of gender roles to show how we expect men and women to be involved in different roles or in different behavior within roles. At the same time, our notions of femininity and masculinity are at least partially constructed by these expectations of role performance and occupational preferences.

One of the more clear conceptualizations of the importance of roles is found in the theory underpinning the Client-Oriented Role Evaluation (Toal-Sullivan & Henderson, 2004). Client aptitudes and environmental factors underpin occupations (self-care, productivity, and leisure), which are organized into multiple roles. In other words, skills and occupations can be cultivated on the assumption that these will eventually be incorporated into roles and will buttress identity, or identity may be broken down into the roles that uphold it and whichever elements of these roles are or are not operating in a satisfying way.

Groups

The literature of the early 1940s is characterized by recognition not only of the occupational nature of humans, but also of their social nature. It was observed that social isolation and occupational dysfunction often went hand-in-hand, and one obvious way to counteract this was to pursue therapeutic activity in groups. In this way, patients could not only learn from one another, but also benefit from the social contact of the group (Kindwall & McLean, 1941; Preston, 1942). The Fundamentals of Interpersonal Relationships model is a basic model that helps to understand the importance of groups. Groups offer members the opportunity for inclusion, control, and affection. When these interpersonal needs are fulfilled, there is considerable reduction in the incidence of anxiety, hostility, and lost productivity (Schaber, 2002).

In the 1960s, the idea of the therapeutic effects of groups was further developed through treatment approaches such as milieu therapy and the therapeutic community. Therapists advanced the notion that OT goals could most effectively be achieved within the dynamic context of groups (Bockoven, 1971; Feuss, 1959; Kielhofner, 1992; McNair, 1959; Opzoomer & McCordic, 1972).

Since 2000, groups have been shown to positively affect outcomes in OT in a number of ways. Group members validate the experience of disability and reinforce the notion that one is not alone with one's problems. Groups share coping strategies and resources and provide both tangible and emotional support to one another (Bazyk & Bazyk, 2009; Hyde, 2001; Olson, 2006). Cowls and Hale (2005) provide advice about the importance of the activities undertaken by groups and the necessity to assess readiness for different levels of group participation.

One of the key groups that shape the occupation of individuals is the family. Although there have been references to the importance of family throughout the literature in OT, since 2000 there has been an emphasis on the role of the family in OT. The family is appreciated not only as a social unit, but also as a cultural unit, with pervasive effects on members and their occupations. Family-centered therapy is an extension of client-centered therapy that focuses on the whole family rather than simply the individual who is referred (Kyler, 2008). Families have been shown to be influential in the recovery and occupational performance of children, adults, and elders, with each age group having unique challenges and considerations (Hanna & Rodger, 2002; Klein & Liu, 2010; La Corte, 2008; Schaber, 2002).

Social Responsibility

Another theme that is prevalent in the OT literature is the idea of therapy as a social good or a social responsibility. This theme hearkens back to the humanistic ideology of the Moral Treatment era. In 1937, Humphreys appealed for a social vision for OT, one that extends beyond the doors of the institution and sees patients restored to meaningful life in the community. He defined the profession's social mission as follows:

> "[Occupational therapy is] a social medium by means of which an individual may be brought more closely into constructive contacts with persons and objects through the use of cultural and industrial techniques."
>
> Humphreys, H. (1937). The value of occupational therapy to the developmentally deficient child. *Occupational Therapy & Rehabilitation*, 2.

Over the subsequent decades, this vision of OT as a calling or vocation in service to society is reiterated in the language of each generation of therapists. In the 1960s, Roberts (1962) talked about both the responsibility and the privilege of contributing to healing for the individual and for society. In the 1970s, Bockoven revived the spirit of the Moral Treatment ideology to address the ills of urban industrialized society. In the 1980s, Yerxa (1980) appealed to occupational therapists to fulfill their destiny as agents of social change by creating a culture of caring in the health care system and in society. More recently, the concept of occupational justice has expressed the theme of social responsibility in OT. *Occupational justice* refers to the right to meaningful occupation for all people and the role of occupational therapists in promoting and protecting that right (Galvin, Wilding, & Whiteford, 2011).

Culture

There is virtually no mention of the concept of culture prior to the 1980s, when geopolitical changes led to an increased awareness of culture in OT. *Culture* is defined as a system of learned values and behaviors that provide a shared way of understanding and relating to the self and the world (Krefting & Krefting, 1991; Mirkopolous & Evert, 1994). Culture consists of assumptions about the self, others, and society. These assumptions can be ethnically specific, or they can relate to other groups in which individuals participate, such as the family, the community, or the nation. Krefting and Krefting (1991) portray these groups as concentric circles of culture, all of which are internalized and reconciled to a greater or lesser degree by the individual.

Since the 1980s, occupational therapists have been interested in how culture affects occupation as well as how it influences the therapeutic relationship. This area of theory began with recognition of culture as a filter through which clients and therapists view the world in general and issues related to therapy in particular. Various authors focused on cultural variations in key concepts, such as independence (Rogers, 1982); self-care, productivity, and leisure (Levine, 1984); learning (Jamieson, 1985); pain (Baptiste, 1988); illness (Levine, 1984); and roles (Iannone, 1987).

This discussion led to a focus on the culturally competent therapist and the skills required to practice in an environment characterized by cultural diversity. To underline the importance of this issue, then-presidents of the American Occupational Therapy Association and the Canadian Association of Occupational Therapists collaborated on an article entreating therapists to take account of the philosophical assumptions and "worldview" of their clients (Mirkopolous & Evert, 1994). Issues where cultural sensitivity is required include communication styles, gender roles, illness beliefs, roles expectations, and therapy outcomes, to name a few (Fitzgerald, Mullavey-O'Byrne, & Clemson, 1997). Bonder (2004) and colleagues recommended that therapists cultivate careful attention, active curiosity, and self-reflection as means of becoming more aware of the cultural overlay in therapeutic interactions.

Beginning in the late 1990s, a literature emerged that critiqued OT for a bias toward Western middle-class cultural values. Paul (1995) initially noted this bias in assessments and clinical evaluations. Since 2000, occupation itself has been seen by some as ethnocentric. Commentators have criticized definitions of self-care, productivity, and leisure; independence; self; and identity as Eurocentric and biased toward the developed world (Darnell, 2002; Hammell, 2009; Hocking, 2000; Whiteford & Wilcock, 2000). Specific values characterize this bias: future orientation, achievement orientation, emphasis on individual choice, mastery over nature, and active observable occupations (Kantzartksis & Molineaux, 2011; Rudman & Dennhardt, 2008). At the same time, however, others were focusing on the universality of occupation, the cultural neutrality of occupation, and the biological need for occupation—in other words, occupation as inherent to humanity (Clark, 1997; Wilcock, 1993; Yerxa, 1998).

One response to this perceived Western bias has been the Kawa model (Iwama, 2003, 2006; Iwama, Thomson, & MacDonald, 2009). The word *kawa* means "river" in Japanese, and Iwama draws on his own cultural heritage to suggest the river as a metaphor of life. Rocks and logs represent obstacles and resources, the river bank represents the environmental context, and the flowing water represents the passage of time across the lifespan. The model has intuitive appeal for many occupational therapists, but it has also been critiqued as being too abstract and substituting Eastern cultural imperialism for Western. The Kawa model offers no explicit guidance for intervention other than to overcome barriers and employ resources in the flow of life.

There is relatively little discussion in the OT literature of the culture of disability or of the relationship of occupational therapists to the notion of disability. The OT literature has implicitly adopted the social model of disability, with its emphasis on participation and barriers found in the environment (Law, 1991). Taylor (2007) challenged occupational therapists with survey data, suggesting that they employ an implicit hierarchy of disability, with perceptual and sensory disabilities at the top and mental illness at the bottom. Further qualitative research to validate and understand this hierarchy would be most helpful.

Spirituality

Perhaps the latest concept to receive attention in the sociocultural area in OT is spirituality. The literature in this area has arisen primarily since 2000. It first appears in the Canadian Model of Occupational Performance in 1983 (Department of National Health and Welfare & Canadian Association of Occupational Therapists, 1983), and the literature has increased exponentially since then.

Egan and DeLaat (1994) defined *spirituality* as "our truest selves" expressed in our occupations. Since 2000, a number of articles followed that all attempted to grapple with the issue of definition of spirit and spirituality (Hammell, 2001; Kang, 2003; McColl, 2000; Unruh, Versnel, & Kerr, 2002). At the root of any definition of spirituality is an understanding of *spirit*. Unruh et al. (2002) offered that there are three ways of thinking about spirit found in the literature: *religious*, referring to a particular faith tradition; *sacred*, referring to forces that exceed our understanding but do not belong to a specific faith tradition; and *secular*, referring to something that exists within human beings and can be understood as humanistic.

One of the main concepts with which spirituality has been linked is "meaning." In 1994, Urbanowski and Vargo tackled the issue of defining spirituality by suggesting that it referred not to the cosmic "meaning of life" but rather to the everyday experience of "meaning in life." This idea had enormous intuitive appeal for occupational therapists and resulted in numerous articles looking at the meaning of particular occupations to particular groups of people. *Meaning* became virtually synonymous with *spirituality*, failing to acknowledge that not all meaning is spiritual meaning. As Persson and colleagues pointed out, some occupations derive meaning for practical reasons—because they produce a valued outcome, avoid a negative consequence, or are simply enjoyable (Persson, Erlandsson, Eklund, & Iwarsson, 2001). These cannot be considered spiritual meanings. On the other hand, some occupations have symbolic value, hidden meanings that derive from attributions about the occupation. These symbolic meanings may be personal, relating to the individual and his or her unique characteristics and background.

Symbolic meanings may also be social or cultural, relating to what is valued by the family, the peer group, the community, or the society; or they may be spiritual, reflecting universal or cosmic meanings that relate to issues such as the nature of our humanity, the purpose of our lives, the relationship to each other and to the world, or the possibility of a divinity or Supreme Being (McColl, 2000, 2011; Persson et al., 2001).

Much of the literature on spirituality in OT consists of surveys of therapists, asking them what they think spirituality is, how they witness it in practice, and how comfortable or prepared they feel to deal with it. The consensus is that although the rhetoric is strong, the use of spirituality in practice lags behind (Beagan & Kumas-Tan, 2005; Belcham, 2004; Collins, Paul, & West-Frasier, 2001; Engquist, Short-DeGraff, Gliner, & Oltjenbruns 1997; Johnson & Mayers, 2005).

Summary

The sociocultural determinants of occupation are those socially and culturally constructed abstract concepts that affect who we are and what we do. Factors such as culture, time, values, roles, and spirituality all shape how we select and enact our occupation. In order to effectively help clients overcome obstacles to full and satisfying occupational performance, and thereby health and well-being, occupational therapists need to understand how these abstract ideas can affect occupation.

Where do these ideas come from? For the most part, they come from the concentric circles of society and culture that we participate in. They originate in the proximal circles of the family, peers, and community. They are shaped and moderated by the more distal groups that we belong to—the region, the country, the religious tradition, the ethnic and cultural situation. All of these ideas are pressed on us by external forces, and to the extent that we take them on board or internalize them, they affect our choices, our methods, and our approaches to occupation.

The sociocultural determinants of occupation are part of the *person*—they exist within the beliefs, values, and ideologies that individuals express every day in every choice or determination that they make. The challenge for occupational therapists is to understand the relationship between these abstract sociocultural factors and occupation and to use that understanding to help clients to optimize their occupational performance and thereby their health.

A short list of sociocultural factors has dominated the literature in OT since its inception at the beginning of the 20th century. Factors such as the use of time, the need for a balance in activities, and the importance of habits and routines have formed the foundation of the profession of OT. Over the years, additional factors have been added, often migrating from the social sciences into the health sciences—ideas such as roles, values, culture, and spirituality. Each of these has been explored for its relationship with occupation and for its potential to act as a therapeutic strategy in improving occupation.

10

The Psychological-Emotional Determinants of Occupation

Terry Krupa, PhD, OT Reg. (Ont.), FCAOT
With an Introduction by Mary Ann McColl, PhD, MTS

Introduction

Theory associated with the psychological-emotional determinants of occupation examines the concepts listed in the box and their effects on occupation. Theory classified in this "drawer" of the filing cabinet (Figure 10-1) helps us understand how each of these concepts affects occupation. These psychological and emotional factors affect what we do and how we do it.

The psychological-emotional determinants of occupation refer to individuals' thoughts and feelings and how these affect their occupations. An occupational therapist might "open this drawer of the filing cabinet" in situations like the following:

- A client is referred to occupational therapy (OT) because his persistent lack of affect and motivation prevents him from participating in work or relationships.

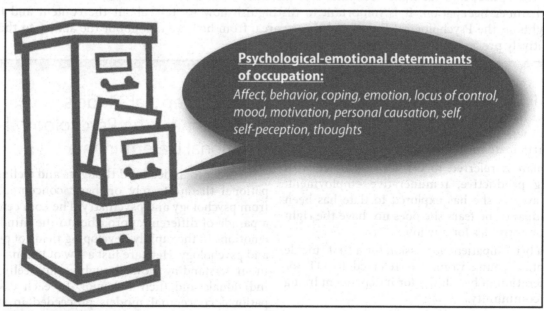

Psychological-emotional determinants of occupation:
Affect, behavior, coping, emotion, locus of control, mood, motivation, personal causation, self, self-peception, thoughts

Figure 10-1. The occupational therapy filing cabinet.

McColl MA, Law M, Stewart D.
Theoretical Basis of Occupational Therapy, Third Edition (pp. 81-90).
© 2015 Taylor & Francis Group.

Concepts and Definitions

- *Affect/mood*: The words *affect*, *emotion*, and *mood* are all used to talk about feelings. They refer to a mental state and usually to an accompanying physiological response, and they can have profound effects on occupation. Emotions tend to reactive and immediate, whereas affect and mood tend to be more sustained, and typically characterized as either positive, negative or absent. Occupational therapists need to understand how emotions can interfere with healthy, satisfying occupation.

- *Behavior*: Behaviors refer to overt expressions or activity. Behaviors can be observed as responses or reactions to a situation. Occupational therapists are particularly interested in those behaviors that constitute occupations or occupational performance.

- *Coping*: Coping refers to a conscious process aimed at dealing with stress. Coping may be designed to address the stressor itself, the perception of the stressor, or the emotional reaction to the stressor. Coping skills may be learned and may be employed to enable occupation in stressful situations.

- *Locus of control/personal causation*: These two terms refer to a belief system about what forces are responsible for the outcome of events. Someone with an internal locus of control believes that he or she is ultimately responsible for how things turn out, whereas someone with an external locus of control believes that fate, chance, or powerful others control his or her destiny. Neither extreme is compatible with health or satisfying occupational performance.

- *Motivation*: Motivation refers to the energy associated with human activity—a particular goal, activity, or outcome. Occupational therapists are interested in motivations for particular occupations, as they are one of the key forces that shape the occupations in which people participate. To understand motivation is to assist clients in discovering the energy that will help them accomplish the occupations they desire.

- *Self*: The self is an image constructed by an individual of who he or she is, how he or she appears and relates to others. The self can be understood both subjectively and objectively. The self is perceived to have preferences, strengths and weaknesses, and these are highly influential in determining occupational choices.

- *Self-perception*: Self-perceptions include a number of beliefs and attitudes about the self, such as self-esteem, self-image, and body-image.

- *Thoughts*: The form and content of thoughts mediate occupation. To the extent that they are constructive or adaptive, they facilitate occupation; to the extent that they are maladaptive or interfering, they may hamper occupation. It is important to distinguish how we talk about the content and form of thoughts in the Psychological-Emotional theory area, from how we talk about the ability to think and cognitively process in the Cognitive-Neurological area.

- Following a divorce, a young man seeks OT because he is not able to cope with the pressure from others to meet someone new, start dating, and participate in couples activities.

- A woman is referred to OT for assistance with finding productive, remunerative employment. Every avenue she has explored to date has been blocked, and she fears she does not have the right skills or aptitudes for any job.

- After a brief inpatient admission for a first suicide attempt, a young woman is referred to OT for consideration of her ability for independent living in the community.

Basic Conceptual Models Underpinning the Psychological-Emotional Determinants

In order to understand thoughts and feelings, occupational therapists rely on basic conceptual models from psychology and psychiatry. The 20th century saw a parade of different approaches to the mind and the emotions in the rapidly developing fields of psychiatry and psychology. Here are just a few of the major trends in understanding how thoughts and feelings affect individuals and their behavior. In each case, occupational conceptual models proceeded in step with these basic conceptual models. In other words, occupational therapists responded to the current schools of thought with attempts to interpret what they meant for occupation and OT.

Sometimes referred to as the father of modern psychiatry, Sigmund Freud had ideas about the mind that dominated the early part of the 20th century. At the root of Freud's psychoanalytic approach was the belief that psychological dysfunction originated in the unconscious mind, and the way to heal was to bring conflict to a conscious level where it could be understood and dealt with. Psychoanalysis was a lengthy process aimed at revealing and interpreting subconscious expressions and discovering the seat of past conflicts that continue to affect the patient. Occupational therapists in the mid-20th century developed the Object Relations approach based on the notion that individuals reveal secrets of the unconscious mind in their interactions with media and objects in their environment. By relating to objects, individuals satisfy needs and desires and express symbolic content.

As a direct response to the psychoanalytic approach, in the 1950s, Skinner and colleagues developed the behavioral approach. The behavioral approach rejected the notion that lengthy analysis was needed to understand behavior. Instead they insisted that behavior could be understood as a function of what was reinforced, learned, and conditioned. The behaviorists were not interested in probing the unconscious but rather in exploring the system of incentives and disincentives in the environment that shaped behavior. Occupational therapists responded to this development with the Action-Consequence approach based on operant conditioning. The contention was that skills for living could be taught by promoting adaptive behavior and extinguishing unwanted behavior through selective reinforcement.

Also in the 1950s, Abraham Maslow offered a developmental approach to how humans think and feel that remains one of the most influential ideas of psychological and emotional therapy. He contended that human behavior is motivated by the drive to meet basic needs and that these needs are hierarchical and developmental: survival needs, safety needs, love and belonging, self-esteem, and self-actualization. At the same time, a number of other developmental approaches were advanced to help occupational therapists understand the psychological and emotional determinants of occupation. Piaget suggested four stages of cognitive development from sensorimotor to formal operational learning. Erikson advanced eight stages of social development, each characterized as a challenge associated with a particular life stage and a tension between a lower and a higher level of development. Kohlberg proposed six stages of moral development, from rule based to universal ethical stages. In response, occupational therapists explored a number of developmental approaches to explain how development affects occupation. Perhaps the best known is Mosey's Recapitulation of Ontogenesis. She suggested that occupation is affected by development in seven skill areas: perceptual motor, cognitive, drive-object, dyadic, group interaction, self-identity, and sexual identity.

Growing out of the social learning theories, Beck and Bandura proposed cognitive approaches to understand and intervene with psychological-emotional problems. Behavior was seen as shaped by three types of negative thoughts: about the self, about the world, and about the future. If the individual could harness the power of the conscious brain to confront these negative thoughts, he or she could overcome the negative messages that interfered with positive relationships with the self, others, and the environment. OT embraced these ideas and developed a number of approaches, including the psychoeducational approach, the teaching of life and social skills, the stress-coping approach, verbal mediation, and self-regulation approaches. All of these have in common the reliance on cognitive strategies to overcome psychological and emotional obstacles to occupation.

Finally, in the latter part of the 20th century, in concert with rights movements among a number of disadvantaged citizen groups, consumers of psychiatric services formed a movement to resist the influence of psychiatry and psychiatric medication, characterizing them as instruments of oppression. Institutionalization was viewed as incarceration, and large-scale social changes resulted in the closing of thousands of psychiatric hospitals in North America and the corresponding, but slow, development of community-based supports and services. Consumer groups developed to exert pressure to maintain the change agenda and to provide peer support and independent living supports to mental health consumers. People with lived experience of mental illness were instrumental in the development of a recovery movement that informed how service providers and systems could work with consumers to enable their full participation. Occupational therapists began to focus on psychosocial rehabilitation, specifically the restoration of community functioning and well-being, vocational rehabilitation, social support, and the personal journey toward hope, meaning, identity, and social inclusion.

Occupational Conceptual Models Associated With the Psychological-Emotional Determinants of Occupation

Terry Krupa, PhD, OT Reg. (Ont.), FCAOT

The psychological and emotional determinants of occupation provide a framework for understanding why and how human beings are innately motivated toward occupation. The profession of OT is founded on the assumption that humans have an inherent drive to engage in occupation to meet many dynamic needs that are elicited by both internal and external factors. In addition to basic physiological needs, humans engage in occupations that satisfy needs related to safety and security, growth, belonging, self-esteem, and self-actualization and ultimately instill life with meaning. All of these needs are considered fundamental to survival and well-being. Participation in occupation is believed to promote adaptation to meet human needs, wants, and expectations in changing contexts and environments.

Psychological and emotional determinants refer to specific mental processes of human function. Motivation, drive, and meaning are psychological and emotional processes that are foundational to participation in occupation. There are, however, a broad range of other psychological and emotional determinants of occupation, including self-perceptions, thoughts, feelings, interpersonal relations, and coping. These are all the focus of this chapter.

Disruptions in psychological and emotional determinants can have a profound impact on occupational participation:

- Sometimes problems related to psychological or emotional determinants are a primary dysfunction of a health condition. For example, problems of mood and drive are central features of clinically diagnosed depression. People can experience depression as a primary disorder of health, or it can co-occur with other health conditions such as stroke or Parkinson's disease.
- Sometimes problems related to psychological and emotional determinants are secondary to a health condition or disability. For example, people with disabilities often experience low self-esteem and self-efficacy as a consequence of life experiences that compromise their self-perceptions, and this can affect their occupations.
- Finally, psychological and emotional processes can be significantly disrupted as a response to particular occupational contexts. A good example is when individuals participate in occupations that are demeaning, unreasonably demanding, and/or without opportunities for control and their self-perceptions, feelings, and coping abilities are seriously affected.

Occupational therapists often emphasize that the expected outcome of their services is improved *performance* of occupation. The notion of performance suggests that the focus is on enabling the functional ability of people to successfully participate in occupations in a way that is needed, desired, and expected. Students of OT will be familiar with the performance aspects of their own academic role. It can include, for example, acquiring and applying the knowledge base of the profession, modeling professionalism, and demonstrating specific competencies to a level expected of entry-level practitioners. Beyond performance, however, the profession is also concerned with occupational *engagement* and occupational *experience*. Both concepts refer to the subjective sense of participating in occupations, and they are closely related to the psychological and emotional determinants of occupation. In the student role, success and satisfaction demands a level of engagement or absorption and commitment. The student occupation might include experiences of interest and satisfaction, a sense of uncertainty about one's abilities, moments of anxiety and joy, and the experience of developing strategies to cope with novel demands and high expectations.

Occupational therapists use their theory and knowledge about the psychological and emotional determinants of occupation to understand how occupation is influenced by these mental processes and, in turn, how occupation influences them. The knowledge base of OT helps us to conceptualize how we might intervene to enable occupation when issues emerge related to self-esteem, sense of agency and control, mood, thought processes, awareness, and coping. Occupational therapists look to other fields, particularly psychology and its sub-disciplines of social, cognitive, and community psychology, to draw on basic theories about the psychological and emotional nature of humans and how these affect human behavior.

In the early 20th century, the founders of OT were often employed in services that focused on treating people with mental illnesses. In this work they became intimately familiar with how disruptions in psychological and emotional functioning affected occupation. They also observed how the societal response to these health conditions, specifically care in asylums, contributed to the deterioration of occupation. As discussed in detail in Chapter 9 about sociocultural determinants, these early champions of the profession recognized that separating people from the normal rhythms and patterns of occupation contributed to mental ill health. The Mental Hygiene movement developed largely in response to personal accounts of the horrible conditions experienced within institutions for those with mental illnesses. It developed the importance of occupations in the relief and cure of conditions of poor mental health and advocated for the opportunity for individuals to receive the services they require to engage in these occupations within the community.

The curative properties of occupation described in these early years included the potential of occupation to place limits on introspection and replace gloomy and unwholesome thoughts and feelings. Occupations also ground people in reality, have a calming influence, induce self-reliance and a sense of accomplishment and mastery, and enhance psychic energy. The approach to occupations in these early times was prescriptive. There was an effort to match occupations to individual dispositions and temperaments. The motivating aspects of occupation were considered to ensure therapeutic benefits, but even though matching activities was in the interests of patients, in practice it was constrained by the institutional context of treatment.

During the First World War, OT was involved both with rehabilitation of returning veterans and with preparing military personnel to return to the battlefield. OT practices integrated attention to the physical injuries experienced by the military and capitalized on the motivating aspects of activity to sustain efforts toward physical remediation. In addition, activities were also used to address the psychological and emotional consequences of war, a therapeutic process that was further developed in World War II and has extended to present combat situations.

The psychoanalytical theories proposed by Freud and his followers, which gained prominence in OT theory in the 1950s and 1960s, had a profound influence on the development of theory related to psychological and emotional determinants of occupation. These theories highlighted the influence of intrapsychic factors on occupational behavior. They provided explanations for how participation in occupations was influenced across the life span by a broad range of psychological and emotional processes that could be either subject to conscious awareness or were unconscious. The OT practice that evolved from these psychoanalytic theories established therapeutic processes that used activities as a means to develop greater self-awareness, strengthen positive psychological and emotional capacities, and ultimately support occupational performance and experience. Early psychoanalytic theories in OT tended to be highly reductionist, focusing on psychological and emotional aspects of the individual rather than on occupation.

In the 1970s, several important ideas and assumptions underlying analytic theory evolved and were integrated into OT theory. These included such important concepts as self and object relations. They also included specific OT interventions such as the therapeutic use of self, therapeutic milieu, projective techniques, and the therapeutic use of groups. In addition, these psychoanalytic theories contributed greatly to the evolution of the nature of the therapeutic relationship between the occupational therapist and the client.

OT's understanding of the factors associated with the motivational properties of occupation was influenced by the development of psychological theories of motivation in the 1960s. These theories provided a foundation for the understanding of both intrinsic and extrinsic motivation, enabling the development of such important concepts as sense of competence and the drive for mastery. The ideas underlying these psychological theories were applied in OT to understand the motivational issues associated with a broad spectrum of disabilities.

In the 1960s OT witnessed the beginnings of the application of behavioral theories. These theories were based on the idea that many of the behavioral problems associated with psychological and emotional disorder (or disruptions in mental health) could be conceptualized as learned behaviors. Thus the processes and principles of learning were integrated into OT practice to enable occupational performance. With its focus on the objective aspects of human behavior, the therapies were particularly attractive to OT as the profession began to address issues of accountability and outcome measurement.

In the 1970s and 1980s behavioral theories evolved to include a focus on behavior in interaction with thoughts and affect. These cognitive-behavioral theories were applied in structured programs in OT to improve occupational performance and psychological well-being. Cognitive-behavioral approaches engaged individuals in actively reflecting and acting on their own thoughts and feelings in relation to desired goals.

Since the 1990s, two large-scale movements related to psychological and emotional determinants have influenced OT practice. The first is the global movement to raise the profile of mental health. The following is a popular definition of mental health: "[A] state of successful performance of mental functioning resulting in productive activities, fulfilling relationships with other people and the ability to adapt to change and cope with adversity" (U.S. Department of Health and Human Services, 1999). This definition suggests that mental health depends on mental processes, including those that are psychological and emotional, in the context of daily life occupations and social interactions and their many challenges. The global mental health movement emerged largely because of the history of marginalization of issues of mental health and mental illness within societies, evidenced by such things as the relative underfunding of services for problems of mental health, and the stigma and discrimination associated with problems of mental health. The impact of this global movement on OT has been to broaden the practice context so that psychological and emotional determinants of occupation are addressed within a range of community environments (schools, workplaces, housing supports, neighborhoods, etc.) and treatment contexts (primary care, private practice, community clinics, etc.) with a view to preventing, treating, and minimizing their negative impact on daily life.

The second contemporary movement has been the growing focus within health care to capitalize on the psychological and emotional capacities of individuals (including awareness, autonomy, empowerment, and coping) so that they can develop a personal understanding of their health and well-being, become empowered to take greater control over the course of their health conditions, and ultimately choose and live a life that is less defined by the illness experience. This movement has been referred to in a number of ways, as "chronic disease management" when applied to individuals with serious and persistent physical health conditions and as "recovery" when applied to people living with mental illnesses.

A broad range of concepts may be included as psychological-emotional determinants of occupation. Many are common concepts that we use in our day-to-day worlds to converse about our psychological and emotional states and to interpret our behaviors and the behaviors of others. For example, many readers will have had the experience of using the word *depression* to describe feeling gloomy or will have felt a lack of "self-confidence" before engaging in an important and challenging task. On the positive side, this familiarity enhances our ability as occupational therapists to communicate with clients and with the public about these ideas. On the negative side, familiarity with key concepts does not necessarily mean there is always a shared understanding, and because they are so familiar, they can easily be taken for granted. This can be

a problem if it leads to dismissing or trivializing the impact of psychological and emotional issues.

One of the goals of this chapter is to provide a framework for organizing these psychological-emotional concepts, with a view to promoting understanding and shared meanings. The concepts are organized in six dimensions, presented in the following discussion, and linked conceptually to occupation and the growing knowledge base of the profession. Motivation and meaning are presented first, reflecting their position as overarching concepts explaining directed and sustained engagement in occupation.

A wide range of distinct psychological and emotional concepts or factors have been linked to directed and sustained human engagement in occupation. Although they appear in the early OT literature, they were discussed in a very general manner, and there was little effort to develop these concepts precisely. This changed in the 1980s and beyond with the rapid rise in scholarly literature that focused directly on specific psychological and emotional determinants of occupation. Carswell-Opzoomer (1990) suggested that shifts in health care systems from a largely biomedical orientation to a more holistic paradigm of health that included attention to social and psychological determinants such as those presented here set the stage for OT contributions in these areas.

Motivation and Meaning

Motivation and meaning provide the foundation for understanding the *why*, *what*, and *how* of any individual's participation in occupation. The term *motivation* typically refers to the impetus or drive for occupations, but it is often used to explain a range of behaviors that suggest this drive. For example, "motivation" can be used to describe occupational behaviors that have a direction or purpose, that are sustained over time and in spite of challenges, and that illustrate preferences for particular types and styles of involvement (Wlodkowski, 2008).

The concept of motivation appeared regularly in the very early literature (1920s-1940s) of the profession and focused largely on the importance of facilitating the sustained commitment of individuals in therapy with a view to working toward their personal well-being. At that time, therapy was largely situated in institutional settings, and activities offered were limited to craft, technical, or creative activities; thus, difficulties associated with motivating clients were often noted. Only a very limited number of publications related directly to motivation and occupation appeared in the 1950s and 1960s, but they did introduce important ideas about how individual motivation could be enhanced through occupation. Dunton (1951), for example, suggested the importance of personal interests and past education and training to engage the "mental excitement" required to sustain attention to occupation, and Dyer (1963) described the potential of strengthening motivation by imagining the future through the setting of goals relevant to the individual's cultural and socioeconomic factors.

In the 1970s motivation in OT was linked to theories of intrinsic motivation. Florey's (1969, 1970), work was seminal in this area. Unlike extrinsic theories of motivation, which posit that human motivation is a response to external incentives, or drive theories that suggest that human behavior is directed to reduce internal tensions, theories of intrinsic motivation advance the notion that humans experience internal rewards through the process of doing. Given its central position in human occupation, disruptions in intrinsic motivation are associated with problematic occupational patterns such as disengagement, learned helplessness, and hopelessness. Identifying how to address these issues was important for occupational therapists, and efforts were made to identify what therapeutic processes might best elicit intrinsic motivation related to occupations. Doble (1988), for example, integrated findings from multidisciplinary scholarship to develop a model that identified four determinants of intrinsic motivation that could be applied to OT practice: organizing the task environment to arouse interest, exploration, and mastery; including occupations with personal meaning; ensuring personal control and choice in occupations; and facilitating perceived and real competence through doing.

Although meaning has emerged relatively recently in OT scholarship, it has received much attention over the past decade. As mentioned previously, meaning in occupation is closely connected to motivation in that the extent to which an occupation is personally meaningful will positively influence sustained motivation. Occupations that are personally meaningful are considered by an individual to be significant, important, and valued. Not all meanings associated with occupations are psychological and emotional in nature, but those associated with affective states of pleasure and enjoyment or closely linked to expressions of the self can certainly be included. Hasselkus (2011), who has written extensively about meaning in OT practices, noted that humans find meaning in activities that allow for self-expression and the development of selfhood. Whalley-Hammell (2004) described how, for people with significant health problems or disability, occupations can influence and be influenced by the meanings ascribed to these life disruptions. Occupations associated with such experiences as self-worth, redevelopment of identity, and control can influence an individual's perception of a life as worth living.

Related to motivation and meaning, the concept of flow, which emerged in the psychology literature in the 1980s, has been identified as highly relevant to the OT concern with intrinsic motivation in occupation. *Flow* describes the experience of being totally involved in an activity, so much so that the individual experiences very focused attention, an altered sense of time, and a loss of self-consciousness (Csikszentmihalyi & Csikszentmihalyi, 1988). OT literature has developed the importance of creating occupational opportunities and conditions that would be likely to lead to experiences of flow (Emerson, 1998; Jonsson & Persson, 2006; Rebeiro & Polgar, 1999), such as ensuring that activities hold meaning for the person and offer an optimal amount of challenge.

Self-Perceptions

Individuals hold insights, awareness, views, evaluations, and judgments about their selves that influence their participation in occupation. Of the very broad range of concepts related to self-perception, those that most often appear in the OT scholarship are self-esteem, self-efficacy, personal causation or a sense of agency, self-awareness, and self-identity.

Concerned about the apparent gap that often existed between an individual's potential capacity and actual occupational engagement and performance, occupational therapists have looked to the work of well-known social psychologists such as Bandura to understand this discrepancy. Gage and Polatajko (1994) highlighted how the people served by OT frequently have a) low self-esteem, meaning that they are vulnerable to holding views of themselves that are negative, based on social comparisons of factors such as bodily appearance and competence; and b) compromised self-efficacy, meaning that they frequently hold negative evaluations of their ability to succeed in particular situations or to reach particular goals. The related concept of personal causation, developed within the Model of Human Occupation (Kielhofner, 1995), suggests that low self-esteem and self-efficacy are connected to a sense of having limited control to affect the desired outcomes while participating in occupations. The result is a personal disposition and self-awareness that can lead to a condition of learned helplessness and seriously interfere with the motivation required for healthy occupational participation. A core assumption of OT is that participation in occupation (i.e., the actual doing of the activities associated with occupations) has the potential to enhance self-esteem and self-efficacy if particular conditions are met. For example, occupations that are constructed to enable success and provide opportunities for control will enhance self-efficacy but may have little impact on self-esteem if they are not perceived by the individual as personally and socially meaningful (Gage & Polatajko, 1994).

The psychological concept of self-identity refers to the overarching sense that humans have of their distinctiveness, of the features that make them unique from others. The work of Christiansen (1999) has been particularly instrumental in developing the concept of identity as applied to OT. Christiansen defined *identity* as having multiple elements, including "an interpersonal aspect (e.g., our roles and relationships, such as mothers, wives, occupational therapists), an aspect of possibility or potential (that is, who we might become), and a values aspect (that suggests importance and provides a stable basis for choices and decisions)" (p. 548). Although identities are complex, people experience their personal identities as integrated and coherent over time. Christiansen highlighted the link between identity and meaning, suggesting that the emotional connections people make to their activities will depend on the extent to which they are interpreted as consistent with their self-identity. According to Christiansen's description, identity is also a social phenomenon in that identities become expressed through our social interactions and influence our relations with others.

The concept of identity has resonated with occupational therapists who often work with people who have identity-related issues, for example, identities that have been disrupted by experiences related to persistent illness and disability and related limitations in occupations. In such cases, participation in occupations is considered integral to the process of identity building—in particular, an identity that is not dominated by illness and disability but rather includes a range of elements associated with purpose, meaning, and well-being. This link between occupation and identity has deep roots in the profession. As far back as 1923, Bassoe, a physician, noted that OT helped people to become "the architect of their own reconstruction" (p. 607). Building on these ideas, Unruh and Elvin (2004), Kielhofner (2002), and others have put forward the notion that *occupational identity* may be considered a distinct form of self-identity.

Affect/Mood

Mood and affect refer to human emotional experiences. Whereas *moods* are the internal subjective experience of human experience, *affect* is the external expression of these moods. Moods are typically considered positive or negative in their nature. Common positive human emotions include pleasure, happiness, joy, satisfaction, happiness, and contentment. Those that are negative are experienced as unpleasant emotions and include anxiety, fear, anger, hate, sadness, grief, unhappiness, and discontentment. The relationship of moods to human occupation is complicated. It makes sense that positive human emotions associated with an occupation are likely to contribute to sustained motivation, and negative emotions are likely to interfere with sustained and committed involvement. Yet we also know that some unpleasant moods such as anxiety and anger can actually be catalysts for personal investment in occupation and actually enable occupational performance. For example, students getting ready for an exam will know that a moderate level of anxiety can positively influence efforts to meet the challenge.

Since its earliest years, OT services were provided to individuals with disturbances of mood and affect. The assumption in these early years was that activities could be used therapeutically by matching activities with individual needs to elicit particular types of affective responses. The activity options, however, in these early times were limited given the constraints of institutional therapy settings. With the advent of psychodynamic approaches, activities were used to elicit emotional responses as a means to promoting self-awareness. In the 1970s and 1980s several scholars focused their work on identifying affective responses and meanings associated with different activity conditions (e.g., sharing or not sharing, group or parallel project; Adelstein & Nelson, 1985; Nelson, Peterson, Smith, Boughton, & Whalen, 1988). Contemporary perspectives of the profession suggest that it is unlikely that affective responses can be attributed to any specific occupation without an understanding of the transaction between the person, the occupation, and the environmental context of the occupation.

Thought Processes

Thought processes refer to the content and form of thoughts and, of particular interest in this chapter, to the relationship of these to participation in occupations. These include, for example, an individual's perceptions and interpretations of situations and the flexibility of these thoughts—their logic, coherence, and reasoning. How we think about people, events, situations, etc., affects our participation in occupations in a variety of ways. Problematic thought processes can, for example, interfere with full attention, influence affective responses, and complicate sound reasoning in context. Although people can show an amazing level of self-awareness and insight with respect to their thought processes in occupation, their efforts to adapt can take considerable energy and effort.

In its early years, the profession viewed participation as a means to divert attention from "unhealthy" thoughts and to provide direction for thoughts that could promote adaptation. While notions of occupation as "diversion" have been largely eliminated from the profession because of the association of the word with entertainment and recreational pastimes, the power of occupations to direct the attentions of people in a purposeful and structured way while offering experiences of choice, autonomy, and meaning continue to be developed within the profession. For example, a recent publication by Reid (2011) applied the notions of flow and mindfulness to consider the processes by which occupational engagement promotes health and well-being. She argued that these psychological concepts capture the connection and awareness that are inherent qualities of occupational engagement that absorb attention.

Furthermore, participation in occupations is also believed to have a "grounding" affect when limitations in thought processes exist. By providing real-life task and interpersonal demands in real-world contexts, occupations press for occupational behaviors that are consistent with social norms. Thus they are believed to provide the context to test out, evaluate, and refine perceptions, judgments, and interpretations (see, for example, Krupa, 2004).

Interpersonal Processes

Interpersonal processes refer to those functions that support human relationships and interactions. Occupational therapists have long been aware that success and satisfaction in participation involves not only task demands, but also the social demands of occupations. Attention to social interactions in OT emerged as a focus in the 1970s and 1980s and was initially based on the use of therapeutic groups and milieu communities structured to develop social interaction opportunities and skills. With the growing focus on addressing occupational participation in natural life contexts, efforts were made to identify and describe the complex array of interpersonal interactions that occurred within natural occupational contexts. For example, Forsyth, Lai, and Kielhofner (1999) developed a framework for organizing information about social interactions. It included the nature of the social interaction (i.e., open, one-to-one, parallel, cooperative), the explicit identification of the environmental context of the interaction (i.e., natural setting, simulated setting, setting unrelated to life role), and dimensions of social interaction to be considered.

In 1992 Doble and Magill-Evans introduced a Model of Social Interaction to guide OT practice in response to a lack of explicit development of the area in general models of occupation. The model describes social interaction as a process of receiving and interpreting social messages and the planning of output, ultimately leading to social enactment skills. The model categorizes a broad range of influences on the process, and this is meant to help structure observations and

interpretations relative to any individual's occupational context. These categories of influence include, for example, volition, sensory organs, cognitive abilities, emotional and affective states, motor planning, and interactional style. By conceptualizing social interaction as an open system, the model acknowledges the influence of feedback on the social interaction process. In their more recent review of occupation therapy and cognate models of social competence, Lim and Rodger (2008) commented that any model of social skills and social interaction for the profession needs to include the fact that social competence may include other task-related social behaviors, such as following instructions or responding to authority.

Coping

Coping in this chapter refers to the psychological and emotional processes that are used by people to successfully engage in occupations in the face of internal or external demands or stressors. The concept of coping is considered distinct but related to human adaptation. Zeidner and Endler (1996) differentiate these terms by suggesting that *adaptation* is a broad term that refers to all modes of adjusting while continuously interacting with the environment, whereas *coping* always refers to managing in the context of some sort of stress. The concept of coping is applied in those situations where, if left unchecked, the person is at risk for being overwhelmed emotionally. Processes of coping can include, for example, regulating emotions and impulses, adapting to change, responding to frustrations and stresses, monitoring personal responses, and seeking support.

Gage (1991) developed an Appraisal Model of Coping to guide OT practice. The model was based on foundational work developed by seminal stress and coping scholars Lazarus and Folkman as well as Bandura's social cognitive theory. In addition, Gage conducted a literature review to identify a broad range of factors influencing the coping process. The model integrates many of the key concepts and ideas from the related scholarship to help occupational therapists understand specific coping strategies and to recognize maladaptive coping strategies with a view to assisting individuals dealing with highly stressful situations.

Fine (1991) offered occupational therapists another perspective on coping. Inspired by the remarkable capacity of people served by OT to recover, bounce back, and grow and flourish under conditions of significant losses, adversity, and trauma, she focused on understanding resilience and how people cope under extreme conditions of stress. Fine's analysis is particularly noteworthy as an early example within the profession of developing theory by accessing lived experiences and the voice of people served to understand psychological and emotional phenomenon. Fine highlighted the importance of this approach:

> I believe that as a group we are far more effective at defining reality and assessing and promoting performance then we are at assessing and making use of patients' views of themselves and their situation. Although our clinical prowess has grown greatly, we are too often committed only to present manifest performance. These snapshot approaches to capacity fail to reflect the unique adaptive style and potential of each person. If we are to enhance outcome, we must integrate the patients' experience of their condition and their preexisting patterns of self-regulating activity with our concerns and strategies for functional mobilization. (p. 500)

Summary

This chapter focused on the psychological and emotional determinants of occupation, providing an organizing framework for key concepts. Psychological and emotional determinants have held an important place in OT since its inception, and indeed, the profession's central assumptions about the occupational nature of humans are based on psychological-emotional theory. Although the determinants were loosely defined in the profession's early scholarship, they became more explicitly defined and developed by the 1970s and beyond. These advances were tied to related developments in the cognate fields of social psychology, social cognitive psychology, and community psychology. Over the past 20 years, there has been considerable evidence that the knowledge base of the profession is advancing occupation-specific concepts, definitions, and theory related to psychological and emotional determinants.

Finally, in earlier years there was the assumption within the profession that activities had particular qualities that could be used therapeutically to influence psychological and emotional well-being and to promote function. With the evolution of practice directed to the natural community contexts of occupation, the profession largely focused on enabling function and performance. More recently, this has expanded to include concern with the conditions of occupation that enhance engagement and experience and ultimately influence psychological and emotional well-being. These are presented throughout this chapter and include, for example, control and choice; access to participation in personally and socially important occupational opportunities; affirmation and recognition; and optimal challenge and achievement of competence.

11

The Physical Determinants of Occupation

Debra Stewart, MSc and Briano Di Rezze, PhD, OT Reg. (Ont.)
With an Introduction by Mary Ann McColl, PhD, MTS

Introduction

The physical determinants of occupation are those factors in the musculoskeletal system that affect our ability to engage in occupations. The musculoskeletal system includes bones, joints, muscles, tendons, ligaments, circulation, peripheral nerves, and skin. The key physical concepts affecting occupation include strength, range of motion, endurance, fatigue, mobility, agility, and pain. Theory associated with the physical determinants of occupation examines the concepts listed in the box at the top of this chapter and their relationships to occupation. Theory classified in this "drawer" of the filing cabinet (Figure 11-1) helps us to understand how each of these concepts affects occupation. These physical factors affect what we do and how we do it.

After identifying occupational performance problems that the client wishes to work on, the occupational therapist speculates about the possible reasons for these problems. If the main reason for occupational performance problems appears to be a physical problem or

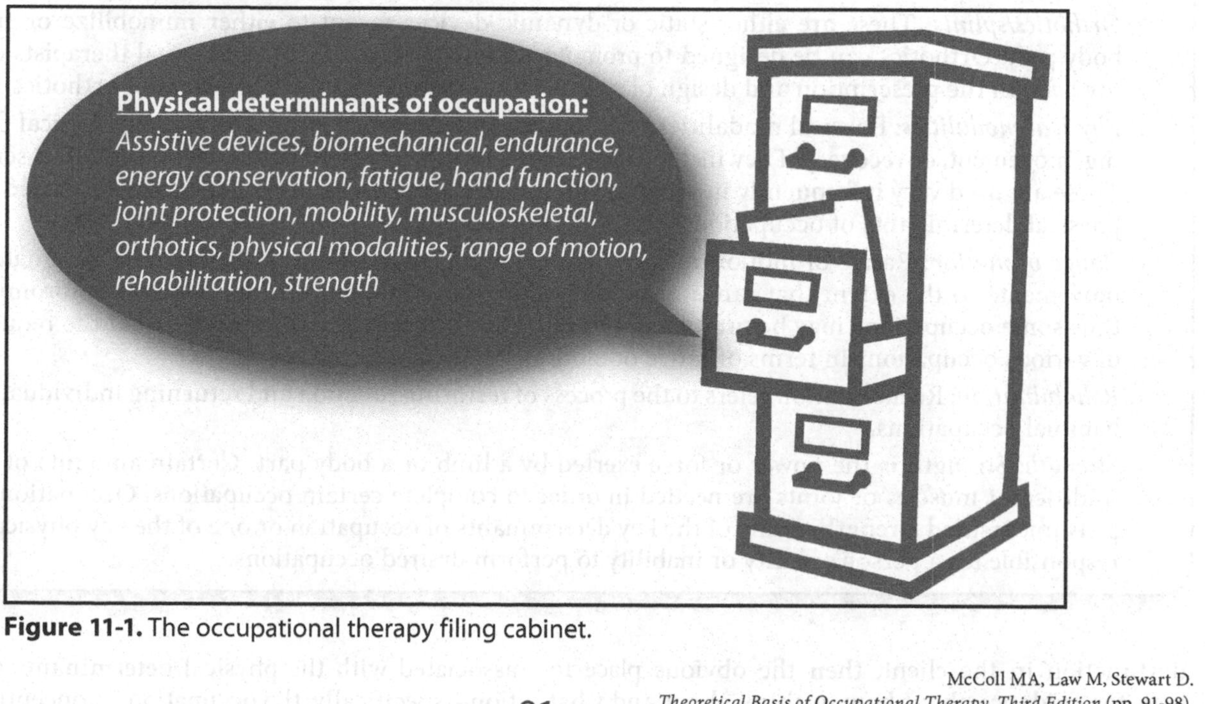

Physical determinants of occupation:
Assistive devices, biomechanical, endurance, energy conservation, fatigue, hand function, joint protection, mobility, musculoskeletal, orthotics, physical modalities, range of motion, rehabilitation, strength

Figure 11-1. The occupational therapy filing cabinet.

McColl MA, Law M, Stewart D.
Theoretical Basis of Occupational Therapy, Third Edition (pp. 91-98).
© 2015 Taylor & Francis Group.

Concepts and Definitions

- *Assistive devices, aids,* and *adaptive equipment*: These are all terms used to refer to equipment used to help people with disabilities to complete specific tasks. Occupational therapists often suggest adaptive devices as a means to enable a particular occupation. For example, there are a number of common devices that assist with activities of daily living, such as a button hook, long-handled shoehorn, or stocking aid.

- *Biomechanical*: Biomechanical means relating to the physics or mechanics of the human body. Biomechanical principles are often used to determine how the physical demands of a task will affect the body and the ability of the body to fulfill the demands of the task.

- *Endurance*: Endurance refers to the ability of an individual to muster stamina to complete a given task. Occupational therapists are often involved in assessing the demands of a task in terms of endurance and assisting individuals to build up their stamina in order to accomplish the occupation they need to do.

- *Energy conservation*: This is an alternative approach to building endurance that consists of a variety of strategies to save energy, maximize endurance, and create efficiencies in the expenditure of energy.

- *Fatigue*: Fatigue refers to a feeling of weariness or exhaustion brought about by exertion. It is associated with a number of conditions commonly seen by occupational therapists, such as multiple sclerosis, arthritis, and pain. Depending on the individual's physical condition, the amount of exertion required to produce fatigue may vary and may, in fact, be quite small.

- *Hand function*: Hand function refers to a number of fine motor tasks, including manipulating objects, grip and pinch strength, and thumb opposition, to name a few. Occupational therapists sometimes specialize in hand function and the many injuries and conditions that may impair it.

- *Joint protection*: Joint protection refers to a battery of techniques, devices, and strategies to save vulnerable joints from pain, dislocation, subluxation, damage, and deformity. Particularly in arthritic conditions, affected joints may be at risk unless good joint protection techniques are mastered.

- *Mobility*: Mobility refers to getting around. It may mean walking with or without supports (human or mechanical), or it may refer to wheeled mobility, such as a wheelchair or scooter. Mobility or movement is one of the key ingredients for successful occupational performance; therefore, occupational therapists are often involved in helping clients optimize mobility.

- *Musculoskeletal*: Musculoskeletal is the name for the system of hard and soft structures that create the basis for form and function of the human body. The musculoskeletal system consists of bones, joints, and muscles and various other related physical structures.

- *Orthotics/splints*: These are either static or dynamic devices meant to either immobilize or support a body part. Orthotics can be designed to promote healing or function. Occupational therapists often are involved in the prescription and design of splints and sometimes in the fabrication of orthotics.

- *Physical modalities*: Physical modalities refer to sensory techniques meant to promote physical functioning, movement, or recovery. They include heat, ice, vibration, ultrasound, or other mechanical sensations. These are used very infrequently in modern OT, and yet they appear in the literature associated with the physical determinants of occupation.

- *Range of motion*: Range of motion refers to the extent of travel of a joint through its designated arc of movement. To the extent that range of motion is limited, some movements may be compromised, and thus some occupations may be prevented. Occupational therapists need to understand the requirements of various occupations in terms of range of motion.

- *Rehabilitation*: Rehabilitation refers to the process of restoring function and returning individuals to their habitual occupations.

- *Strength*: Strength is the power or force exerted by a limb or a body part. Certain amounts of strength in different muscles or joints are needed in order to complete certain occupations. Occupational therapists understand strength as one of the key determinants of occupation or one of the key physical factors responsible for a person's ability or inability to perform desired occupations.

dysfunction in the client, then the obvious place to look for guidance about how to think about and what to do about the client's problems is the theory area associated with the physical determinants of occupation—specifically, the occupational conceptual models and the occupational models of practice that explain the physical factors associated with occupation. This is the fourth drawer of the filing cabinet. An occupational therapist might "open this drawer of the filing cabinet" in situations like the following:

- The client wishes to return to work but does not have the endurance or stamina for his or her previous job.
- The client has experienced a peripheral nerve injury and experiences paralysis in the affected arm.
- Because of prolonged bed rest, an elderly client is significantly deconditioned and unable to do essential occupations.
- A client with inflammatory arthritis has responded well to medication but needs strategies to protect her vulnerable joints and create efficiencies in her movements.
- A young woman has back pain that interferes with her role as a nurse's aide.

These are examples of situations where a client presents for occupational therapy (OT), and the occupational therapist determines that the origins of his or her problems lie in the physical aspect of the person.

Basic Conceptual Models Underpinning the Physical Determinants of Occupation

In order to understand how the physical determinants affect occupation, we must first understand the musculoskeletal system itself—how it operates and what can go wrong with it. To do so we rely on *basic conceptual models* from a number of biomedical sciences, such as anatomy, physiology, kinesiology, biomechanics, and ergonomics. These sciences tell us about how the physical aspect of human beings functions, how it interacts with other systems and with the environment, and finally, how illness or injury can compromise physical functioning. Occupational therapists need an understanding of these basic sciences if they are to understand how the physical aspect of the person affects his or her occupation.

In order to set the stage for a discussion of the physical determinants of occupation, there are three historical themes that provide some perspective for the development of OT theory in this area. In each case, occupational therapists responded to these events with attempts to interpret what they meant for occupation and OT.

Tuberculosis is an infectious disease that is rarely seen in the developed world today, although it is endemic in the developing world and affects approximately one-third of the world's population. Tuberculosis was a major public health threat in North America in the early 20th century until the discovery of a viable vaccine in 1946. The common treatment for tuberculosis (or "consumption") was to enter a sanatorium. This effectively segregated infected individuals from the population and attempted to optimize conditions leading to recovery. Sanatoria were usually located outside major population centers, often at higher elevations or in desert areas. They specialized in rest cures, consisting of fresh air, sunlight, nutrition, and good hygiene. Occupational therapists were associated with many of the major sanatoria in North America, and for patients capable of some level of activity, therapists proposed the "work cure" to take the place of the rest cure. The work cure further extended the ideal milieu for recovery by adding a balanced regimen of meaningful work to occupy the mind and body and promote overall health.

Another trend in the early 20th century that contributed to the development of OT theory was related to another infectious disease, polio myelitis. Polio was endemic in Europe and North America in the 19th century, leading to a level of natural immunity in the population; however, with improvements in public health in the early 20th century, epidemics of polio began to appear. There were a number of major epidemics between 1900 and the mid-1950s, until a vaccine was discovered and made available to the public in 1955. Typically, 10% to 15% of polio victims died, and the remainder experienced varying degrees of permanent paralysis after six to eight months of recovery. The field of rehabilitation generally, and OT specifically, responded to the need for treatment of polio survivors with a variety of treatment modalities that have become mainstays in modern physical rehabilitation.

Finally, the 20th century was marked by international conflicts that changed the way we thought about disability and rehabilitation. World War I, World War II, and the Vietnam War each produced huge changes in the way society related to disabled people, in particular to veterans of those wars. Technical, surgical, and pharmacological improvements in the care of injured soldiers led to the survival of large numbers of disabled citizens. These were not the typical demographic of disabled individuals; they were young men and women who had been injured in the service of their country. In World Wars I and II, these casualties were a part of the cost of victory, and public sentiment was so strong that society needed to do everything in its power to honor their service and their sacrifice. They still had the bulk of their adult lives ahead of them, and rehabilitation was central to the societal response to these individuals. The Vietnam War also produced a significant number of casualties; however, the response of the society to which these veterans returned was considerably more ambivalent. Again, however, rehabilitation was at the center of programs to return them to productive lives.

Occupational Conceptual Models Associated With the Physical Determinants of Occupation

Debra Stewart, MSc and Briano Di Rezze, PhD, OT Reg. (Ont.)

Current OT textbooks use different terminology to describe and categorize the physical determinants of occupation (Crepeau, Cohn, & Schell, 2013; Pendleton & Schultz-Krohn, 2013; Radomski & Trombly, 2011). The International Classification of Functioning, Disability and Health (ICF; World Health Organization, 2001) can provide a common language to describe areas of physical function. The physical determinants of occupation fall mainly under the categories of body functions and structures. *Body functions* are physiological in nature, and *body structures* are the anatomical parts of the body (World Health Organization, 2001). The specific body functions and structures in the ICF that fit with the physical determinants of occupation include the following:

- Functions and structures of the cardiovascular system
- Functions and structures of the respiratory system
- Functions and structures of the joints and bones
- Muscle functions and structures
- Functions and structures of the skin

In the ICF, the term *impairment* is used to describe problems in body structure and function. An impairment can be "temporary or permanent; progressive, regressive or static; intermittent or continuous" (World Health Organization, 2001, p. 12). Physical impairments can be caused by injury or trauma but can also be congenital or acquired over time. Any type of physical impairment in body structures or functions (e.g., problems with muscles, joints, skin, or the heart) can affect daily occupations that require movement, strength, and endurance. Conditions such as arthritis, hand injuries, amputations, soft tissue injuries, burns, and cardiac and pulmonary conditions are often the cause of impairments of the physical determinants of occupation. Occupational therapists therefore need to be familiar with the physical functions and structure and related impairments in the body that can influence the performance of occupation.

This chapter reviews the international peer-reviewed OT literature about the physical determinants of occupation. A historical perspective of relevant theories is presented first, after which the current literature from the year 2000 on is reviewed. The final section of this chapter discusses the trends in theory about the physical determinants of occupation.

The literature on the physical determinants of occupation starts near the end of the First World War in response to the needs of returning veterans. Occupational therapists worked in hospital workshops and industrial therapy to help veterans resume their former work or learn new trades (Hall, 1917). These new programs stressed the importance of adapting the physical components of activities, such as slowly increasing the amount of physical exertion or strength required, to gradually improve a patient's functioning and movement (Barton, 1917). Activities were analyzed for their therapeutic value with the goal of finding the best fit for the patient's needs. The primary outcome of interest in these early days of OT was to return the patient to some type of work.

In the 1920s the "biomedical" or "medical model" of health care began to emerge, in which the biological and medical aspects of human functioning were most important (Hall, 1921). As the medical model developed, occupational therapists focused more of their efforts on the treatment of physical problems (Green, 1922; Hall, 1921; Lull, 1926). The field of physical rehabilitation became stronger but, at the same time, more reductionistic and less holistic. The term *activity analysis* emerged to describe a unique and systematic form of analysis used by occupational therapists to determine the physical demands of different activities. Activity analysis began in military hospitals after World War I and continued to evolve over time (Creighton, 1992). The importance of work for the health of the individual and a return to a productive life after injury remained key driving forces for OT in this decade (Brown, 1923; Swaim, 1921).

With societal developments in automation and urban industrialization, the use of physical rehabilitation, primarily in hospitals, increased throughout the 1930s to treat physical disabilities from industrial and motor accidents. The influence of the medical model was more pronounced in the literature of this decade, as the term *exercise* was used more often than *activity*. Graduated exercise (through the grading of activities) was an important treatment modality for the restoration of physical function (Hurt, 1939; Merritt, 1938). Prevocational and vocational training were common in OT practice (Elton, 1934; Kidner, 1932; Shimberg, 1936), with the goal of returning a person to productive life. The role of OT in the treatment of tuberculosis through the use of physical modalities was prevalent in this decade as well (Banyai, 1938; Heaton, 1937; Spector, 1936). At the end of the 1930s, Patterson (1939) wrote about the expanding opportunities for occupational therapists to work outside of hospitals in homes, schools, and communities.

The second World War had a strong influence on the field of physical rehabilitation and OT (Grossman, 1946; Licht, 1944). With an increase in the prevalence of physical disability and chronic conditions, OT practice broadened to include more physical techniques such as kinetic analysis (Covalt, Yamshon, & Nowicki, 1949; Licht, 1947). Another interesting development noted in the literature of the 1940s was the suggested division of OT practice that separated physical from psychological treatments (Franciscus, 1946).

As medical science advanced, the OT literature about physical function and dysfunction in the 1950s focused more on techniques and less on theory (Gordon, 1954; Krusen, 1954). Specific treatment areas included kinetics, orthotics, self-help techniques, work evaluation and retraining, and energy conservation (Hendrickson, Anderson, & Gordon, 1960; Hood, 1956; Howard, 1956; Klinger, 1965; Patterson, 1963; Reilly, 1956; Sutherland, 1964). This continued into the 1960s; however, toward the end of that decade some authors began to call for a more holistic approach to OT practice connecting physical and psychological components (Fiorentino, 1966; Johnson & Smith, 1966). Spackman's (1968) review of OT practice for physical function identified the need for a clearer definition of OT with an increased focus on activity to enable a person to become more independent.

OT literature of the 1970s and 1980s placed more emphasis on theory than on techniques in all areas of practice. However, very little was written specifically about physical rehabilitation theory in these two decades, and it was noted that few theoretical models in OT were based on physical concepts alone (Llorens, 1984). In the 1980s, the role of the occupational therapist appeared to be moving beyond the assessment and treatment of physical skills to view the whole person within the context of his or her daily environments and occupations (Bing, 1981; Rogers, 1982). The goals of OT in the area of physical disability were shifting toward independence and quality of life rather than focusing strictly on such components as endurance, range of motion, and strength (Frieden & Cole, 1985; McCuaig & Iwama, 1989).

This evolution continued through the 1990s, with authors supporting a shift in priorities in OT assessment and treatment: occupation and role performance were the first priorities, and physical components played a secondary or supporting role (Mathiowetz, 1993). An example of this was seen in a position paper on physical agent modalities from the American Association of Occupational Therapy. The paper stated that physical agent modalities, including the use of heat, cold, and ultrasound, were adjunctive methods of treatment that should be used by occupational therapists only to "support and promote the acquisition of the performance components necessary to enable an individual to resume or assume the skills that are a part of his or her daily routine" (McGuire, 1997, p. 870). In other articles, concepts of occupation and principles of client-centered care were applied to the assessment and prescription of assistive devices and technology for people with physical disabilities (Bailey, 1994; Smith, 1995).

In the last decade of the 20th century, occupational therapists wrote more about the theoretical foundations of OT practice in the area of physical function and dysfunction (Trombly, 1995). Two primary approaches or frames of reference for OT were described in the literature:

1. The *biomechanical framework* is based primarily on principles of physics, kinetics, and biomechanics (Colangelo, 1999). It is typically considered to be a remedial approach to improve physical components such as strength and range of motion using exercise and other physical modalities.

2. The *rehabilitative approach* is primarily based on principles of compensation and adaptation (Trombly, 1995). This approach focuses on adaptation of activities and compensatory strategies, such as the use of assistive devices when necessary, to help a person maintain his or her ability to perform daily occupations when there are residual physical problems (Dutton, 1995; Kielhofner, 1997; Pedretti & Zoltan, 1996).

Very little contemporary OT literature is theoretical or conceptual about the physical determinants of occupation. Most of the current literature in this area is practical, applied, evidence based, and not theoretical. The theoretical literature is older and appears in interdisciplinary journals to which therapists refer, because much of the work in these areas is interdisciplinary. Within this more practical literature, the underlying concepts and ideas about physical determinants have shown some progression theoretically in the past decade, and these trends are influencing OT practice. The remainder of this chapter reviews current OT literature (since the year 2000) that describes concepts and theories about the physical determinants of occupation. The findings of this literature review are organized under three main "categories" of physical determinants:

1. *Musculoskeletal determinants*—This section includes ICF categories of joints, bones, and muscle structures and functions. Related concepts include extremity training, strengthening, and physical modalities. Some examples of the types of conditions that would fit under this category would be arthritis, joint replacements, and traumatic injuries to the body's musculoskeletal system.

2. *Cardiorespiratory determinants*—This section includes ICF categories of cardiovascular and respiratory structures and functions. Related concepts include fatigue, endurance, and energy conservation. Some examples of conditions within this category are chronic obstructive pulmonary disease (COPD) and cardiac disease/impairment.

3. *Skin determinants*—This section includes burns and other traumatic or chronic impairments associated with the skin and related structures and functions.

These three traditional categories are used to provide the reader with some structure in thinking about physical determinants of occupation. The themes of physical determinants that populate these categories from the current literature include training and strengthening as well as physical modalities, support, and taking control. Some of these concepts relate to all three categories, but based on the evidence, they were grouped accordingly. A fourth category was dedicated to the description of physical activities that address physical determinants of occupation.

Musculoskeletal Determinants

The literature that represents musculoskeletal determinants focuses on areas such as the skeletal system, muscles, and joints, as well as common injuries seen by occupational therapists (i.e., hand and upper extremities). This section describes the current literature related to musculoskeletal determinants of occupation and has been categorized as follows: extremity training and strengthening; modalities; and other key considerations in physical muscle systems.

Extremity Training and Strengthening

Movement, strength, and range of motion are key physical determinants of good physical health and, in turn, of successful occupation. One recent paper described how physical limitations affect occupation within a population of older women with upper extremity fractures (Dekkers & Nielsen, 2011). In this population, occupations that required strength in bilateral activities were most frequently reported as being problematic (i.e., cleaning, hygiene, and cooking).

Other papers have identified the impact of musculoskeletal factors on occupation by demonstrating how occupation-based interventions have improved physical function outcomes and hence enhanced occupational performance. One study examining functional outcomes in clients who had upper-extremity injury or surgery demonstrated improvements in functional gains when receiving OT (Case-Smith, 2003).

Some research in hand therapy demonstrated improved physical functioning after occupation-based interventions (Colaianni & Provident, 2010). A final consideration in the intimate relationship between occupation and physical functioning is the importance of considering the complexity of an occupation because of its potential influence on the forcefulness and smoothness of motor functioning (Ma & Trombly, 2004). These works emphasize the challenges of physical function within the context of occupation and how physical functioning is addressed in OT to improve occupational performance.

Physical Modalities

Physical agent modalities have been defined as "those modalities that produce a physiological response through the use of light, water, temperature, sound, electricity, or mechanical devices" (AOTA, 2003, p. 650). They can be integrated into an OT intervention program to enhance improvements in physical function (McPhee, Bracciano, Rose, Brayman, & Commission on Practice, 2003). In a systematic review, the use of physical modalities in OT interventions has a positive impact on client physical skills for upper extremity issues in work-related injuries (Amini, 2011). In some situations, physical modalities are used primarily to reduce symptoms of pain, such as joint pain, that is the result of physical dysfunction, such as arthritis. It is important to note here that no articles were found about theories or models that support the use of physical modalities, and yet they continue to be a part of physical rehabilitation.

More recent modalities that extend beyond the traditional definition of physical modalities involve the potential use of computers to aid in addressing physical issues within intervention. One particular study demonstrated that a computer interface (or video game) for wrist movements produced improvements in physical function and demonstrated promising new approaches to addressing physical determinants in OT (Jarus, Shavit, & Ratzon, 2000).

Cardiorespiratory Determinants

The cardiorespiratory determinants of occupation include fatigue and endurance. They are often relevant to specific conditions, such as COPD and multiple sclerosis. Within the current OT literature, the key themes related to cardiorespiratory determinants include disability education and support as well as taking control of the disability. Literature in the area of COPD demonstrates the importance of addressing issues related to the disability that affect occupation. Some examples include the need to increase knowledge of the disability, to empower clients in disability management, and to increase support from their personal and health care team (Chan, 2004). The importance of educating and empowering clients on the cardiorespiratory determinants of their disability to improve occupational performance has been identified in other literature. Migliore (2004) provided more specific recommendations (e.g., dyspnea management and energy conservation) to improve physical function in adults with COPD. These studies highlight the importance of understanding the physical impairment issues related to the disability in order to improve occupational performance.

Skin as a Determinant

Although the skin is the largest organ of the human body, and skin conditions such as burns, sensory impairments, and wounds are important areas within the context of OT practice, the current OT literature does not describe papers that identify novel or updated evidence on skin determinants affecting occupation.

Physical Activities Impacting Physical Determinants

Within the current OT literature, several articles describe the importance of engaging in physical activities as ways to address the physical determinants that limit occupational performance. Studies that examined the effects of exercise on occupational functioning in a well elderly population demonstrated that participants in regular exercise functioned more independently (Venable, Hanson, Shechtman, & Dasler, 2000). Related work by Wagstaff (2005) reported that well elders participating in exercise improved physical health and abilities in activities of daily living. Similar research in child and adult populations with physical disabilities has demonstrated how adaptations in occupations (Bontje, Kinébanian, Josephsson, & Tamura, 2004) and physical activities (Sharp, Dunford, & Seddon, 2012) addressing physical determinants of the disability can influence occupations.

Summary

This chapter demonstrates the progression of the theoretical basis of physical determinants of occupation. The OT literature shows how theory has been influenced by societal events such as two world wars and industrialization. The strong influence of the medical model from the 1920s into the present day has guided OT practice in this area to focus on physical modalities to treat problems with musculoskeletal, cardiopulmonary, or skin structure and function. The influence of the medical model resulted in occupational therapists focusing more on one physical component, such as muscle strength or endurance, and rarely looking at the whole person. Since the 1970s, increased attention on occupation and occupational performance has led occupational therapists working with people with physical dysfunction to adopt a more holistic approach that addresses all aspects of the person (Cole & Tufano, 2008). Less emphasis is paid to just the physical components individually and more on how these physical components influence occupational performance—that is, the physical determinants of occupation.

Review of the OT literature since the mid-1990s highlights some common themes or trends regarding the theoretical basis of the physical determinants of occupation:

- Occupational therapists are now using a combination of remedial and compensatory approaches for improved occupational performance (Cole & Tufano, 2008).

- There is an increased understanding that physical activity (occupations) not only influences physical function but can also influence everyday functioning or overall health and well-being. This concept of what one can do in everyday life acknowledges the interaction between components of the person and occupational performance and general health, and fits with current OT models, such as the Person-Environment-Occupation model (Law et al., 1996), Model of Human Occupation (Kielhofner, 2008), and the model of functioning that is described in the ICF (World Health Organization, 2001).

- More attention is being paid to patient experiences and illness perspectives as well as symptom and disease management. Recent articles have demonstrated the significance of meaning in helping an individual optimize occupational performance (Dubouloz, Laporte, Hall, Ashe, & Smith, 2004) and the use of motivating occupations that address mind and spirit as well as physical functioning (Chan & Spencer, 2004) for clients with different physical conditions.

The theoretical basis of physical determinants of occupation will no doubt continue to evolve as our understanding increases about related concepts of health, functioning, disabilities, and occupation. Recent trends in OT literature indicate an ongoing shift toward holistic, occupation-based practice that places more emphasis on physical activity and exercise as occupations and the strong connection between mind, body, and spirit. Furthermore, new concepts related to client experiences and illness perceptions may provide occupational therapists with a broadened view of health and occupational performance that will enhance their practice with people with physical challenges.

12

The Cognitive-Neurological Determinants of Occupation

Michelle Villeneuve, PhD, MSc, BSc OT

With an Introduction by Mary Ann McColl, PhD, MTS

Introduction

The cognitive-neurological determinants of occupation are those features of the central nervous system (CNS) that affect occupation. This is the fourth category of determinants of occupation covered in this book. It developed largely from the 1950s onward as technology permitted more and more sophisticated understanding of the brain and the CNS.

Theory associated with the cognitive-neurological determinants of occupation examines the concepts listed in the box and their relationships to occupation. Theory classified in this "drawer" of the filing cabinet (Figure 12-1) helps us understand how each of these concepts affects occupation. These cognitive and neurological factors affect what we do and how we do it. Theory in the cognitive-neurological area attempts to explain how the CNS and the brain relate to occupation.

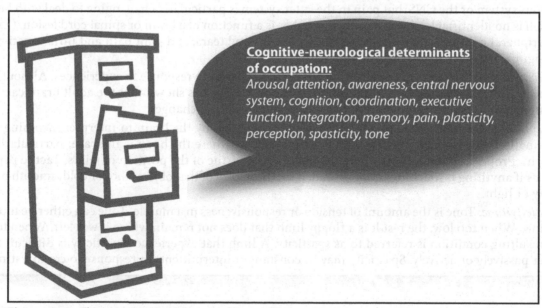

Cognitive-neurological determinants of occupation:
Arousal, attention, awareness, central nervous system, cognition, coordination, executive function, integration, memory, pain, plasticity, perception, spasticity, tone

Figure 12-1. The occupational therapy filing cabinet.

99

Concepts and Definitions

- *Arousal, attention, awareness*: All three of these concepts refer to a state of readiness in the CNS to receive input and consciously process incoming information. Arousal simply refers to a state of consciousness, from unconscious to hyperaroused. Awareness refers to a general state of being able to appreciate and interpret one's surroundings. Attention refers to a selective focus on a particular subset of stimuli from the environment. A moderate level of all three is required for most occupations, and occupational therapists need to be aware of these states as either helping or hindering the performance of occupation.

- *CNS*: The CNS refers to the brain and the spinal cord. Its function is to integrate and coordinate incoming and outgoing signals from and to the body. It is distinguished from the peripheral nervous system in that it cannot regenerate damaged tissue.

- *Cognition*: The reader will remember that we spoke about cognition in the psychological-emotional theory area as well. There we were interested in the content of thoughts; here we are interested in the process of cognition. Is the brain capable of basic cognitive functions, such as memory, learning, problem solving, and reasoning? Most occupations require a certain level of cognitive function, so an occupational therapist would need to be able to assess not only the cognitive abilities of the client, but also the cognitive demands of the task.

- *Coordination/integration*: To be able to produce smooth, purposeful movements, the CNS must be capable of managing a number of different functions and assembling them in a coherent whole. For example, some parts of the body need to be stabilized, whereas others have to move in specific patterns relative to one another. Furthermore, the two sides of the body, governed by different sides of the brain, need to be brought together.

- *Executive function*: Executive functioning is a term referring to a number of important operations typically located in the frontal area of the brain. These functions include planning, regulation, problem solving, and sequencing, to name a few. Executive functions are often impaired by a brain injury. The more complex the occupation, the more important executive functions are to its successful execution.

- *Memory*: Memory is the process of encoding, storing, and retrieving information resulting from the senses and from experiences.

- *Pain*: Pain is a noxious experience usually associated with a specific location in the body. Pain motivates individuals to withdraw both physically and psychologically. Pain may originate in either the peripheral nervous system or the CNS, but pain in the latter system is particularly challenging to deal with because it often has no identifiable physical cause but rather is a function of a brain or spinal cord lesion. (Examples of peripheral pain include wounds, soft tissue strains and tears, and joint pain and inflammation.) Pain is a significant deterrent to occupation.

- *Plasticity*: Plasticity refers to the ability of the brain to change in response to experiences. Although much of the brain is hard wired by adulthood, recent brain science has shown that the adult brain can develop collateral pathways resulting both in functional and structural changes.

- *Perception*: Perception refers to a number of processes used by the brain to interpret incoming sensory information. For example, vestibular perception tells us where the body is in space, particularly if it is upright. Proprioception tells us where the limbs are by virtue of the position of joints. Tactile perception tells us if anything is touching the body and, if so, the nature of that object—hot or cold, smooth or rough, heavy or light.

- *Spasticity/tone*: Tone is the amount of tension or responsiveness in a muscle. Tone can either be too high or too low. When too low, the result is a floppy limb that does not remain where it was left. When too high, the resulting condition is referred to as spasticity. A limb that experiences spasticity is difficult to move either passively or actively. Spasticity may be constant or intermittent (in response to certain stimuli).

An occupational therapist might "open this drawer of the filing cabinet" in situations like the following:

- A client is referred to occupational therapy (OT) because she has had a stroke and is experiencing paralysis of the nondominant hand and leg, and difficulties with activities of daily living.

- A young man has had a cycling accident and, with it, a brain injury. He has difficulties managing his money, his temper, and his energy.

- A child is referred to OT by her teacher, who has noticed that she has difficulties with things the other children master easily, such as using scissors, holding a pencil, and riding a bike.

Basic Conceptual Models Underpinning the Cognitive-Neurological Determinants of Occupation

Prior to the mid-20th century, only the most basic understanding of brain function as electrical impulses was available. In the 1930s and 1940s, the science of cybernetics represented a search for organizing principles of the brain. This led to early computer science in the 1940s and 1950s, which sought to simulate brain function mechanically. The 1950s brought the breakthrough studies of Wilder Penfield and others, who began to map the human cortex and localize functions in the brain. This led to a rudimentary understanding of the regionalization of brain functions, the lateralization of neural activity, and the effects of lesions in the motor and sensory cortex.

Also beginning in the 1950s, interest was stirred about the process of recovery from a lesion in the CNS. It was already clear that peripheral nerve injuries could be healed, but the process for central nerve lesions was different. The nerve did not simply grow back, restoring previous function. Instead, another process of recovery seemed to be afoot. Theories abounded about how this process unfolded, with stroke recovery as a natural experiment and a living laboratory.

Along with each of these theories of recovery came an intervention approach for promoting, hastening, and securing recovery.

Brunnstrom (1970) was the first to describe a predictable pattern of recovery with a fixed sequence of developments that simulated normal neural development in the fetus, infant, and child. Functional electrical stimulation attempted to mimic normal electrical impulses from the muscles, with the hope of eliciting movement responses. Proprioceptive neuromuscular facilitation involved stretching and handling techniques with a similar aim—to produce passive and active movements that would send signals to the brain. Rood (1958) and others developed cutaneous sensory techniques such as brushing, icing, and vibration to encourage motor responses. Neurodevelopmental therapy (NDT), designed by Karel and Berta Bobath (1864), was a complex approach based on proximal stabilization (trunk and large joints) to permit distal purposeful movement. Finally, in OT, Jean Ayres (1972) proposed sensory integration therapy (SIT), focusing on vestibular, tactile, and proprioceptive inputs to stimulate motor outputs.

Over the next 40 years, increasingly sophisticated technology permitted more and more detailed understanding of the brain and its processes. The role of language in mediating brain function, the operation of neural networks, and the complexity of brain function all made huge strides forward. In the 21st century, with the advent of functional imaging technology, a new wave of brain science has been developed and popularized that focuses on plasticity and the seemingly endless potential for adaptation.

Occupational Conceptual Models Associated With the Cognitive-Neurological Determinants of Occupation

Michelle Villeneuve, PhD, MSc, BSc OT

The cognitive-neurological area of OT theory contributes to our understanding of how components of the person including sensation, perception, cognition, and movement shape occupational performance. This chapter focuses on theory that informs OT practice with clients who have experienced damage to the CNS. In CNS damage, neural communication is often preserved, but it becomes disordered because of disease or trauma (Shumway-Cook & Woollacott, 2012).

Theories informing how cognitive-neurological factors influence occupation are based on interdisciplinary concepts about how information coming into the body through our senses is received, communicated, stored, and used to engage in activities. This theory area includes understanding about how people use information from the body together with information coming from the environment to initiate, control, and monitor the performance of occupation. Theoretical work in this area supports our understanding about the following:

- The nature and control of movement for optimal performance of occupation
- The forms of learning that support performance, generalization, and maintenance of skills for optimal occupational functioning
- The role of sensory-perceptual processing in supporting and maintaining meaningful interaction within the environment for the performance of occupation
- The influence of cognitive processes on planning, initiating, and monitoring our engagement in meaningful occupation

In examining this theory area, it is important to distinguish it from theory about the physical determinants of occupation that emphasizes musculoskeletal constraints affecting occupational performance. The cognitive-neurological area draws on theory about the central processing of internal and external stimuli. However, musculoskeletal components are important to the analysis of occupational performance because biomechanical factors (e.g., strength, range of motion) influence the ability to use our muscles and joint movement for action.

Theoretical understanding in this area has experienced notable development since the 1950s. Practitioner-scientists in rehabilitation therapy were instrumental in shaping early theory development,

giving rise to neurodevelopment treatment (NDT) (Bobath, 1978) and SIT (Ayres, 1972) therapy approaches that remain prominent in OT practice today. In this way, clinical practice informed scientific inquiry about cognitive-neurological impairments and the impact of dysfunction on occupational performance. There are several accounts of the parallel developments between theory and clinical practice in the literature (e.g., see Gordon, 1987).

Developments in basic neuroscience research in the 1950s and 1960s enabled occupational therapists to hypothesize about the relationship between the cause of cognitive-neurological dysfunction and ways to act therapeutically (Doubt, 2003). Medical science knowledge and techniques for diagnosis and treatment of acute illness developed rapidly during these decades, and the OT profession responded with an increased focus on science and acute illness in education, practice, and research. In keeping with the biomedical model of disability, OT literature of this era emphasized therapy techniques to change performance components, rather than a holistic approach to understanding occupation. During these decades, there is also evidence of a dramatic increase in writings related to neurological, sensorimotor, and cognitive-perceptual function. Publications by authors such as Ayres (1954, 1955, 1961), Brunnstrom (1961), Llorens et al. (1964), and Rood (1956) tended to focus on neurophysiological explanations and strategies for assessment and intervention to improve motor performance. Little theory was developed to explain the relationship between occupation and neurological or cognitive function.

In the 1970s and 1980s rapid expansion of knowledge in the neurosciences and understanding of the neuromuscular system became increasingly available to occupational therapists. However, the biomedical model, characterized by technological discoveries, quantifiable measurement, and acute medical care, continued to dominate in the health disciplines, making it difficult to rationalize occupation-based therapies. OT practitioners were left to bridge the gap between emerging neurological theories and occupation. At this time, there was a persistent focus on assessment and treatment of components of occupation rather than occupational performance.

Consistent with the emerging interest in understanding disability as a biopsychosocial interaction and the development of sociopolitical models of disability, the 1980s and 1990s brought a shift from institutional-based service delivery to community-based practice roles for occupational therapists. The literature of this time began to reflect an increased interest in developing ideas about occupation. Articles encouraged the integration of OT knowledge and neurobehavioral sciences, and exploring the role of theory in neurodevelopmental treatment approaches became more prevalent. By the end of the 1990s, a growing body of research literature aimed at understanding the relationship between cognitive-neurological deficits and occupational performance problems became available to students. Of particular interest to the OT profession was increased scientific support for the importance of meaningful engagement in occupation for clients with CNS deficits. Emerging research has studied the contribution that performance of everyday tasks and activities plays in shaping recovery and compensation in clients with CNS impairments.

At the turn of the century, we saw a steady development of occupation-based approaches in the literature, illustrating increasing confidence of the profession in using occupation to influence recovery for clients with CNS dysfunction. Advances in neuroscience knowledge and increasing interdisciplinary developments informing research and practice are firmly grounded in systems theory thinking about the impact of CNS dysfunction, in interaction with the environment, on the performance of occupation. At the end of the first decade of the 21st century, understanding about the complex and multidimensional nature of CNS processing and recognition of the important influence that the environment and occupation have on both planning and performance encouraged the OT profession to attend to the importance of meaningful occupation as a medium for intervention.

A sound understanding of the relationship between cognitive-neurological theory and functional performance of occupation allows us to better understand how OT intervention supports meaningful outcomes for clients with disorders affecting the CNS. Two questions guided the development of this theory chapter:

1. What do we know about cognitive-neurological determinants of occupation?
2. What cognitive-neurological factors affect occupation, and what do we know about how they affect occupation?

This chapter is organized into three sections:

1. Motor control and motor learning theory
2. Cognitive-perceptual theory
3. Sensory processing theory.

Each of these sections provides an overview of the theory area and discusses OT research of the past decade that has applied the theory to address occupation.

Motor Control and Motor Learning Theory

Motor control refers to the ability to direct and control the movements of one's body. Efficient motor control relies on coordinating movements of the trunk, head, and limbs to maintain balance (Shumway-Cook & Woollacott, 2012) and is important for the performance of occupation (Kielhofner, 2004). *Motor learning theory* is concerned with the acquisition of movement while recovery or motor relearning focuses on the reacquisition of movement skills following injury (Shumway-Cook & Woollacott, 2012). Occupational therapists work with children and adults who have CNS dysfunction in order to facilitate motor relearning and the development of postural control and mobility needed to perform daily occupations.

The next section provides an overview of motor control (reflex-hierarchical and dynamical systems) and motor learning theory that has evolved over the past century. These theories are informed by an interdisciplinary body of knowledge about the nature and control of movement and the (re)acquisition of motor control in people who experience CNS dysfunction, thus it is not possible to provide a comprehensive review in this chapter. Rather, emphasis is placed on the relevance of this theory area to OT. Recent OT research on the application of motor control and motor learning theory to influence occupation is integrated throughout.

Reflex-Hierarchical Theory

The *reflex-hierarchical* theory of motor control has been influential in shaping OT practice for clients with CNS dysfunction. This theory gave rise to neurofacilitation intervention approaches such as NDT, which was originally developed to address movement problems in children with cerebral palsy (Kielhofner, 2004). It has also been used to treat adult hemiplegia (Levit, 2008). NDT is grounded in traditional (reflex-hierarchical) theory about the nature and control of movement. These older models of motor control emphasize the importance of sensory input for the production of patterned movement responses (or reflexes) that are biologically determined and hierarchically organized within the CNS (Shumway-Cook & Woollacott, 2012). Reflex patterns emerge in the course of normal development as the nervous system develops and matures. The reflex-hierarchical model of motor control assumes that development and reorganization of the CNS results in the progressive integration of reflexes into voluntary control over movement.

According to this theory, the CNS is the primary source of movement. Voluntary movement control emerges as higher centers of the CNS develop and gain control over primitive reflex movements generated by lower levels of the CNS hierarchy. Furthermore, this model assumes that normal development of movement control in infants proceeds through a predictable sequence from head to foot (cephalocaudal) and from trunk to extremities (proximodistal). From this theoretical perspective, reflexive movement patterns are thought to support motor development of infants who are born without the voluntary control needed for skilled movement. Many of the instruments used to assess infant development are based on reflex-hierarchical theory that was used to explain the numerous developmental progressions seen in infants and young children (Shumway-Cook & Woollacott, 2012).

Reflex theory has also been used to explain the importance of reflexes on our adaptive functioning. For example, if we accidentally step on a sharp object, we automatically withdraw our foot from the source of pain. The flexion of that leg causes a reflexive extension of the opposite leg so that we do not lose our balance and fall over. Similarly, touching a hot stove will result in reflexive (flexor) withdrawal of our hand before the pain message is even received by higher levels of the CNS. In this way, reflexes serve a protective function. Reflex theory helps us understand how sensory input can influence stereotypical or patterned motor behavior. Hierarchical control of the CNS allows us to override our protective responses to act voluntarily. For example, we can override our reflexive withdrawal response in order to enter a burning building to save a loved one. Hierarchical control also supports the production of planned movement patterns that enable the most efficient movement patterns as we engage in occupation. Together, reflex-hierarchical control by the CNS supports our adaptability in the performance of a range of occupations.

Reflex-hierarchical theory has been applied both to children and adults with CNS damage. Motor dysfunction after brain damage involves changes in muscle tone (e.g., spasticity) and results in abnormal patterns of posture and movement that interfere with the coordination needed to perform occupations (Kielhofner, 2004). Reflex-hierarchical theory has been used to explain the stereotypical movement synergies seen in individuals with CNS damage (Shumway-Cook & Woollacott, 2012). Following a lesion to the brain, higher centers are less able to exert control over lower levels of the nervous system that organize reflexes. Consequently, individuals with brain damage are constrained to stereotypical movement patterns. When movement patterns and postures are impaired, sensory input reflects these abnormalities and provides incorrect information to the CNS (Kielhofner, 2004). This can result in inaccurate perception needed for skilled movement. These movement synergies (abnormal

movement patterns or reflexes) constrain voluntary movement control and limit one's adaptability to engage in everyday occupations. Hemiplegic postures seen after stroke, for example, influence one's ability to coordinate two sides of the body for effective weight shifting to rise from sitting or to climb stairs. It can also interfere with the bilateral hand movements needed for effective performance of many daily occupations (e.g., dressing, bathing, cooking, and cleaning). CNS dysfunction disrupts the communication of information between the brain and the muscles of the body; thus motor control impairments can influence the timing, speed, and accuracy of movement in clients with damage to the CNS, as seen in some clients with multiple sclerosis. CNS impairment can also affect one's ability to initiate movement or to sustain and control a movement sequence once initiated, as in Parkinson's disease.

The reflex-hierarchical model of motor control implicates the CNS as the key system responsible for the development and reacquisition of movement control. It assumes that the CNS is a flexible system that has the potential for reorganization (often referred to as plasticity) as a result of experience.

Dynamical Systems Theory

Dynamical systems theory is based on interdisciplinary concepts about the nature and control of movement that have developed from earlier reflex-hierarchical models of motor control. These newer models do not replace reflex-hierarchical theory but rather expand our understanding of motor control and learning to consider the dynamic interrelationship between the CNS and musculoskeletal systems of the person in interaction with the environment.

From a dynamical systems perspective, movement patterns are not the sole responsibility of the CNS, but rather, they are developed in response to task characteristics and environmental demands. Motor control is learned through a process of seeking optimal solutions for accomplishing one's occupations. In this way, the CNS and musculoskeletal systems cooperate to produce the most effective movement given specific task and environmental demands. This results in preferred patterns of movement to accomplish occupational goals (Shumway-Cook & Woollacott, 2012). Dynamical systems theory assumes that movement patterns can change in response to changes in variables within the person (CNS and musculoskeletal systems), the task, or the environment (Kielhofner, 2004). Interdisciplinary research supports dynamic systems theory and advocates the use of task-oriented models for intervention to improve motor control in clients with neurological conditions (Kielhofner, 2004; Shumway-Cook & Woollacott, 2012). Task-oriented models of motor control intervention are consistent with goal-directed, occupation-based practice advocated by occupational therapists.

Contemporary theory of motor control provides a different explanation for the typical progression of motor development in infants. From a dynamical systems perspective, postural control emerges through the progressive ability of infants to stabilize their body posture and coordinate the many joints of their bodies to interact with objects and move through their environment. Maturation of the CNS in combination with physiological growth and development explain how infants develop postural control and progress in their ability to move off of this stable posture to interact with people and objects. A classic example of infants controlling the numerous joints of their bodies is when they are first learning to walk. Babies will constrain the movements of their arms by retracting their shoulder blades and holding their arms in a "high-guard" position. Similarly, they control the degrees of freedom of their lower extremities by widening their base of support and fixing their knees and ankles. The resulting block-like posture supports them to maintain their balance while taking their first steps; however, they are not particularly adaptable and can easily fall. As infants practice controlling their bodies, they are gradually able to "release" their joints and move through space with improved coordination and adaptability. Dynamical systems theory recognizes that musculoskeletal growth influences the selection of movement strategies, and that infants and young children alter their strategies to accommodate changes in body size and muscle mass throughout development (Shumway-Cook & Woollacott, 2012).

More recently, ecological theory has contributed deeper understanding about the role of perception in motor control, further expanding our knowledge about the importance of task characteristics to motor control (Shumway-Cook & Woollacott, 2012). Ecological systems theory acknowledges the importance of the task demands in shaping motor performance. For example, we may adjust our movement patterns when reaching for a cup depending on whether the cup is empty or full. We may also adjust our grasp to accommodate the type of cup (e.g., paper vs ceramic), and we may adjust the force of our grip to accommodate other features such as condensation on the glass (suggesting that it might be slippery).

Dynamical systems theory recognizes that although disorders of movement are related to CNS deficits, they are not the direct consequence of those deficits. Like reflex-hierarchical theory, dynamical systems theory views the CNS as flexible, with potential for reorganization. However, neuroplasticity is shaped by experiences with occupations in response to environmental demands. Therefore, changes in the person, the task, or the environment all have the potential to affect motor performance and learning (Bass-Haugen, Mathiowetz, & Flinn, 2008). When applied to children and adults with CNS dysfunction, task-oriented theory views movement disorder as the result of the individual's attempt to compensate for CNS impairments in order to accomplish occupation under specific environmental circumstances. The emphasis of task-oriented therapy approaches is therefore placed on goal-oriented occupational performance (Mastos, Miller, Eliasson, & Imms, 2007). The aim of task-oriented therapy is to support clients in developing effective strategies for performing their occupations safely and effectively. Hence, emphasis during intervention is on the performance of occupations rather than discrete movements or movement sequences (Kielhofner, 2004). Dynamical systems theory helps us recognize the importance of experimentation and problem solving so that clients are actively involved in developing their own solutions to motor problems (Shumway-Cook & Woollacott, 2012).

Motor Learning

Motor learning refers to a set of processes associated with practice or experience that lead to a relatively permanent change in the capability for skilled movement (Shumway-Cook & Woollacott, 2012). Dynamical systems theory contributed understanding about motor (re)learning. Four motor learning principles that support occupational therapists to facilitate motor learning in clients with CNS dysfunction include stage of learning, task characteristics, practice conditions, and feedback (Zwicker & Harris, 2009). These strategies are thought to affect performance, generalization, and maintenance of learned skills, which in turn contributes to one's occupational functioning. These principles are used by occupational therapists to support the design of intervention sessions by analyzing task demands and structuring feedback on performance (Bass-Haugen et al., 2008).

Fitts and Posner's (1967) stage theory of motor learning suggests that proficiency with motor learning proceeds through a series of stages from cognitive to associative to autonomous. In the *cognitive* stage, the individual may have an idea of the movement to be performed, but performance is highly variable and requires conscious cognitive attention to task requirements. This results in more effort and movement than needed, making performance less efficient. At the *associative* stage, motor skills become refined, and performance becomes more consistent. Movements are more accurate, and errors can be used to adjust subsequent movements for improved accuracy in performance. Learners at this stage can benefit from practice and feedback from the therapist on their performance to further refine their movement. Once at the *autonomous* stage, little cognitive effort is needed to perform the movement. Fewer demands on attention allows for skilled motor performance while engaging in other tasks.

Motor performance and learning are affected by the occupation to be learned. Schmidt and Lee (2005) classified tasks as *discrete* (recognizable beginning and end, like putting on a pair of socks); *continuous* (no inherent start or finish, as when walking); *serial* (series of discrete tasks, such as cooking a meal); *open* (where responding to changes in the environment is required, such as playing volleyball); and *closed* (where the environment is relatively stable, enabling more predictable performance, such as bowling). In the OT literature, Nelson (1988) provided a detailed conceptualization of the relationship between occupational form and performance relevant to consideration of the features of tasks on performance of occupation. Two occupational forms, materials-based occupation and imagery-based occupation, are thought to promote motor performance within the context of occupational tasks (Nelson & Peterson, 1989). *Materials-based occupation* involves the use of everyday objects to elicit and shape motor performance, whereas *imagery-based occupation* uses verbal or visual stimuli to elicit an imagined or visualized activity in the absence of materials. A number of studies have examined the influence of goal-directed materials-based occupation on the performance of reaching in participants with neurological impairment (Trombly & Wu, 1999; van Vliet, Sheridan, Kerwin, & Fentem, 1995; Wu, Trombly, Tickle-Degnen, & Lin, 1998, 2000) and those without neurological impairment (Lin, Wu, & Trombly, 1998; Ross & Nelson, 2000; Wu, Trombly, & Lin, 1994). Findings support the relationship between task features and contextual demands on efficiency of reaching, amount of force generated, and speed of movement. An exploratory study by Fasoli, Trombly, Tickle-Degnen, and Verfaellie (2002) tested the assumption that materials-based occupation would elicit significantly better movement than imagery-based occupation by comparing individuals with and without stroke. They found that individuals with and without stroke adjusted their movement to the affordances of the task. Their findings reinforced the relationship between motor performance and context, and provided further support for the use of goal-directed materials-based occupation for both discrete and continuous tasks (Fasoli et al., 2002).

The conditions under which one practices a motor skill can influence learning. Practice schedules may include massed or distributed, blocked or random, and part or whole task practice (Bass-Haugen et al., 2008; Shumway-Cook & Woollacott, 2012). *Massed practice* occurs when the practice sessions are greater than the rest period, whereas *distributed practice* incorporates rest periods of equal or greater duration. *Blocked practice* involves repetition of the same task before altering the task demands, whereas *random practice* involves varying the task demands over the course of the practice session. Random practice introduces an element of contextual interference that is thought to place greater demand on the learner. Each condition can have a different influence on learning. Massed and blocked practice, for example, may improve performance in the short term, allowing the individual to progress through cognitive to autonomous stages of learning more quickly (Shumway-Cook & Woollacott, 2012). However, greater retention and transfer of learning may occur with distributed and random practice. Similarly, practicing *parts* of a task may support performance during early stages of learning, but *whole-task* practice will facilitate the use of the skill in context (Bass-Haugen et al., 2008).

Feedback is important to motor learning. Feedback can be intrinsic (sensory feedback on how the movement was performed) or extrinsic (e.g., instructions or verbal prompts about the quality of performance; Shumway-Cook & Woollacott, 2012). Extrinsic feedback, provided by the therapist, can be provided during movement, after the completion of a task, or after a delay. It is used to augment intrinsic feedback and to support clients in their evaluation of both the outcome of the movement and the quality of performance.

Cognitive-Perceptual Theory

Cognitive-perceptual theory is based on understanding about how information is processed by the brain. Occupational performance is based on the ability to perceive and evaluate sensory-perceptual information and the ability to conceive of, plan, and execute purposeful action (Kielhofner, 2004). When applied to people with CNS dysfunction, cognitive-perceptual theory focuses on how impairment in sensation, perception, and cognition restricts occupational performance.

Cognitive-perceptual dysfunction is associated with a range of clinical conditions and can occur across the lifespan. The cognitive-perceptual theory area is used most commonly when working with clients who have acquired brain injury or traumatic brain injury (TBI) and conditions affecting learning (Kielhofner, 2004). This theory area comprises a collection of concepts and approaches informed by interdisciplinary knowledge from the fields of neuropsychology and neuroscience (Kielhofner, 2004). Although discussed together with perception as cognitive-perceptual theory in this chapter, it is important to recognize the broader field of cognitive rehabilitation and the multidisciplinary research base that has informed the development of assessment and intervention approaches in this area of practice.

Sensation, perception, and cognition lie on a continuum (Kielhofner, 2004; Shumway-Cook & Woollacott, 2012). Sensation is at one end of the continuum, involving awareness of information received by different systems of the body. Perception involves interpretation of sensory information. At the other end of the continuum is cognition, which involves abstract reflective action and awareness of thinking (metacognition).

Perception involves taking sensory input from the body and the environment and combining that information with previous experiences to make psychologically meaningful interpretations of the information (Quintana, 2008). Sensations from our visual system, vestibular system, and body or somatosensory system (e.g., skin and joints) are processed within the CNS to give us an awareness of our body and make us conscious of our body with respect to the environment. Combining of sensory information enables complex discrimination and interpretation of information coming from multiple systems of the body. Impairments in perception have been categorized into taxonomies of perceptual abilities (Kielhofner, 2004). One such taxonomy describes perceptual impairments in three areas: *discrimination problems* (recognizing and discriminating forms using vision; touch discrimination); *body scheme disorders* (e.g., recognizing body parts; unilateral neglect of body, tasks, or environment); and *problems with praxis* (e.g., planning and performing purposeful movements) (Zoltan, 2007). Other taxonomies have been used to describe cognitive and perceptual functions and include visual foundation skills (e.g., Quintana, 2008; Radomski, 2008).

Cognition refers to the ability of the brain to process, store, retrieve, and manipulate information. Cognition is typically divided into 1) *basic cognitive processes,* such as orientation (knowing who we are, where we are, and having a sense of time), attention (which allows us to register, sustain, and alternate our focus on information), and memory (including short-term, working memory and long-term storage of information) and 2) *executive functions* that enable more complex planning, adaptive problem solving, self-monitoring, and self-awareness (Radomski, 2008). Cognitive dysfunction can affect basic and executive processing of information and interfere with the performance of occupation.

Learning is an important concept in this theory area because the expectation of cognitive-perceptual intervention is for the clients to generalize what they have learned to similar tasks outside of treatment sessions and to transfer what they have learned to new activities and situations (Kielhofner, 2004). *Metacognition,* which refers to awareness and control of one's cognitive processes and capacities, is an important factor in determining a client's ability to transfer learning.

Metacognition includes knowledge of one's cognitive abilities (self-awareness) as well as the capacity to appraise task difficulty, select and implement appropriate cognitive strategies, and monitor one's performance (Toglia, 1998). Self-monitoring and self-correction of errors during performance are important components of metacognition (Toglia & Kirk, 2000). Learning interventions that target client-identified occupational goals through problem solving and metacognitive strategies are therefore central to this theory area.

It has long been recognized that quality of performance provides important information about how cognitive-perceptual deficits influence the performance of occupation. Within the cognitive-perceptual theory area a number of intervention approaches have been developed to support and guide occupational therapists in their interventions (e.g., Dynamic Interactional Approach, Toglia, 2005; Cognitive Disabilities Model, Allen, Earhart, & Blue, 1992; Cognitive Rehabilitation Model, Averbach & Katz, 2005; and Cognitive Orientation to Daily Occupational Performance, Polatajko & Mandich, 2005) (American Occupational Therapy Association, 2014). These approaches draw on two major categories of intervention strategies: remedial and functional approaches.

Remedial Approach

The *remedial approach* seeks to restore specific cognitive-perceptual abilities and assumes that the brain has the capacity to reorganize and improve its information processing capacity following injury or disease (Kielhofner, 2004). Remediation uses tasks that require the brain to process information in specific ways that target impaired information processing abilities (Neidstadt, 1990). Remedial training often involves repetition of cognitive tasks, such as paper and pencil or computerized tasks, many of which replicate assessment tasks as exercise drills to develop cognitive and perceptual abilities (Kielhofner, 2004; Radomski & Davis, 2008). The expectation is that remedial gains will translate into improved performance of occupations requiring those skills (Radomski & Davis, 2008).

Remedial tasks are also used by occupational therapists as a means to increase self-awareness of cognitive-perceptual impairments and provide feedback to clients concerning the impact of impairments on performance. As a component of metacognitive training, feedback interventions have been used to improve self-awareness, self-monitoring, error correction, and strategy use in individuals following traumatic brain injury (TBI) (Fleming, 2009). Feedback interventions have emphasized direct verbal feedback provided by the therapist on a client's performance of remedial tasks (Fleming & Ownsworth, 2006). However, the effectiveness of these interventions has not been established (Dirette, Plaisier, & Jones, 2008). An alternative approach to improving self-awareness uses feedback interventions in the context of engaging in familiar occupations, where the effects of impairments can be seen (Fleming, 2009; Toglia & Kirk, 2000). Different forms of feedback interventions have been used in the context of occupation-based metacognitive training for individuals following TBI including verbal, video-recorded, and experiential feedback (Schmidt, Fleming, Ownsworth, Lannin, & Khan, 2012). OT research in this area is emerging. Schmidt et al. (2012) recently published a randomized, controlled trial protocol to evaluate the effectiveness of these three different forms of feedback interventions on self-awareness in people with TBI. More research is needed to understand the efficacy of different forms of feedback interventions and their impact on function.

Functional Approach

The *functional approach* consists of both *compensation* and *adaptation,* which capitalize on the clients' existing abilities to support occupational functioning despite cognitive-perceptual impairment. *Compensation* focuses teaching strategies to bypass clients' cognitive or perceptual impairments so that they can perform occupations safely and effectively. For example, a client with left hemiplegia who neglects one half of space because of unilateral inattention may be taught to visually scan the environment on the affected side (Zoltan, 2007). Compensation requires that clients have a degree of self-awareness of their limitations in order to compensate for them (Kielhofner, 2004). Understanding clients' metacognitive awareness may be helpful in determining whether they will benefit from compensatory approaches to intervention (Kielhofner, 2004).

Adaptation refers to changes in the environment that enable one's performance of occupation despite the persistence of cognitive or perceptual impairment. For example, if the client has problems discriminating among objects in a cluttered environment, such as finding the appropriate utensil in a kitchen drawer, the therapist would work with the client and family to unclutter the environment to make locating objects easier. Adaptations also refer to accommodations made by others to support a client's performance (such as providing verbal prompts and memory cues or allowing more time for a response; Zoltan, 2007). The functional approach may also attempt to circumvent deficits by teaching functional tasks and establishing routines for performance. For example, an individual with dressing apraxia (problems planning and performing dressing) may be taught a particular pattern for dressing and be engaged in daily practice of the dressing routine (Zoltan, 2007).

Sensory Processing Theory

Sensory processing theory is concerned with how CNS processes of receiving, registering, modulating, organizing, and interpreting sensory information influence functional behavior. This theory area addresses problems that individuals have with sensory processing in the absence of physical damage to the CNS (Kielhofner, 2004). Sensory processing dysfunction has been used to explain the challenges that some children have with occupational performance, such as paying attention, organizing themselves, participating in social play activities with peers, and learning new skills (Pollock, 2009).

This theory area views tactile, vestibular, and proprioceptive sensations as a foundation for complex occupations (Parham & Mailloux, 2010). *Tactile* sensations provide input about physical contact with the external world. *Vestibular* sensation provide information about one's position with respect to gravity. Located in the inner ear, vestibular receptors detect movement of the head and elicit compensatory head, trunk, and limb movements in order to maintain orientation with respect to the environment (Shumway-Cook & Woollacott, 2012). *Proprioception* is the perception of position of the body in space and includes perception of joint movement. Together, *vestibular-proprioceptive sensation* provides information about the active movement of one's own body and acts as a reference point for interpretation of other sensory information and for monitoring and controlling movement (Kielhofner, 2004). Two other senses, *visual* and *auditory,* also provide information from the external environment and are considered important for accurate processing and integration of sensory information for use (Bundy & Murray, 2002).

This theory area gave rise to SIT, developed by Jean Ayres. Since its development, it has been widely applied through direct and indirect intervention approaches with children with developmental disabilities, learning disabilities, developmental coordination disorder, attention-deficit/hyperactivity disorders, and autism spectrum disorders (Koeing & Rudney, 2010; Pollock, 2009; Schaaf & Miller, 2005). As a therapeutic approach, carefully constructed sensory experiences are used to support children in organizing their goal-directed actions on the environment (Parham & Mailloux, 2010). Ayers called this an *adaptive response,* which is made possible when the brain is able to organize and use sensory information effectively (Kielhofner, 2004). Bicycle riding provides an excellent example of the integration of vestibular and proprioceptive sensations together with visual information to successfully balance and steer often in unpredictable environments. Adaptive responses are thought to support development and contribute to the performance of increasingly complex occupations through improved processing of sensory information by the brain. The process is thought to be mutually reinforcing, such that sensory integration enables adaptive responses and adaptive responses promote sensory integration (Kielhofner, 2004).

Winnie Dunn (2001) contributed conceptual understanding about sensory processing and developed a framework for understanding the role of sensory processing in performance. Dunn's (1997) sensory processing model described the relationships between neurological thresholds for processing sensory information (e.g., high/low) and behavioral responses (e.g., sensory seeking, sensory avoiding). This framework recognizes the importance of self-regulation strategies as an important feature of adaptive functioning. Dunn's model has contributed important theoretical understanding concerning key constructs that affect how young children respond to sensory events in their daily lives (Dunn, 1997). Indeed, an important component of sensory processing theory has been the identification of types of sensory processing impairments and explanation of their impact on function.

Parham and Mailloux (2010) summarized the general literature on sensory processing theory and identified four major ways that sensory integrative dysfunction can manifest: 1) sensory modulation problems, 2) sensory discrimination and perception problems, 3) vestibular-proprioceptive problems, and 4) dyspraxia. Each of these is discussed briefly here; however, the reader is encouraged to consult the numerous textbooks available to occupational therapists that describe sensory integration approaches and provide detailed information about the application of this approach in practice.

Sensory Modulation

Sensory modulation refers to the nervous system's ability to regulate its own activity (Bundy & Murray, 2002). Individuals with sensory modulation problems have difficulty maintaining the normal limits of registering and responding to sensations (Kielhofner, 2004). Certain behaviors characterize modulation problems. These individuals may respond in different ways, such as avoiding sensory stimulation, seeking sensation, overreacting, or underresponding to sensory input (Parham & Mailloux, 2010). Modulation problems may also interfere with the individual's ability to register relevant sensory information. The literature on SIT has described the functional consequences of each of these behaviors. For example, individuals who fail to attend to relevant environmental stimuli may experience problems with classroom learning. Being able to attend to what the teacher is saying while filtering out other extraneous sensory information (e.g., artwork on the classroom wall, noises in the hallway) is important for learning.

Parham and Mailloux (2010) gave examples of children who exhibit underresponsiveness to incoming sensory stimuli. These children may appear to seek intense movement (vestibular) and stimulation (e.g., swinging, spinning) and yet do not react to it to the degree that most children do (i.e., they don't get dizzy from the experience). Others may seek proprioceptive input and may appear to bump, push, or fall into other people and objects in an attempt to seek active resistance to their muscles and deep pressure stimulation through their skin and joints (Parham & Mailloux, 2010). Children who experience hyporesponsivity to sensory stimuli may appear restless and driven to thrill-seeking behavior and be perceived as disruptive or inappropriate in social situations (Parham & Mailloux, 2010). In learning contexts where these behaviors are discouraged, these children may be labeled as having social, emotional, or behavioral problems. Occupational therapists may use SIT as a lens for understanding these behaviors and developing strategies for the children to obtain the level of sensory stimulation they seek without being socially disruptive.

Another type of modulation problem involves overresponsiveness to sensory stimuli (Parham & Mailloux, 2010). Commonly discussed modulation challenges include tactile defensiveness that produces a "fight-or-flight" reaction in response to ordinary touch sensation (Parham & Mailloux, 2010) and *gravitational insecurity*, which refers to fear of movement or being placed in an unstable position. Gravitational insecurity has been associated with hyperresponsivity to vestibular sensory input. Both tactile defensiveness and gravitational insecurity can present as fear, anxiety, or avoidance in the context of performing daily living activities (e.g., descending stairs, playing on playground equipment; Parham & Mailloux, 2010). Dunn's (1997) widely used Model of Sensory Processing provides a conceptual framework for describing patterns of sensory modulation problems and interpreting behavioral responses observed in clients.

Sensory Discrimination and Perception Problems

Sensory discrimination and perception problems describe sensory integrative disorders that involve inefficient or inaccurate organization of sensory information (Parham & Mailloux, 2010). Sensory discrimination is needed to distinguish sounds, objects, and shapes for efficient use of that information in the performance of daily occupation. For example, being able to discriminate among objects or parts of objects based on touch sensation supports efficient motor performance (e.g., fine manipulation of objects) without having to rely on vision to orient objects for use (e.g., buttoning clothes, tying shoes, playing games, and constructing objects out of small, manipulative toys). Being able to discriminate visually the letter *b* from the letter *d* supports learning to read and write, and auditory discrimination of sounds supports language development. Proprioceptive information provides information about the position of joints of the body; thus unreliable processing of proprioceptive information makes it difficult to determine the position of the body needed for the performance of tasks. Performance of daily occupations requires the integration of sensory information and discrimination of meaningful details to support performance. As a result, children with sensory discrimination and perception problems may appear clumsy or awkward and are at a disadvantage when learning and performing motor tasks because inaccurate sensory feedback interferes with efficient motor performance (Parham & Mailloux, 2010).

Vestibular-Proprioceptive Problems

Vestibular-proprioceptive problems are characterized by mild motor dysfunction that results from poor balance and coordination, lower than average extensor muscle tone, poor postural stability, and difficulty coordinating the two sides of the body (bilateral integration; Parham & Mailloux, 2010). These challenges affect performance of tasks such as playing sports and engaging in activities that require substantial balance (e.g., skating, bicycle riding). Since the development of SIT, impaired sensory processing of vestibular and proprioceptive information has been implicated in these differences observed in children who experience these forms of mild motor dysfunction.

Praxis

Praxis is the capacity to plan new movements. *Dyspraxia* therefore refers to dysfunction in the ability to conceptualize, plan, and execute nonhabitual movement (Parham & Mailloux, 2010). Dyspraxia may result from problems processing tactile information (somatodyspraxia) or deficits in bilateral integration, such that the individual has problems with sequencing and coordinating movements—especially those involving both sides of the body. Some individuals have problems with generating the idea for movement in a novel situation, whereas others have difficulty with the execution of the movement despite having a reasonable plan for action. Consequently, skills typically attained in childhood (e.g., tying shoes, managing utensils, jumping rope, writing) are remarkably difficult for children with dyspraxia and require substantial motivation and practice on the part of the child (Parham

& Mailloux, 2010). These children are typically aware of their differences, and their participation in sports and school tasks can be frustrating and embarrassing. Consequently, it is important to address these challenges in a way that supports the child's confidence and motivation (Pollock, 2009).

This theory area has held a consistent focus on the relationship between sensory processing and occupational performance since its inception. For occupational therapists, *sensory integration* is a term with specific meaning that expands beyond the neurophysiological understanding of synaptic connections in the brain for processing of sensory information to include the relationship of these neural processes to functional behavior (Parham & Mailloux, 2010). This understanding is evident in Ayers' (1972) definition of sensory integration as "the organization of sensation for use" (p. 1). A central principle of SIT is that increased efficiency with processing sensory information will support occupational functioning. However, empirical evidence of the impact of sensory processing dysfunction on occupational performance is lacking (Baranek et al., 2002).

In the early 2000s, researchers explored the relationship between sensory processing dysfunction and occupation, including children with genetic disorders and autism in their research (Baranek et al., 2002; Bundy, Shia, Qi, & Miller, 2007; Walz & Baranek, 2006; White, Mulligan, Merrill, & Wright, 2007). Findings from this emerging body of research are consistent with dynamic systems theory, which proposes a more complex understanding of the relationship between sensory processing dysfunction and occupation. A recent study by Bagby, Dickie, and Baranek (2012) used a grounded theory approach to explain how sensory experiences of children with and without autism affect family occupations. They concluded that sensory experiences of children affect what families choose to do, how the family prepares for activities and outings, and the extent to which experiences, meaning, and feelings about family occupations are shared.

Summary

A substantial breadth of research informs this theory area. Common across all areas reviewed in this chapter is the role of ecological and dynamic systems theory in supporting our understanding about the relationship between cognitive-neurological impairments and occupation. Occupation-based approaches used by OT practitioners to enable occupational functioning in clients with CNS dysfunction is a key feature of this theory area and is supported by current understanding about the nature and control of movement. Emerging research reinforces the importance of occupation for learning and recovery after CNS damage. Recent research findings provide further encouragement for occupational therapists to utilize occupation-based approaches with confidence. Future research that addresses the question of how occupation contributes to neurophysiological changes for individuals with CNS dysfunction will be an important contribution to this theory area.

13

The Environmental Determinants of Occupation

Mary Law, PhD, FCAOT

With Introduction by Mary Ann McColl, PhD, MTS

Introduction

The environmental determinants of occupation are those factors outside of the individual that affect his or her occupation. Unlike the previous four chapters, where we looked inside the person for the source of occupational performance problems, in this theory area we focus exclusively on factors outside the person. As an arbitrary boundary, we take anything beyond the skin to be part of the environment. (The one exception to this was discussed in Chapter 9 on the physical

determinants, where we considered things applied directly to the skin, such as an orthotic, prosthetic, or mobility device, to be part of the physical aspect of the person rather than part of the environment.)

Because of the close alliance of occupational therapy (OT) with the health sciences throughout its professional development over the 20th century, we are naturally inclined toward the biomedical model. Our default expectation, if we are perfectly honest with ourselves, is to seek the source of occupational performance problems INSIDE the person—in his or her

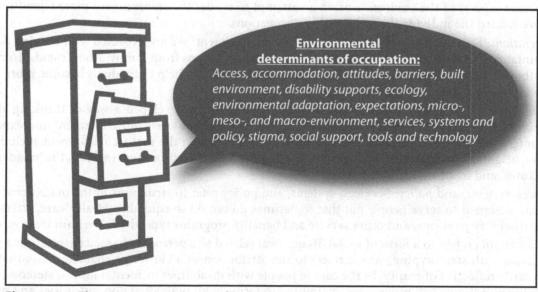

Environmental determinants of occupation:
Access, accommodation, attitudes, barriers, built environment, disability supports, ecology, environmental adaptation, expectations, micro-, meso-, and macro-environment, services, systems and policy, stigma, social support, tools and technology

Figure 13-1. The occupational therapy filing cabinet.

McColl MA, Law M, Stewart D.
Theoretical Basis of Occupational Therapy, Third Edition (pp. 113-122).

Concepts and Definitions

Theory associated with the environmental determinants of occupation examines the concepts listed in the box at the beginning of this chapter and their relationships to occupation. Theory classified in this "drawer" of the filing cabinet helps us to understand how each of these concepts affects occupation. These environmental factors affect what we do and how we do it. Theory in the environmental area attempts to explain how aspects of the environment relate to occupation. Here are some working definitions of these important concepts:

- *Access*: Access refers to the ability to approach, enter, and use facilities, services, and equipment. In OT, we are usually talking about accessibility considerations for people with disabilities.

- *Accommodation*: An accommodation refers to an adjustment or adaptation to a task or an environment that affords an individual an equal opportunity to participate, regardless of his or her disability or special needs.

- *Attitudes*: Attitudes are the demeanors or dispositions of individuals or groups toward a person, an action, or an idea. Attitudes can exert a powerful influence on behavior, either negatively or positively. Attitudes are sometimes communicated in words but are often communicated subtly and can be difficult to overcome.

- *Barriers*: Barriers are obstacles that inhibit participation and restrict access. Occupational therapists use a variety of means to help their clients overcome barriers and seek solutions that result in enablement.

- *Built environment*: The built environment refers to those human-made structures that constitute a major part of our physical environment. The built environment is traditionally designed to a normative standard, and often does not take account of the needs of people who move through the world differently.

- *Disability supports*: Disability supports refer to financial, instrumental, and information supports needed to live fully with a disability. Disability supports acknowledge the extraordinary costs of living with a disability as well as the need for specialized information and products, for example, knowledge about available programs or products such as wheelchairs or other assistive devices.

- *Ecology*: Ecology is the science of organisms in their environment. When applied to human beings, it refers to the study of humans in relation to their environment, particularly their structures and institutions. An ecological approach is an organic, holistic approach that acknowledges the interdependence of all things in a given environment.

- *Environmental adaptation*: One of the ways that occupational therapists can help to make a difference in occupation for their clients is to plan, negotiate, and execute environmental adaptations, or adjustments to various aspects of the environment, in an attempt to render the environment more friendly and supportive toward the individual and his or her occupations.

- *Expectations*: Expectations are everywhere in our environment. We are expected with varying degrees of accountability to respond to many different types of expectations from family, from friends, from people in authority, or from society as a whole. Occupational therapists help individuals become more aware of expectations and manage them effectively.

- *Micro-, meso-,* and *macro-environment*: Bronfenbrenner (1979) developed a way of thinking about the environment as a series of concentric circles, each with different levels of involvement and expectation. The micro-environment involves close or intimate connections; the meso-environment includes work, school, neighborhood, friends, and community; and the macro-environment includes the broader society, structures, and institutions.

- *Services, systems,* and *policy*: Services, systems, and policy refer to structures in the macro-environment that are designed to serve people but that sometimes do not do so equitably. Health care, attendant services, disability pensions, and other service and benefits programs typically fall within this category.

- *Stigma*: Stigma refers to a form of social disapproval related to a personal characteristic. Stigma is closely associated with stereotyping, which refers to the attribution of a cluster of characteristics that are not necessarily reflective of reality. In the case of people with disabilities or mental illness, stereotypes about disability and stigma can prove severely limiting in terms of an individual's opportunities and prospects.

(continued)

Concepts and Definitions (continued)

- *Social support*: Social support refers to the perception that one is cared for and loved, valued and esteemed, and able to count on others should the need arise. Support may be instrumental or practical, informational, or emotional.
- *Tools and technology*: Tools and technology refer to the many articles and instruments used in human occupation. Occupational therapists may recommend specialized tools or technology, may fashion customized tools, or may adapt existing tools to assist individuals with occupational performance.

---

physical, psychological-emotional, sociocultural, or cognitive-neurological makeup. We ask, "What is the underlying impairment or disorder in the person that is responsible for the difficulties he or she is having?" Even the biopsychosocial model, although more holistic than the biomedical model, still locates the source of the problem inside the person.

This area of theory—the environmental determinants of occupation—requires a radically different way of thinking about the causes of occupational performance problems. We begin with the assumption that the person is not responsible for his or her problems. Instead, it is an environment ill-suited to the individual that is responsible for the occupational performance problems he or she experiences. We look for the cause of problems in an environment that provides inappropriate or inadequate support for occupation. By extension, we seek to address occupational performance problems not by asking the person to change in any way, but rather by modifying or supplementing the environmental supports to permit the desired occupation.

An occupational therapist might "open this drawer of the filing cabinet" (see Figure 13-1) in situations like the following:

- A client wishes to return to work after the onset of a disability, but she is aware that her previous workplace will now be inaccessible for her. Both the building itself and her work station will need considerable adaptation for her to be able to use it.
- A long-standing client is frustrated by his inability to navigate the bureaucracy of disability pensions, supports, attendant care, and equipment purchase.
- A client experiences stigma and discrimination in her workplace when she returns from a hospital admission for a mental health problem.
- An elderly client experiences repeated falls and is deemed unsafe to remain in her home. Unless the occupational therapist can devise strategies to keep her safe, she will be forced to enter long-term care.
- A child is referred for difficulties participating in classroom activities and completing his school work.

Basic Conceptual Models Underlying the Environmental Determinants of Occupation

The basic conceptual models underlying OT theory about the environmental determinants of occupation come from such diverse fields as architecture, anthropology, geography, sociology, political science, economics, art, and design. From these disciplines, we learn how humans are affected by the physical, social, cultural, and the political-economic environments they live in. In particular, three environmental movements affected the development of OT theory.

Beginning in the 1960s, an increasing awareness of inequities in society led to a movement to ensure that the rights of all people were equally protected under the law. In the United States, the civil rights movement sought to correct longstanding inequities toward African Americans. Over the next 20 years, this movement spread to address rights of other oppressed minorities. In Canada, the Quiet Revolution sought freedom from oppression by the Church. Particularly in Quebec, the government proceeded to nationalize the development of natural resources and to secularize a number of public institutions, such as education, health care, and labor law. All over the world, women sought equality under the law, and fair and equal treatment in employment and civic participation. Aboriginal groups sought justice for historical inequities, and gay, lesbian, bisexual, and transgender groups sought recognition for their sexual orientations and personal identities.

Sometimes referred to as the "fifth civil rights movement," people with disabilities in the early 1980s advocated for a legal framework that would allow them full participation and citizenship. In 1981, the United Nations declared the International Year of Disabled Persons, and in 1983 it passed its Declaration of the Rights of People with Disabilities, kicking off the "Decade of Disabled Persons." The Independent Living Movement expressed the sentiment of the disability movement: that disabled people themselves were the experts in disability, not medical and health professionals. The health care system represented a source of oppression for disabled people. Advocates in Britain and the United States coined the notion of the social model of disability, in which disability was not seen as a shortcoming of the individual but rather of an environment that was designed without a thought for people who engage the world in unconventional ways.

At approximately the same time, the 1970s and 1980s, the environmental movement was drawing our attention to the limited supply of natural resources, to the proliferation of greenhouse gases, and to the impact of an ever-increasing human population on the world we live in. The environmental movement spanned a number of physical sciences and entreated citizens and industry to preserve the wilderness, prevent pollution, promote healthy and sustainable development, conserve natural resources, and resist nuclear energy. The idea of ecology was popularized, the ideas that

all things are interconnected, that every action has a multitude of ripple effects, and that we cannot always appreciate the consequences of human intervention.

Finally, in the worlds of architecture, art, and design, the idea arose of the possibility of creating environments that were simple, equitable, and flexible so that they presented no barriers to anyone and all could participate equally. The universal design movement, or barrier-free design movement as it was sometimes called, embraced the utopian idea of perfect inclusiveness and equitable use of space. Instead of the previously held assumptions about the average user of space and technology, the principles of universal design attempt to do away with those assumptions and instead replace them with a creative approach to ensuring physical, sensory, and linguistic access by all types of users.

Occupational Conceptual Models Associated With the Environmental Determinants of Occupation

Mary Law, PhD, FCAOT

The environmental determinants of occupation are factors within the physical, social, cultural, and institutional environments that either facilitate or impede occupation. As stated earlier in the book, using environmental theory leads to a structural analysis of issues of occupation. Occupational functioning, according to environmental theorists, is understood by examining environmental forces that act on occupation. Using this viewpoint, dysfunction in occupation is seen to be the result of an inadequate, inaccessible, hostile, or indifferent environment. Basic sciences that contribute to our understanding of the environment include anthropology, architecture, art and design, ecology, geography, sociology, political science, and economics.

For the purposes of this book, *environment* refers to everything outside the individual. The study of human ecology is concerned with human beings and their relationship with their environment. Environmental theorists have studied and documented the impact of environment on behavior for many decades. For example, Barker (1978) investigated environments and their effects on children in a small Midwest American town from the 1950s to the 1970s. Using streams of behavior recording to measure daily activities, he discovered that an environmental setting such as a coffee shop, dance hall, or bowling lane has a significant effect on behavior. There are persistent behaviors that remain constant over years in particular settings.

A concept prevalent in the environmental literature is person-environment congruence or environmental fit (Law et al., 1996; Wahl, 2001). Person-environment congruence is the ongoing relationship between human beings and the environment, with neither dominating the other. Several taxonomies of the environment have been created to assist in studying the interaction between individuals and the environment. Shalinsky (1986) described environmental factors as *physical* (the built and natural environments) and *psychosocial* (the psychological and social factors such as attitudes, family, and government).

Over the past three decades, disability advocates have stressed that disability is a problem in the relationship between the individual and the environment (Hahn, 1984; Jongbloed & Crichton, 1990). If environments create barriers to everyday functioning, the most appropriate solutions are to focus on modification of these environmental barriers. The fundamental principle of this approach is the recognition of the ecological nature of disability—that disability is caused by interactions with the environment, not by the impairment itself. This point of view has challenged society, including health services, to see disability in a new way. For occupational therapists, this point of view has fostered a renewed interest in examining how different types of environment influence participation in everyday occupations.

Another important development in this area is the International Classification of Functioning, Disability and Health from the World Health Organization (2001). The purpose of this classification system is to provide a framework by which to understand the impact of a health condition on people's participation in daily life. It provides a dynamic and interactive view of the connections among body function and structure, activity, participation, personal factors, and environmental factors. The inclusion of environmental factors in this framework highlights the potential impact of factors such as physical access, family structure, and social supports on participation.

OT, within the environmental framework, focuses intervention at the environment rather than the person. Environments can facilitate or limit participation in everyday occupations. The relationship between people, the occupations they choose to do, and the environments in which they live, work, and play ultimately determines the person's occupational performance (Law et al., 1991). Change in occupation is facilitated through change or accommodation of the environment rather than the person. Although this area of OT was traditionally less active than other areas of theory, the focus on environmental determinants of occupation has increased dramatically since the 1990s.

In the early decades of the OT profession from 1910 until 1930, very little was written specifically about the environment or environmental determinants of occupation. The only references to environment within the OT literature at this time discussed the need for healthy hospital environments. For example, Crane (1919) discussed the utilitarian, remunerative, and educational aspects of OT and proposed the establishment of healthy hospital environments based on these principles. During the 1930s, although there were no specific writings about environmental theory, the literature discussed how a patient relates to the environment and how OT could provide environments that were conducive to recovery and promoted skill development. It was during this decade as well that occupational therapists began outpatient clinics as a means to assist patients in their readjustment to the community environment.

The decade of the 1940s focused primarily on the rehabilitation of soldiers. In the literature, the mental aspects of rehabilitation and the importance of looking at the whole person within the physical and social environment was stressed. Discussion focused on how occupational therapists could modify the environment to influence person's behaviors. In the context of psychiatric treatment, Anderson (1942) stated that occupational therapists must modify the environment to direct patients' reactions into more acceptable channels of expression. The success of an OT program is dependent on the social atmosphere of the therapy environment. The increased emphasis on the environment continued through the 1950s, but with the influence of the medical model, references to the environment always separated it into the physical and social dimensions. An exception to this influence was an article by O'Reilly (1954) in which she discussed person-environment interaction and the need to fit patients into the environment, so that their community lives could be resumed with minimal stress. Other authors continued to talk about the effects of the environment on human behavior, particularly the effects of color and the effects of the physical environment on older adults.

From 1960 until 1975, the literature on the specific application of environmental theory to different areas within OT practice increased substantially. There was a growth in the use of environmental adaptations to promote independence for people with disabilities (Hopkins, 1960; Takata, 1971). Occupational therapists were part of the creation of "prosthetic environments" in the institutions for older adults as a means of minimizing the disabling factors that cause stress (Pincus, 1968). Prosthetic environments focus on ensuring easy discrimination among environmental stimuli to ensure that older adults are able to respond to their environments with increased success. The role of the environments on behavior in the area of mental health, and the development of a community-oriented conceptual approach to treatment in this area was emphasized. As well, enrichment of the environment was seen as a way to modify behavior in pediatrics. Occupational therapists also began to view the environment as having many interactive variables affecting clients and discussed the need for people to alter or improve the environment to maximize independence. In the early 1970s, there was increased interest in OT about minimizing architectural barriers and in the role of OT in this area. The importance of the environment in the development of play and other skills in children was articulated in a seminal article by Dunning (1972), who discussed environmental OT, in which the person is viewed within his or her total environmental context. Dunning developed a classification system to analyze the environment by its parts: space, people, and tasks. She used this system to develop an environment questionnaire that therapists could use to determine the relationship between environment and behavior.

In the 1980s and 1990s, there were several important theoretical developments in the discussion of environment and its impact on occupations and occupational performance. Hagedorn (1995) described the growing recognition of the physical, social, and cultural environments and their influences on the individual. She also theorized about the ability of the environment to enhance or impede occupational performance and the need for occupational therapists to employ environmental analyses.

Barris (1982) explored the idea of incorporating environmental themes into models of occupation in order to broaden the concept of occupational performance. An individual's relationship to the environment is discussed in three areas: 1) properties of the environment that influence personal causation and the development of interests and values; 2) the demands of the environment for performance and their influence on the development of roles, habits, and skills; and 3) factors affecting a person's participation in an expanding range of settings. Howe and Briggs (1982) proposed that the ecological systems model could help conceptualize the theoretical and practice goals of OT. *Ecology* is the study of the relationship between organisms and their environment. States of health and illness are viewed as reflections of ecological adaptation. A human being is viewed as an open system participating as part of the ecosystem. Humans and the environment are interconnected and shape each other. Function and dysfunction are defined in terms of clients' effectiveness in achieving their goals for quality of life in their interactions with the ecosystem.

Kiernat (1982) proposed a focus on the environment as an effective treatment modality. She concluded that the environment must be viewed as an integral part of any rehabilitation program and that therapists must assess the client's psychosocial and physical environment and use this information as another modality in order to facilitate independence. In 1990, Christenson discussed the importance of designing living environments that promote optimal "adaptation levels" for older adults, which are balances between the person's competence and environmental demand. The author encourages the occupational therapist to use the environment in her or his overall treatment plan. Baum and Law (1998) encouraged the profession to shift its thinking from a biomedical to a sociomedical context and to take an active role in building healthy communities in response to society's changing definition of health. In this new context, occupational therapists can help change the environment and social policy rather than the person.

Several authors described shifts in theoretical perspectives on disability and the implications of that for OT. Jongbloed and Crichton (1990) and Craddock (1996) described changes to a sociopolitical definition of disability from an individualistic one. Because the sociopolitical definition of disability stresses the importance of environmental barriers in determining disability outcomes, therapists need to pay greater heed to environmental contexts and view clients as consumers of service. In 1991, Law explored how several factors, including the physical environment, production of space, classification of individuals based on norms, labeling of disability as deviance, power imbalances between health care professionals and clients, and increased bureaucracy in institutions have led to disabling environments that limit occupation for people with disabilities. Ideas about occupation are explored and an approach to OT intervention to change disabling environments, with the active participation of people with disabilities, was proposed. Grady (1995) challenged occupational therapists to consider an expanded view of the environment with a focus on environment-person relationships.

Ecology, Environment, and Behavior

In 1938, Murray wrote about environmental press, describing it as a condition outside of individuals that affects the way in which the environment is interpreted and influences behavior. Thirty-five years later, Nahemow, Lawton, and Center (1973) extended Murray's work to create an ecological theory of adaptation and aging. They theorized that behavior results from ecological transactions between a person's skills and abilities and the level of environmental press. As people age or encounter health issues, increasing limitations on skills and abilities result in greater environmental press.

The work of Nahemow and colleagues has influenced occupational therapists who have explored barriers within the environment that influence participation in occupations. The importance of easy access to environmental supports, whether these are physical, social, or institutional in nature, has been emphasized. For example, Andonian (2010) explored environmental facilitators and barriers for persons with mental health issues. Supports such as availability of friendship, community programs, and transportation were important for community participation. Community attitudes about mental illness, lack of availability of housing, and supports for disease management were felt to be important barriers to occupation. Environments can provide opportunities for participation as well as barriers. Rebeiro and Cook (1999) theorized that environments

that enable people with mental illness to experience belonging and support will enhance participation in occupations.

For older adults, negotiating self-care occupations even within a familiar environment can take precedence over community participation (Vik, Lilja, & Nygård, 2007). Environmental factors that help community participation include support from family and friends and the availability of assistance. Andresen and Runge (2002) explored the transactional relationship between older adults and their living accommodations. Their findings indicated that participation in occupations is highly influenced by the relationship between their physical and social environment. The choices that older adults are able to make about occupation often need to be modified because of restrictions within their environment.

The home environment is considered to be an important environment to support daily occupations and provide meaning to those who live there. Cipriani et al. (2009) found that older adults constructed a meaningful home environment through the retention of objects that held importance from past roles (work, family, leisure). She theorized that understanding the occupations of older adults is enhanced through the exploration of objects within their home. Haak, Ivanoff, Fänge, Sixsmith, and Iwarsson (2007) focused on how the environment can shape participation experiences of adults over 80 years of age. With increasing age, older adults spend more time within their homes. The home environment becomes "the locus and origin for participation." With this change in environment over time, older adults participate in fewer physically based occupations and communities and take on more of a spectator role from within their home.

Others have focused on community environments. Hand, Law, McColl, Hanna, and Elliott (2012) examined themes from studies of older adults with chronic health conditions in terms of the influence of neighborhood environments. Several factors within a neighborhood, such as availability of services, income level, physical accessibility, social cohesion, and safety have been shown to influence participation in occupations. Beagan and Etowa (2009) described the impact of racism on the way in which African Canadian women engage in daily occupations. Even though racism may be subtle in nature, it can have a substantial impact on the way in which women experience occupation and find meaning. This is an example of how characteristics of the social environment influence performance of occupation.

Few authors have focused on the workplace environment. Dyck and Jongbloed (2000) explored work for women diagnosed with multiple sclerosis and found that factors within the social and institutional environments had important influences on their ability to continue working. In particular, the ability to modify work conditions, the attitudes of employers, and the ability to share household tasks enhanced employment experience. They also highlighted the need for occupational therapists to analyze environmental factors as part of any assessment and intervention plan.

Person-Environment Transaction

The concept of person-environment transactions is discussed much more frequently in the theoretical literature since 2000. Law (2002) described how information about patterns of occupation across people, locations, and lifespan helps occupational therapists understand complex person-environment transactions. Theoretical perspectives from sociology and geography (O'Brien, Dyck, Caron, & Mortenson, 2002) are useful for environmental analysis to examine characteristics of the environment that influence occupation. They highlight the theoretical background of social constructivism in terms of how both physical and social spaces are evaluated. Person-environment transactions have substantial influences on how people perceive environments, so it is important to understand different perceptions about how space is understood and used. For example, individuals with a disability may have different experiences with the same space, some finding it welcoming, whereas others finding it excluding. The specific meaning of a place to an individual is fundamental to its perception as a support or barrier.

Dickie, Cutchin, and Humphry (2006) critiqued the individualism present within occupational science. They believed that scientists had not embraced the concept of person-environment transactions and so tend to view person and environment separately. The use of the concept of transaction as put forward by Dewey is suggested as a way in which occupational scientists can study the complexity inherent with persons within their environment. Shank and Cutchin (2010) put forward two concepts about older adults "aging in place." The first concept holds that older adults create meaning in their lives through participation in occupations. The second concept focuses on the transactional relationship between older adults and occupation as they experience changes through aging.

Scholars within occupational science have also examined how theory of occupational justice, with its focus on participation in occupations, justice, and environment, can provide stronger linkages between theory and practice. For example, Aldrich (2008) compared the utility of complexity theory with transactionalism in terms of their ability to support the development of theories and understanding of behavior in occupational science. Complexity theory has emerged from mathematics and physics and focuses on the complex, nonlinear relationships between person and environment. Behaviors, including occupations, emerge from the ongoing dynamic relationships among many factors. An example of an OT conceptual model based on complexity theory is the most recent version of the Model of Human Occupation (Kielhofner, 2008). In contrast, Cutchin (2004) has criticized complexity theory because it continues to separate person from environment. He argued that a transactional approach in which people are considered within their environment is more appropriate for OT. Aldrich (2008), following a critical analysis of both theoretical approaches, concluded that Dewey's theory of transactionalism was more suited to occupational science theory development than complexity theories.

Space and Place

Graham Rowles (2008), a geographer, has written about the importance of places for people as they participate in everyday occupations. He believed that the ongoing relationships between people and place are fundamental to finding meaning through occupation. The search for meaning involves "four overlapping domains: achieving a sense of worth through occupation, experiencing fulfillment through interpersonal relationship, exercising the ability to choose one's course of action, and, through the process of simply 'being,' developing understanding and acceptance of one's place in the cosmos" (p. 127). Cutchin (2007) discussed how occupations are informed and created by habits or everyday routines that are complex and social in nature. These habits are influenced tremendously by the places and landscapes in which we live, work, and play: "Places and landscapes cannot be taken out of the equation; individuals or societies cannot exist without place, nor can we usefully consider them without considering place" (Cutchin, 2007, p. 57S).

Zemke (2004) discussed the way in which the OT profession considers time and space as part of the external environment. She posited that it is equally important to consider the experiential characteristics of time and space and how they influence the meaning of everyday occupations. Through engagement and occupation, humans experience the rhythm and meaning of time, beyond the typical clock-based time. For example, when a person is very engaged in an occupation, his or her experience of how time passes can change. Humans' sense of space does not focus only on external space but also on the space taken by our bodies. Through moving in space, humans create a sense of place, with both physical and symbolic characteristics. Zemke also discussed "placemaking" as "the act of creating and maintaining places—a human occupation often in collaboration with others" (p. 613). Time and place come together to influence our occupations and daily routines in a complex, ever-changing fashion.

Universal Access

Within North America, there have been significant legislative changes to support universal access for all people (Americans With Disabilities Act, 1990; Government of Ontario, 2005). Although there has been little theoretical writing about universal access in the community by occupational therapists, there has been work focused on access within the home. Using qualitative methods and content analysis, Barstow, Bennett, and Vogtle (2011) identified five categories of home safety for older adults with vision loss: 1) lighting, 2) contrast, 3) visual distractions, 4) glare, and 5) compensation strategies. In order to understand the dimensions of home that influence decisions about home modifications, Aplin, de Jonge, and Gustafsson (2013) thematically analyzed interviews from 55 adults and older adults who had been involved in a home modification process. Four dimensions of the home environment were most influential in decisions about home modification—the personal, societal, physical, and temporal aspects of the home. The complex relationship among personal preferences, societal standards and policies, physical space, and future plans influenced the home modifications that were made or used. The use of flow modifications was also influenced by personal preferences for occupations and social expectations of others within the home environment. These works pointed out the complexity of making changes within the home environment and the need to address these issues in the decision-making process.

Cultural Environment

Few authors have written theory about the cultural environment specifically, although consideration of this environment is included in all of the key conceptual models. One example of work in this area is the writing of Nayar, Hocking, and Wilson (2007), who focused on the experiences of Indian immigrant women of New Zealand society. The daily challenging experience of living in a unique and unfamiliar cultural environment is initially compensated for through the performance of familiar activities. As the women become comfortable enough to explore their new cultural environment, they begin to try out new activities more common to New Zealand ways of life. Nayar, Hocking, and Giddings (2012) argued that occupational therapists can help with this process by using knowledge about person-environment-occupation interactions.

Social Environment

The importance of the social environment in supporting a person's ability to carry out daily occupations has been increasingly recognized. Availability of social support from family, friends, and community members is considered one of the most important environmental supports across all age groups (Coutinho, Hersch, & Davidson, 2006; Isaksson, Lexell, & Skär, 2007; Lund & Nygård, 2004). For older adults who acquire dementia, the availability of social support is considered to be a key environmental support for participation (Teitelman, Raber, & Watts, 2010). The authors discussed the need to consider the social environment as a potentially powerful means of intervention. Lund and Nygård (2004), in themes emerging from a constant comparative analytic study, highlighted the importance of social support as a means to enable performance of occupations in the home that have been disrupted by physical disability. Social support is fundamentally important for people with newly acquired disability. For example, Isaksson and associates employed a grounded theory approach to examine environmental supports of women from 25 to 61 years of age with spinal cord injury. They theorized that social support provided an important means to enhance motivation as well as sustain participation in occupations.

Coutinho, Hersch, and Davidson (2006) examined literature about informal caregiving to explore the concepts inherent in this occupation. They highlighted the complexity of caregiving and how the home and community environment influence whether this role is deemed to be meaningful. Informal caregiving is a lengthy, adaptive process in which the caregiver works within the environment and also adapts it to meet the needs of their charge. Environmental modifications and the development of daily routines are theorized to improve person-environment fit both for the caregiver and the person in care.

Technology

There has been an increase in the work focused on the use of technology by persons with health conditions. However, most of this work is quantitative research rather than explicitly theoretical in nature. Engström, Lexell, and Lund (2010), following a qualitative study of use of technology by persons with acquired brain injury, theorized that challenges lay at the transaction between technology, the occupation, the person, and the environment. In addressing the use of technology, occupational therapists must consider it an integral part of the person, environment, and occupation relationship. Bain (1998) theorized that occupational frames of reference that consider "consumer-task-environment-device" (p. 498) are useful for the provision and evaluation of assistive technology.

Environment as a Change Agent

A final area of the environment as a determinant of occupation is consideration of environment as a change agent or the focus of OT intervention. There are only a few evaluation studies that focus on the impact of environmental interventions, and the majority of environmental interventions are focused on the physical or social environment (McColl & Law, 2010). Thus, there is a need for increased theory focused on the development of environmental interventions that recognize the dynamic and transactional nature of person, occupation, and environment relationships (Law, 2002).

O'Brien, Dyck, Caron, and Mortenson (2002) have written about the way in which the meanings of cultural, physical, social, and institutional environments are constructed based on the environmental characteristics that either help or hinder daily occupations. Based on case studies and theoretical constructs from geography and sociology, they posited that the meaning of environments can change over time in a dynamic fashion. They recommended that occupational therapists employ a broader range of assessment and intervention strategies to more fully understand the transactional relationships between individuals and their environments. Information gathered through a broader, more dynamic analysis of environmental factors can support OT interventions to change environments within the home, workplace, or community.

Hand, Wilkins, Letts, and Law (2013), following a metasynthesis of qualitative research about adults with chronic disease, discussed the way in which environments are renegotiated to enable participation in daily occupations. Based on the concepts emerging from this analysis, they recommended that OT interventions focus on enabling social supports and changing institutional environments to improve policies and access.

Summary

There are several important theoretical ideas about the environmental determinants of occupation. This area of theory locates the source of occupational performance problems entirely outside of the person—that is, in the environment. The environment consists of physical, social, cultural, institutional, political, and many other aspects. It may be considered as three concentric spheres, with the most proximal representing the immediate family and the most distal representing society as a whole.

Occupational conceptual models help us understand how the environment acts on individuals and their occupation performance. Models of practice in this area of OT need to be developed that focus exclusively on change in the environment; because the problem is located in the environment, therapeutic interventions must address the problem in the environment. Environmental models of practice do not seek to bring about any change in the person.

Section IV

Occupational Models of Practice

Determinants of Occupation

- Physical
- Psychological-Emotional
- Sociocultural
- Cognitive-Neurological
- Environmental

Occupation

- Self-care
- Productivity
- Leisure

Consequences of Occupation

- Health
- Well-Being
- Participation
- Community integration

14

Occupational Models of Practice
Interventions

Mary Ann McColl, PhD, MTS and Mary Law, PhD, FCAOT

Now, the moment you have all been waiting for: the part where we tell you what you need to DO in order to be an occupational therapist. It is no surprise that you are focused on *doing*, given your chosen profession. However, if you have learned anything by this stage in this book, it should be that *doing* is not as simple as it often looks! Therefore, telling you what to do as an occupational therapist is not as simple as you might hope. On the other hand, it is that very complexity of occupation and of human beings that keeps life interesting over a whole career as an occupational therapist.

Basically, what occupational therapists do with every client is help them to make changes they seek to make in their occupational performance. Clients come to us when they are having trouble *doing* something, and we consult the body of knowledge contained in the filing cabinet, and employ the tools stored in the toolbox to help them overcome their difficulty. We use the telescope to help us better understand their problems. Then we use our conceptual models to help us to know how to *think* about the problems they bring to us and our models of practice to help us know how to *act* to facilitate change. This chapter is about the final piece of the puzzle: the models of practice that occupational therapists have at their disposal.

Remember that models of practice are made up of two components: assessments and interventions. In this chapter we focus on *interventions*, meaning those maneuvers that therapists perform to facilitate change in occupations. The challenge of defining and describing interventions is a common issue across disciplines, including occupational therapy (OT). Whyte and Hart (2003) articulated the need to accurately define the

"active ingredients" of intervention procedures. Krupa (2010) recently referred to OT interventions as the "black box of therapy," and Bright, Boland, Rutherford, Kayes, and McPherson (2012) referred to them as a "Russian doll" with many layers hidden from view.

Occupational therapists typically promote changes in occupational performance using three major processes (McColl et al., 2003):

1. *Remediation*—directly addressing dysfunction to alleviate it
2. *Compensation*—addressing the task or the way the individual approaches the task to optimize function
3. *Advocacy*—seeking changes in the environment to permit optimal function

When occupational therapists believe there is the opportunity for function to actually change, for the individual to recover, develop, or improve, they tend to act first in a *remediation* capacity to improve function to its optimal level. This type of OT intervention focuses on the **person**.

When occupational therapists discern that actual changes in the person are unlikely, they intervene at the level of the **occupation**. They adapt tools, methods, or supports to *compensate* for lost function.

When occupational therapists see that the environment is the primary impediment to occupation, they *advocate* on behalf of their clients to seek the necessary accommodations and supports. This type of OT focuses on the **environment**.

In a scoping review of the international OT literature, eight types of interventions were differentiated and detected (Table 14-1; McColl & Law, 2013):

McColl MA, Law M, Stewart D.
Theoretical Basis of Occupational Therapy, Third Edition (pp. 125-130).

Table 14-1

Eight Types of Occupational Therapy Interventions Found in the Literature

Occupational Therapy Interventions	Description	
1. Training	Enhancing performance of physical, psychological, cognitive, and social components—non-purposeful activities associated with performance components; often seen as exercises, practice with no explicit occupational outcome	Person
2. Skill Development	Improving performance of specific tasks, development of purposeful tasks that are the building blocks of occupation; may refer to cognitive, physical, psychological-emotional, or social skills	
3. Education	Learning more about one's condition, options for improvement, ways of preventing difficulties, or improving function	
4. Task Adaptation	Modifying a task to permit it to be accomplished in a different manner given personal limitations; includes proximal adaptations and adaptive media	Occupation
5. Occupation Development	Optimizing participation in integrated occupations such as vocational training, leisure programs, activities of daily living	
6. Environmental Modification	Modifying the nonhuman environment to enhance function; may include distal adaptive equipment, cueing, accessibility	Environment
7. Support Provision	Provision of physical or psychological support by the therapist to enhance occupational performance	
8. Support Enhancement	Enhancing the ability of the family or caregivers and support system to provide support for occupational performance	

- Three types of intervention focus on the person: training, skill development, and education.
- Two types of intervention focus on occupation: task adaptation and occupational development.
- Three types of intervention focus on the environment: environmental modification, support provision, and support enhancement.

An example is offered to illustrate the breadth of possibilities among which occupational therapists can choose when selecting intervention approaches. Imagine a client who has lost the ability to dress him- or herself due to paralysis of the dominant arm following a stroke. The client might be offered any of the following interventions:

- The therapist might engage in training of the affected upper extremity to alter tone and promote recovery (training).
- He or she might teach specific skills, such as buttoning a shirt with one hand (skill development).
- He or she might provide information and suggestions about stroke, the course of recovery, and the various options available for assistance with dressing (education).
- The therapist might teach an adapted form of the activity, such as dressing the affected side first or using a button hook (task adaptation).
- Dressing might be approached in the context of the broader occupational perspective, including

<u>Table 14-2</u>
Summary of Intervention Approaches Found in the Literature (1980-2010)

	Focus*	Self-Care	Productivity	Leisure	Total
Occupational Development	O	7	6	2	15
Skill Development	P	7	3	2	12
Training	P	6	5		11
Education	P	3	6		9
Task Adaptation	O	5			5
Environmental Modification	E		1	2	3
Support Enhancement	E	1		1	2
Support Provision	E			2	2
Total		29	21	9	59

*Focus of intervention: P = person; O = occupation; E = environment.

returning home and resuming social activities (occupational development).

- The patient's environment might be modified so that clothes are left out the night before within reach of the bed and in the proper order of dressing (environmental adaptation).
- The therapist may provide support, encouragement, and cueing needed for the client to be able to take on the goal and process of dressing (support provision).
- The therapist may intervene with the support system (e.g., partner, family) to provide social cues, assistance, and encouragement toward dressing (support enhancement).

These eight categories are used in the remainder of the chapter to describe and classify interventions found in the OT literature during the years 1990 through 2010 (for more detailed descriptions of methodology and results, see Law & McColl, 2010). It should be noted that programs found in the literature often used interventions from more than one category—that is, they were not a pure representation of a single intervention type, but rather, they included elements of a number of intervention approaches. In carefully reading each paper, however, it was usually evident that one intervention approach dominated or was central to the overall intent of the program. Therapists may have an inherent preference for one or more of these types of intervention; in fact, readers may have a strong reaction that some of these approaches are considerably more likely to be successful than others.

We found 59 studies that described 57 programs offered by occupational therapists aimed at promoting self-care, productivity, or leisure among adults and seniors (two programs were featured in two articles each) (Table 14-2). Of these, nine articles focused on leisure outcomes, 21 on productivity outcomes, and 29 on self-care outcomes. Approximately half of the interventions evaluated focused on self-care, whereas only about 15% focused on leisure, even though for many people with disabilities, mental or chronic illnesses, the satisfactory use of leisure time is a major issue. It was also somewhat limiting that many of the studies on productivity focused exclusively on paid work. The most common intervention approaches were occupational development, skill development, training, and education, accounting for 80% of all programs described.

Occupational Development

Fifteen occupational development programs were found in the literature. These programs focused broadly on a range of activities in one or more occupational categories (self-care, productivity, or leisure). They are distinguished by their macro-level approach to all aspects of involvement in occupation. Many of these programs were multidisciplinary, including OT. They included both inpatient and outpatient programs and were a mixture of individual and individual plus group formats. Periods of therapy varied from one or two sessions to follow-up periods many months long. These programs involved a wide variety of disability types, including people with musculoskeletal injuries and pain, acquired brain injury, mental illness, stroke, and elderly patients. There were a number of vocational training, activities of daily living, and instrumental activities of daily living programs as well as programs aimed at overall leisure participation and satisfaction.

Skill Development

There were 12 skill development programs, focusing on specific skill sets, such as coping skills, organizational skills, leisure skills, transfers, dressing, mobility, social skills, and communication skills. Frequency and duration of these programs was highly variable, from several sessions to regular meetings over a year. Many of these programs were offered on an inpatient basis, preparing clients for discharge and community living. Most were multidisciplinary. These programs were offered to a range of types of clients, including people with strokes, mobility disabilities, vision impairments, acquired brain injuries, schizophrenia, and chronic fatigue syndrome.

Training

Eleven of the interventions described in the literature related to training. These interventions had as their main focus the remediation of deficits of strength, range of motion, and dexterity. These were often multidisciplinary programs and often run in collaboration with physiotherapists. Most were individually focused, with some also including a group component. These tended to be briefer, more intense interventions, averaging daily contact for 4 to 8 weeks. These training interventions focused on stroke patients, people with Parkinson's disease, and people with back pain and other soft-tissue injuries. They were approximately equally split between inpatients and outpatients.

Education

Nine intervention studies featured education approaches. These were characterized by the occupational therapist providing information that would assist with enabling occupation. Educational interventions typically taught clients about the nature of their condition, recommendations and contraindications for occupation, and specific techniques such as ergonomics, work simplification, injury prevention, and joint protection. Educational approaches were designed for patients with injuries, arthritis, human immunodeficiency virus/acquired immune deficiency syndrome (HIV/AIDS), Parkinson's disease, and chronic obstructive pulmonary disease. They were often multidisciplinary and included group as well as individual components. These programs varied from several days to weekly sessions for many weeks.

Task Adaptation

Five interventions described in the literature emphasized task adaptation, and all were aimed at self-care. Specific techniques included task analysis and problem solving, compensatory strategies, and neurological approaches. These interventions were also targeted toward patients with neurological disorders, such as stroke, Parkinson's disease, and multiple sclerosis. All but one was multidisciplinary, and only one was conducted in a group setting. These programs represented a mixture of inpatient, outpatient, and community programs. They varied from 1 week to several months.

Environmental Adaptation

Only three programs focused on environmental adaptation to accommodate client needs. One was designed for people recently diagnosed with rheumatoid arthritis, and its main focus was inspection and adjustment to the work site as well as the prescription of adaptive equipment. Two others involved home visits to try adaptive devices to enhance leisure participation and remove barriers to leisure participation.

Support Enhancement

Two programs were aimed at enhancing support for self-care and leisure. They focused on arranging the necessary help to allow clients to stay in their homes. This support could come from agencies, health professionals, or community resources, or it could come from informal sources such as partner, family, friends, and neighbors. The occupational therapist acted as a catalyst to marshal the necessary supports.

Support Provision

Finally, two support provision programs were found in which the occupational therapist directly provided support to permit or enhance occupational performance. The examples found in the literature involved home visiting to offer support for leisure involvement and opportunities to try new activities.

Other Classifications of Occupational Therapy Interventions

Several other classifications are also available for understanding what occupational therapists actually

Table 14-3
What Occupational Therapists Do

	Mosey's (1981) Six Legitimate Tools	Ecology of Human Performance (Dunn et al., 1994)	CMOP-E Enabling Skills (Townsend & Polatajko, 2007)	Law & McColl (2010)	AOTA Framework (2014)
Person	Conscious use of self Teaching-learning process Purposeful activities	Establish/restore skills and abilities Shift perspective	Coach Educate Collaborate Engage Specialize Consult	Training Education Skill development	Remediation Maintenance Education Health promotion Preparatory tasks Prevent disability
Occupation	Activity analysis and synthesis	Adapt task Compensate/ substitute/ prevent	Adapt	Task adaptation Occupational development	Occupations and activities Compensation
Environment	Nonhuman environment Activity groups	Alter context/ environment	Design/Build Advocate Coordinate	Environmental modification Support enhancement Support provision	Advocacy Group interactions
AOTA = American Occupational Therapy Association; CMOP-E = Canadian Model of Occupational Performance and Engagement.					

do and how we classify the different approaches that occupational therapists have at their disposal. In this chapter, we feature four:

- In 1981, Mosey identified six legitimate skills that characterize OT interventions in her book entitled *Occupational Therapy: Configuration of a Profession.* These six core skills are the conscious use of self, teaching and learning, purposeful activities, activity analysis and synthesis, the non-human environment, and activity groups.
- Dunn, Brown, and McGuigan (1994) identified five approaches associated with the Ecology of Human Performance Model: adapting the task, altering the environment, preventing barriers, creating positive circumstances, and restoring or establishing capacities.
- The Canadian Model of Occupational Performance and Engagement (Townsend & Polatajko, 2007) offers a model of practice consisting of 10 enabling

skills. These include adapting, advocating, coaching, collaborating, consulting, coordinating, designing and building, educating, engaging, and specializing.

- The third edition of the American Occupational Therapy Practice Framework (American Occupational Therapy Association, 2014) includes both types of intervention (occupations and activities, preparatory methods and tasks, education and training, advocacy, and group interventions) and approaches to OT intervention (health promotion, remediation, maintenance, compensation, and disability prevention).

Table 14-3 compares these four approaches with the taxonomy described earlier in this chapter. Several observations about similarities and differences among approaches follow. We have tried to group them into interventions targeting the person, the environment, or the occupation itself.

The first observation that occurs to most observers is the prevalence of person-focused interventions compared with occupation or environment-focused interventions. Of 29 interventions listed in the table, almost half (14) are person focused. This is probably a function of the longstanding relationship of OT with the reductionistic, biomedical approach that seeks to isolate an underlying problem in the individual and repair, remediate, and resolve it. Within person-focused approaches, all of the classifications include interventions aimed at training and education. Environmentally focused interventions tend to focus on either the human or the nonhuman environment. Finally, although activity analysis does not appear explicitly in any of the later lists, it is a necessary precursor to the task adaptation approach common to the other four.

15

Models of Service
in Occupational Therapy

Mary Ann McColl, PhD, MTS

We talked in the previous chapter about *models of practice* in occupational therapy (OT), meaning theory that helps occupational therapists know what to do. We clarified that models of practice are made up of assessments and interventions. They may be focused on improving occupation (occupational models of practice) or on enhancing a particular aspect of the person or the environment (basic models of practice). In either case, they describe how occupational therapists act to promote the health and well-being of their clients.

In this chapter, we offer a somewhat broader concept called *models of service*. Models of service describe how occupational therapists relate to their clients, the health and social service organizations within which they work, and the systems of governance and funding. Models of service govern how occupational therapists think about the people they serve and the services they deliver.

Occupational therapists typically work in one of four models of service: biomedical, client-centered, community-based rehabilitation, or independent living. Each model is based on a different assumption about who the client is and who the therapist is. Each has advantages and disadvantages. Each has situations in which it is more or less appropriate.

Biomedical

The *biomedical model* of service is based on the assumption that the problems experienced by people who seek OT services can be objectively observed by therapists and remediated using the body of professional knowledge that therapists have acquired. The role of the therapist in this model is to accept referrals from other professionals, assess and analyze problems, identify the locus of the problem within the patient, and treat the focal problem, assuming that more far-reaching consequences of the problem will resolve themselves once the underlying cause is rectified. Therapists, for their part, are expected to act in what they perceive to be in the best interests of the patient and to be guided by benevolence in their relationship with their patients.

Recipients of service in this model are typically referred to as "patients," and they play a relatively passive role in the therapy process. The only other types of professionals who call their customers "patients" are providers within traditional health services, such as doctors and nurses. They expect their patients to respond truthfully to inquiries, accept the diagnosis that is offered, and cooperate with the prescribed treatments and instructions.

As with each of the models discussed, there are situations in which the biomedical model is exactly the correct model of service to meet the needs of some patients. For example, in the most extreme case, the biomedical model is the appropriate model of service when patients are unconscious or otherwise unable to represent their own interests. Often at the onset or early stages of a disability, an overwhelming array of changes and problems may leave patients unable to make good decisions and dependent on health professionals to act in their best interests. Another situation that renders the biomedical model appropriate is a cultural expectation of this type of service relationship. That expectation is often associated with age groups or with cultural groups characterized by greater social distance among social classes.

McColl MA, Law M, Stewart D.
Theoretical Basis of Occupational Therapy, Third Edition (pp. 131-132).
© 2015 Taylor & Francis Group.

Client-Centered

The *client-centered model* of service assumes that people referred to OT can tell us about the occupational performance problems they experience and seek help with. The recipients of service in this model are referred to as "clients" because they effectively engage the services of a therapist and instruct the therapist as to what they seek from the service. This model assumes that clients know what they want from therapy and are able to participate actively in the therapeutic process. If we think about the other professionals who call their customers "clients," it may help us to understand the relationship, for example, lawyers, accountants, decorators. They offer their expertise but would not presume to instruct or order their clients as to what they should or should not do. Instead they advise and act on instruction from their clients.

In OT, the client-centered model of service is felt by many to be preferable to the biomedical model for clients who are seeking to optimize their independence and enhance their participation and integration. It is explicitly preferred by clients who seek to exert their autonomy and control over their own life circumstances. It can be unsuitable for clients who do not wish to take responsibility for their care or who are unable to make reliable decisions.

Most occupational therapists, if asked, would say that they operate within a client-centered model of service. They would say they believe in transferring power to clients and permitting clients to participate in the goal setting and decision making. Yet, the very language of these two statements suggests that these therapists are in fact intrinsically oriented toward a biomedical model but are posing as client-centered because they feel it is expected. From a client-centered perspective, a therapist believes that the client already *has* the power to direct the relationship with the therapist and that it is, in fact, the client who is inviting the therapist to participate in his or her decision-making process.

Community-Based Rehabilitation

A third alternative model of service is *community-based rehabilitation*. Community-based rehabilitation is a model derived for use in under-resourced areas where professional human resources are insufficient to permit one-to-one care. This is a community development approach in which the customer is a whole community. Often one or more members of the community experience disability and have occupational performance problems. The therapist's role is to act as a catalyst to the community development process. He or she assists the community to claim the problems of its members, to identify and marshal resources, and to make plans and execute solutions. Collective community solutions address the needs not only of identified community members, but also of other disenfranchised members now and in the future. They also develop capacity in the community and leave communities better equipped to solve future problems.

Independent Living

The fourth model of service is *independent living*. The independent living model views customers as consumers who are empowered to take control of resources and make rational, informed decisions about the best disposition of resources. The independent living model arose out of the disability rights and psychiatric survivors movements. It is based on the principle of service of, for, and by people with disabilities. The role for therapists is as professional adjuncts to consumer-run agencies and organizations. Community agencies are operated by consumers (or their delegates), and therapists are engaged to contribute their expertise to the consumer-led enterprise.

These four models of service provide a framework for occupational therapists to consider their relationship to their clients, to the organizations within which they work, and to the resources that support service provision. Most therapists will have a preference for one or more of these ways of working with clients, but it does not necessarily follow that one of these models is better or worse than others. Each has circumstances under which it is most appropriate. For example, the biomedical approach is best when patients are unable to make good decisions on their own behalf. The client-centered approach is best when clients seek to assert their autonomy and their agency in solving problems. The community-based approach is best when problems cannot be adequately solved on an individual basis but must be addressed in the context of the community within which they arise. Finally, the independent living approach is best when consumers are empowered to assert control over the resources available to address barriers to full participation and citizenship.

In each of these cases, the recipients of service are called by different titles. In the biomedical model, they are called "patients"; in the client-centered model, they are called "clients"; in the independent living model, they are called "consumers," and in the community-based model, the recipient of service is the community. As stated earlier, throughout this book we have tried to use the appropriate terminology for the model of service being discussed.

16

Conclusion

Mary Ann McColl, PhD, MTS

We began this book by stating that there were five types of knowledge required to be an occupational therapist: about human beings, about our environments, about disability, about occupation, and about the therapeutic use of self. We acquire much of this knowledge during our occupational therapy (OT) education and training. We layer what we learn in OT school on top of the education and life experience we had prior to entering the program. Then we supplement what we learned in school throughout the remainder of our careers and, in fact, our lives by attending courses, reading, working, and living! There is a huge amount of knowledge and information that contributes to being an occupational therapist.

In the absence of a reasonably good filing system, all this knowledge exists in a jumble, something akin to a big box of theory! This book has offered three metaphors for ways to store, organize, access, and use theory to make it readily available for decision making in OT.

The first metaphor is a toolbox (Figure 16-1). The toolbox helps us to sort the knowledge we possess as occupational therapists into four types of tools:

- Tools that help us to think about occupation (occupational conceptual models)
- Tools that help us think about the component parts of humans and about their environments (basic conceptual models)
- Tools that help us to act therapeutically toward clients with regard to their occupation (We are referring to assessments and interventions that focus specifically on occupation [occupational models of practice])

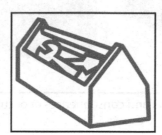

Figure 16-1. OT toolbox.

- Tools that help us to intervene to address the component parts of human beings or their environments—that is, assessments and interventions focusing on the physical, psychological-emotional, sociocultural, or cognitive-neurological aspects of clients or on the environment (basic models of practice)

In this book, we focus on the first quadrant of the toolbox, occupational conceptual models, theoretical tools that help us to think about humans and their occupations.

When we think about occupation, we think not only about occupation itself, made up of self-care, productivity, and leisure; we also think about the determinants and consequences of occupation (Figure 16-2):

- The *consequences* of occupation are those outcomes that occupational therapists seek or help their clients to achieve. Those outcomes are typically health, well-being, participation, and community integration.
- The *determinants* of occupation are those factors that affect occupation and that may be employed therapeutically to help improve occupation. To use those factors effectively, we need to have a detailed understanding of their relationship

McColl MA, Law M, Stewart D.
Theoretical Basis of Occupational Therapy, Third Edition (pp. 133-136).
© 2015 Taylor & Francis Group.

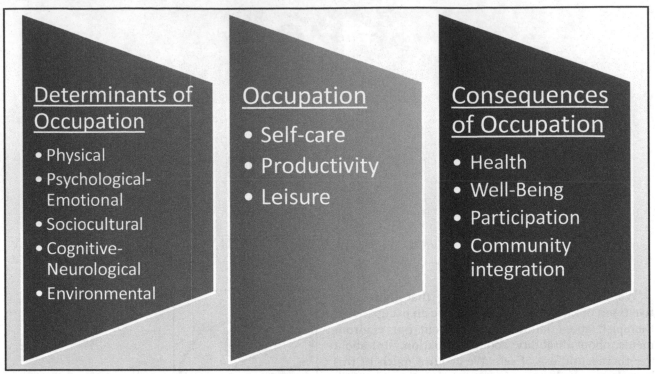

Figure 16-2. The determinants and consequences of occupation.

with occupation. Those factors may relate to the person—physical factors, psychological-emotional factors, sociocultural factors, or cognitive-neurological factors—or they may relate to the environment. For every factor that potentially affects occupation, occupational therapists need to understand the nature, extent, and parameters of its relationship to occupation.

All of this information about determinants and consequences needs to be able to be readily retrieved and applied to daily practice. It needs to be filed and stored in such a way that it can be summoned at a moment's notice and used to understand clients' problems and propose solutions to those problems. It needs to be available to allow therapists to explain to clients, families, and other professionals how they are thinking and what they are doing. It needs to be used to design programs and evaluate outcomes.

As a response to this filing challenge, we proposed a second metaphor, the OT filing cabinet (Figure 16-3). The filing cabinet has six drawers. The top drawer contains information about the consequences of occupation. Specifically it contains information on theoretical models that explain the relationship of occupation to the desired outcomes. In this book, we review six of the most well-known and widely used models that offer different perspectives on the relationship of occupation to health and well-being. In Chapter 6, we discussed these models in some detail; specifically, we reviewed their development and history and tried

Figure 16-3. OT filing cabinet.

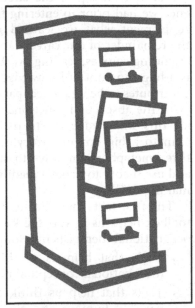

to situate them within the trajectory of intellectual development in OT. We observed a number of commonalities among these models, but we also noted the unique qualities of particular models and the original contributions each has made to our developing understanding of occupation.

The remaining five drawers of the filing cabinet contain information on the five determinants of occupation. Taken one at a time, from oldest to most recent, we offered five chapters on the sociocultural determinants, the psychological-emotional determinants, the physical determinants, the cognitive-neurological determinants, and the environmental determinants of occupation. Each chapter began by offering the reader a snapshot of some ideological developments in the field. These may be considered basic conceptual models derived from other disciplines but important and influential in the development of OT thinking. Some definitions of key concepts in the theory area were also offered. Guest authors have provided detailed summaries in each of these five chapters of the scope and history of OT theory in the area. They have summarized the state of knowledge in the field in relation to key concepts and have emphasized theoretical developments since 2000.

We have devoted a considerable portion of this book to examining in detail the six occupational conceptual models and the information that is filed in each drawer of the OT filing cabinet:

1. *Occupation-focused models*—The top drawer of the filing cabinet contains a number of approaches to understanding the relationship between occupation and health. We featured six specific models that are most prevalent in the literature:

    a. Occupational Behavior and the Model of Human Occupation

    b. The Canadian Model of Occupational Performance (and Engagement)

    c. The Person-Environment-Occupational Performance) model

    d. Occupational Science

    e. Occupational Adaptation

    f. Ecology of Human Performance

2. *Sociocultural determinants of occupation*—Starting with the earliest theoretical developments in the emerging profession of OT, we looked at some of the founding movements and ideas about the sociocultural determinants of occupation, that is, those social and cultural factors that affect how we engage in occupation.

3. *Psychological-emotional determinants of occupation*—The third drawer of the filing cabinet contains theory about the thoughts and feelings that affect our occupation.

4. *Physical determinants of occupation*—The fourth drawer contains knowledge about how physical factors such as strength, endurance, and range of motion affect our ability to engage in occupations.

5. *Cognitive-neurological determinants of occupation*—The fifth drawer includes theory about the functioning of the central nervous system (the brain and spinal cord) and its effect on occupation.

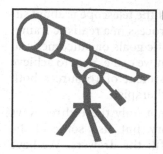

Figure 16-4. OT telescope.

6. *Environmental determinants of occupation*—The sixth drawer of the filing cabinet contains what we know about the environment and its effects on occupation. This emerging theory area looks outside of the person for social, geographic, institutional, and political factors that affect occupation.

The third and final metaphor employed in this book is the telescope (Figure 16-4). The telescope suggests a way of applying OT theory to assist in addressing the problems of an individual client:

- We begin by focusing on his or her occupation and occupational performance problems. Therefore, the first lens of the telescope offers us a rough focus on the stated problems of our client.

- The second lens of the telescope permits us to see the client in a lifespan perspective to understand how his or her age and stage bring with them not only particular challenges, but also skills, experiences, and perspectives that may be employed to promote occupation.

- The third lens of the telescope brings our theory into play. What do we know about the physical, psychological-emotional, sociocultural, or cognitive-neurological aspects of humans that might account for the problems we are seeing in our client? What aspects of the environment might be contributing to the difficulties? This is where we open one or more drawers of the filing cabinet to draw on our knowledge base and our theory to help us understand how these occupational performance problems are affecting health and well-being and how aspects of the person or the environment might be contributing to the problems.

- The fourth focusing lens of the telescope helps us ascertain what tools we have in our toolbox that might assist this client. Which of his or her problems are amenable to therapy, and what assessments and interventions do we have at our disposal to assist? This is where we draw on our knowledge of the relationship between conceptual models and models of practice to help us know not only how to think about the problem, but also what to do.

- The final focusing lens of the telescope is about situating the therapeutic process in a realistic framework consisting of specific goals or outcomes and time frames around what we can expect to achieve with a reasonable investment of resources both from the client and the therapist.

This book has provided not only these three ways of thinking about OT theory, but also some of the substantive information to fill the drawers. We have focused on the filing cabinet to a greater extent than on the toolbox or the telescope. In other words, we have attempted to provide historical and contemporary information about *conceptual models* for occupation, its consequences, and its determinants. We believe the contents of these six drawers to be the theoretical basis of OT, and we are very pleased to have the opportunity to update it again in this third edition.

References

Adelstein, L. A., & Nelson, D. L. (1985). Effects of sharing versus non-sharing on affective meaning in collage activities. *Occupational Therapy in Mental Health, 5,* 29-45.

Aldrich, R. (2008). From complexity theory to transactionalism: Moving occupational science forward in theorizing the complexities of behavior. *Journal of Occupational Science, 15*(3), 147-156.

Alessandrini, N. A. (1949). Play—A child's world. *American Journal of Occupational Therapy, 3,* 9-12.

Allen, C. K., Earhart, C. A., & Blue, T. (1992). *Occupational therapy treatment goals for the physically and cognitively disabled.* Rockville, MD: American Occupational Therapy Association.

American Occupational Therapy Association. (2003). Physical agent modalities: A position paper. *American Journal of Occupational Therapy, 57*(6), 650-651.

American Occupational Therapy Association. (2014). Occupational therapy practice framework: Domain and process (3rd ed.). *American Journal of Occupational Therapy, 68*(Suppl. 1), S1-S48. doi: http://dx.doi.org/10.5014/ajot.2014.682006

Americans With Disabilities Act of 1990, Pub. L. No. 101-336, 104 Stat. 328 (1990). Retrieved June 15, 2014, from www.ada.gov/archive/adastat91.htm.

Amini, D. (2011). Occupational therapy interventions for work-related injuries and conditions of the forearm, wrist, and hand: A systematic review. *American Journal of Occupational Therapy, 65*(1), 29-36. doi:http://dx.doi.org/10.5014/ajot.2011.09186

Anaby, D. R., Backman, C. L., & Jarus, T. (2010). Measuring occupational balance: A theoretical exploration of two approaches. *Canadian Journal of Occupational Therapy, 77*(5), 280-288. doi:http://dx.doi.org/10.2182/cjot.2010.77.5.4

Anderson, C. L. (1942). The social environment of occupational therapy. *Occupational Therapy and Rehabilitation, 21,* 333-336.

Andonian, L. (2010). Community participation of people with mental health issues within an urban environment. *Occupational Therapy in Mental Health, 26*(4), 401-417.

Andresen, M., & Runge, U. (2002). Co-housing for seniors experienced as an occupational generative environment. *Journal of Occupational Therapy, 9*(4), 156-166.

Aplin, T., de Jonge, D., & Gustafsson, L. (2013). Understanding the dimensions of home that impact on home modification decision making. *Australian Occupational Therapy Journal, 60*(2), 101-109.

Ashby, S., & Chandler, B. (2010). An exploratory study of the occupation-focused models included in occupational therapy professional education programmes. *British Journal of Occupational Therapy, 73*(12), 616-624. doi:http://dx.doi.org/10.4276/030802210X12918167234325

Averbach, S., & Katz, N. (2005). Cognitive rehabilitation: A retraining model for clients with neurological disabilities. In N. Katz (Ed.), *Cognition and occupation across the lifespan: Models for intervention in occupational therapy* (2nd ed., pp. 113-138). Bethesda, MD: AOTA Press.

Ayers, A. J. (1954). Ontogenetic principles in the development of arm and hand functions. *American Journal of Occupational Therapy, 8,* 95-99.

Ayers, A. J. (1955). Proprioceptive facilitation elicited through the upper extremities. Part III: Specific application to occupational therapy. *American Journal of Occupational Therapy, 9,* 121-126.

Ayers, A. J. (1961). Development of the body scheme in children. *American Journal of Occupational Therapy, 15,* 99-102.

Ayres, A. J. (1972). *Sensory integration and learning disorders.* Los Angeles, CA: Western Psychological Services.

Ayres, A. J. (1974). *The Development of Sensory Integrative Theory and Practice: A Collection of the Works of A. Jean Ayres.* Dubuque, Iowa: Kendall/Hunt Pub Co.

Backman, C. L. (2004). Muriel Driver Memorial Lecture: Occupational balance: Exploring the relationships among daily occupations and their influence on well-being. *The Canadian Journal of Occupational Therapy, 4*(71), 202.

Bagby, M. S., Dickie, V. A., & Baranek, G. T. (2012). How sensory experiences of children with and without autism affect family occupations. *American Journal of Occupational Therapy, 66,* 78-86. doi:10.5014/ajot.2012.000604

Bailey, D. M. (1994). Technology for adults with multiple impairments: A trilogy of reports. *American Journal of Occupational Therapy, 48,* 341-345.

Bain, B. K. (1998). Assistive technology in occupational therapy. In M. E. Neistadt, & E. B. Crepeau (Eds.). *Willard & Spackman's Occupational Therapy* (9th ed., pp. 498-517). Philadelphia, PA: Lippincott-Raven.

Banyai, A. L. (1938). Modern trends in the treatment of tuberculosis. *Occupational Therapy and Rehabilitation, 17,* 245-254.

Baptiste, S. (1988). Chronic pain, activity and culture. *Canadian Journal of Occupational Therapy, 55,* 179-184.

Baranek, G. T., Chin, Y. H., Hess, L. M. G., Yankee, J. G., Hatton, D. D., & Hooper, S. R. (2002). Sensory processing correlates of occupational performance in children with fragile X syndrome: Preliminary findings. *American Journal of Occupational Therapy, 56,* 538-546.

Barker, R. G. (1978). *Habitats, environments, and human behavior.* San Francisco, CA: Jossey-Bass.

McColl MA, Law M, Stewart D.
Theoretical Basis of Occupational Therapy, Third Edition (pp. 137-148).
© 2015 Taylor & Francis Group.

Barris, R. (1982). Environmental interactions: An extension of the model of occupation. *Canadian Journal of Occupational Therapy, 36,* 637644.

Barstow, B. A., Bennett, D. K., & Vogtle, L. K. (2011). Perspectives on home safety: Do home safety assessments address the concerns of clients with vision loss? *American Journal of Occupational Therapy, 65*(6), 635-642.

Barton, G. E. (1917). The movies and the microscope. *The Trained Nurse and Hospital Review, 59,* 193-196.

Bass-Haugen, J., Mathiowetz, V., & Flinn, N. (2008). Optimizing motor behaviour using the occupational therapy task-oriented approach. In M. Vining Radomski, & C. A. Trombly Latham (Eds.). *Occupational therapy for physical dysfunction* (6th ed., pp. 599-617). Baltimore, MD: Lippincott Williams & Wilkins.

Bassoe, P. (1923). Why one physician approves of occupational therapy in general hospitals. *The Modern Hospital, 20,* 606-607.

Baum, C., & Law, M. (1998). Community health: A responsibility, an opportunity, and a fit for occupational therapy. *American Journal of Occupational Therapy, 52,* 7-10.

Bazyk, S., & Bazyk, J. (2009). Meaning of occupation-based groups for low-income urban youths attending after-school care. *American Journal of Occupational Therapy, 63*(1), 69-80.

Beagan, B. L., & Etowa, J. (2009). The impact of everyday racism on the occupations of African Canadian women. *Canadian Journal of Occupational Therapy, 76*(4), 285-293.

Beagan, B., & Kumas-Tan, Z. (2005). Witnessing spirituality in practice. *British Journal of Occupational Therapy, 68*(1), 17.

Beagan, B., & Saunders, S. (2005). Occupations of masculinity: Producing gender through what men do and don't do. *Journal of Occupational Science, 12*(3), 161-169.

Belcham, C. (2004). Spirituality in occupational therapy: Theory in practice? *British Journal of Occupational Therapy, 67*(1), 39-46.

Bejerholm, U. (2010). Occupational balance in people with schizophrenia. *Occupational Therapy in Mental Health, 26*(1), 1-17.

Bing, R. K. (1981). Eleanor Clarke Sagle Lectureship 1981. "Occupational therapy revisited: A paraphrastic journey." *American Journal of Occupational Therapy, 35,* 499-518.

Black, M. (1976). Adolescent role assessment. *American Journal of Occupational Therapy, 30,* 73-80.

Bluestone, E. M. (1942). The argument for occupational therapy. *Occupational Therapy and Rehabilitation, 21,* 222-225.

Board of Trustees University of Illinois. (2014). Model of Human Occupation: Theory and Application. Retrieved May 18, 2014 from http://www.cade.uic.edu/moho/.

Bobath, B. (1978). *Adult hemiplegia: evaluation and treatment* (2nd ed.). London: William Heinnemann.

Bobath, K., & Bobath, B. (1964). The facilitation of normal postural reactions and movements in the treatment of cerebral palsy. *Physiotherapy, 50,* 246-62.

Bockoven, J. S. (1971). Legacy of moral treatment: 1890s to 1910. *American Journal of Occupational Therapy, 25,* 223-225.

Bonder, B. (2004). Culture and occupation: A comparison of weaving in two traditions. *The Canadian Journal of Occupational Therapy, 68*(5), 310.

Boniface, G., Fedden, T., Hurst, H., Mason, M., Phelps, C., Reagon, C., & Waygood, S. (2008). Using theory to underpin an integrated occupational therapy service through the Canadian Model of Occupational Performance. *British Journal of Occupational Therapy, 71*(12), 531-539.

Bontje, P., Kinébanian, A., Josephsson, S., & Tamura, Y. (2004). Occupational adaptation: The experiences of older persons with physical disabilities. *American Journal of Occupational Therapy, 58*(2), 140-149.

Bouteloup, Z., & Beltran, R. (2007). Application of the occupational adaptation framework in child and adolescent occupational therapy practice. A case study. *Australian Occupational Therapy Journal, 54,* 228-238.

Boyt Schell, B., Gillen, G., Scaffa, M. (2013). *Willard & Spackman's Occupational Therapy* (12th ed.). Baltimore, MD: Lippincott, Williams & Wilkins.

Bränholm, I., & Fugl-Meyer, A. R. (1992). Occupational role preferences and life satisfaction. *The Occupational Therapy Journal of Research, 12*(3), 159.

Bright, F. A. S., Boland, P., Rutherford, S. J., Kayes, N. M., & McPherson, K. M. (2012). Implementing a client-centered approach in rehabilitation: An autoethnography. *Disability & Rehabilitation, 34*(12), 997-1004.

Bronfenbrenner, U. (1979). *The Ecology of Human Development: Experiments by Nature and Design.* Cambridge, MA: Harvard University Press.

Brown, P. K. (1923). The problem of our physically handicapped. *Archives of Occupational Therapy, 2,* 171-178.

Brunnstrom, S. (1961). Motor behavior of adult hemiplegic patients, hints for training. *American Journal of Occupational Therapy, 14,* 6-10.

Brunnstrom, S. (1970). *Movement Therapy in Hemiplegia: A Neurophysiological Approach.* New York, New York: Harper & Row.

Bryant, L. C. (1926). Manual work with the mentally defective child patient. *The Modern Hospital, 27,* 61-63.

Bundy, A. C., & Murray, E. A. (2002). Sensory integration: A. Jean Ayres' theory revisited. In A. C. Bundy, S. J. Lane, & E. A. Murray (Eds.), *Sensory integration: Theory and practice* (2nd ed., pp. 141-165). Philadelphia, PA: F. A. Davis.

Bundy, A. C., Shia, S., Qi L., & Miller, L. J. (2007). How does sensory processing affect play? *American Journal of Occupational Therapy, 61,* 201-208.

Cahill, M., Connolly, D., & Stapleton, T. (2010). Exploring occupational adaptation through the lives of women with multiple sclerosis. *British Journal of Occupational Therapy, 73*(3), 106-115. doi:http://dx.doi.org/10.4276/030802210X12682330090415

Canadian Association of Occupational Therapists. (1997). *Enabling occupation: An occupational therapy perspective.* Ottawa, Ontario: CAOT Publications ACE.

Canadian Association of Occupational Therapists. (2002). *Enabling occupation: An occupational therapy perspective (2nd ed.).* Ottawa, Ontario: CAOT Publications ACE.

Carswell-Opzoomer, A. (1990). Occupational therapy: Our time has come. *Canadian Journal of Occupational Therapy, 57*(4), 197-205.

Case-Smith, J. (2003). Outcomes in hand rehabilitation using occupation therapy services. *American Journal of Occupational Therapy, 57*(5), 499-506.

Chan, J., & Spencer, J. (2004). Adaptation to hand injury: An evolving experience. *American Journal of Occupational Therapy, 58*(2), 128-139.

Chan, S. (2004). Chronic obstructive pulmonary disease and engagement in occupation. *American Journal of Occupational Therapy, 58*(4), 408-415.

Christiansen, C. H. (1999). Defining lives: Occupation as identity: Competence, coherence and the creation of meaning. *American Journal of Occupational Therapy, 53,* 547-558.

Christiansen, C. H., & Baum, C. (Eds.). (1991). *Occupational therapy: Overcoming human performance deficits.* Thorofare, NJ: SLACK Incorporated.

Christiansen, C. H., & Townsend, E. A. (2004). *Introduction to occupation: The art and science of living.* Upper Saddle River, NJ: Prentice Hall.

Christenson, M. A. (1990). Designing for the older person by addressing environmental attributes. *Physical and Occupational Therapy in Geriatrics, 3,* 31-48.

Cipriani, J., Kreider, M., Sapulak, K., Jacobson, M., Skrypski, M., & Sprau, K. (2009). Understanding object attachment and meaning for nursing home residents: An exploratory study, including implications for occupational therapy. *Physical & Occupational Therapy in Geriatrics, 27*(6), 405-422.

Clark, B. (1937). The use of occupational therapy in social stabilization. Results of a recent research. *Occupational Therapy and Rehabilitation, 16,* 143-158.

Clark, F. (1997). Reflections on the human as an occupational being: Biological need, tempo and temporality. *Journal of Occupational Science: Australia, 4*(3), 86-92.

Clark, F.A. (2000). The concepts of habit and routine: A preliminary theoretical synthesis. *OTJR: Occupation, Participation & Health, 20*(supplement), 123-137.

Clark, F., Sanders, K., Carlson, M., Blanche, E., & Jackson, J. (2007). Synthesis of habit theory. *OTJR: Occupation, Participation and Health, 27*(Suppl. 1), S7-S23.

Colaianni, D., & Provident, I. (2010). The benefits of and challenges to the use of occupation in hand therapy. *Occupational Therapy in Health Care, 24*(2), 130-146. doi:http://dx.doi.org/10.3109/07380570903349378

Colangelo, C. (1999). Biomechanical frame of reference. In P. Kramer, & J. Hinojasa (Eds.). *Frames of reference for pediatric occupational therapy* (2nd ed.). Philadelphia, PA: Lippincott, Williams & Wilkins.

Cole, F. (2010). Physical activity for its mental health benefits: Conceptualising participation within the Model of Human Occupation. *British Journal of Occupational Therapy, 73*(12), 607-615. doi:http://dx.doi.org/10.4276/030802210X12918167234280

Cole, M. B., & Tufano, R. (2008). Biomechanical and rehabilitative frames. In M.B. Cole, & R. Tufano. *Applied theories in occupational therapy. A practical approach.* Thorofare, NJ: SLACK Incorporated.

Collins, J. S., Paul, S., & West-Frasier, J. (2001). The utilization of spirituality in occupational therapy: Beliefs, practices, and perceived barriers. *Occupational Therapy in Health Care, 14*(3/4), 73.

Coutinho, F., Hersch, G., & Davidson, H. (2006). The impact of informal caregiving on occupational therapy: Practice review and analysis. *Physical & Occupational Therapy in Geriatrics, 25*(1), 47-61.

Covalt, D. A., Yamshon, L. J., & Nowicki, V. (1949). Physiological aid to the functional training of the hemiplegic arm. *American Journal of Occupational Therapy, 3,* 286-288.

Cowls, J., & Hale, S. (2005). It's the activity that counts: What clients value in psycho-educational groups. *Canadian Journal of Occupational Therapy, 3*(72), 176-182.

Craddock, J. (1996). Responses of the occupational therapy profession to the perspective of the disability movement, part 2. *British Journal of Occupational Therapy, 59*(2), 73-78.

Crane, B. T. (1919). Occupational therapy. *Boston Medical and Surgical Journal, 181,* 63-65.

Creek, J., & Hughes, A. (2008). Occupation and health: A review of selected literature. *British Journal of Occupational Therapy, 71*(11), 456-468.

Creighton, C. (1992). The origin and evolution of activity analysis. *American Journal of Occupational Therapy, 46,* 45-48.

Csikszentmihalyi, M., & Csikszentmihalyi, I. (1988). *Optimal experience: Psychological experiences of flow in consciousness.* Cambridge, UK: Cambridge University Press.

Cutchin, M. P. (2004). Using Deweyan philosophy to rename and reframe adaptation-to-environment. *American Journal of Occupational Therapy, 58*(3), 303-312.

Cutchin, M. P. (2007). From society to self (and back) through place: Habit in transactional context. *OTJR: Occupation, Participation & Health, 27*(Suppl. 1), 50S-59S.

Darnell, R. (2002). Occupation is not a cross-cultural universal: Some reflections from an ethnographer. *Journal of Occupational Science, 9*(1), 5-11.

Dekkers, M. K., & Nielsen, T. L. (2011). Occupational performance, pain, and global quality of life in women with upper extremity fractures. *Scandinavian Journal of Occupational Therapy, 18*(3), 198-209. doi:http://dx.doi.org/10.3109/11038128.2010.510205

Department of National Health and Welfare (DNHW) & Canadian Association of Occupational Therapists (CAOT). (1983). *Guidelines for the client-centered practice of occupational therapy* (Cat. H39-100/1986E). Ottawa, ON: Author.

Dickie, V., Cutchin, M., & Humphry, R. (2006). Occupation as transactional experience: A critique of individualism in occupational science. *Journal of Occupational Science, 13*(1), 83-93.

Dirette, D. K., Plaisier, B. R., & Jones, S. J. (2008). Patterns and antecedents of the development of self-awareness following traumatic brain injury: The importance of occupation. *British Journal of Occupational Therapy, 71*(2), 44-51.

Doble, S. (1988). Intrinsic motivation and clinical practice: The key to understanding the unmotivated client. *Canadian Journal of Occupational Therapy, 55,* 75-81.

Doble, S. E., & Magill-Evans, J. (1992). A model of social interaction to guide occupational therapy practice. *Canadian Journal of Occupational Therapy, 59,* 141-150.

Doble, S. E., & Santha, J. C. (2008). Occupational well-being: Rethinking occupational therapy outcomes. *Canadian Journal of Occupational Therapy, 75*(3), 184-190.

Dodson, D. W. (1959). Occupational therapy for what? A look at values. *American Journal of Occupational Therapy, 13,* 189.

Doubt, L. (2003). The cognitive-neurological determinants of occupation. In M. A. McColl, M. Law, D. Stewart, L. Doubt, N. Pollock, & T. Krupa (Eds.), *Theoretical basis of occupational therapy* (pp. 117-136). Thorofare, NJ: SLACK Incorporated.

Dubouloz, C. J., Egan, M., von Zweck, C., & Vallerand, J. (1999). Occupational therapists' perceptions of evidence-based practice. *American Journal of Occupational Therapy, 53,* 445-453.

Dubouloz, C. J., Laporte, D., Hall, M., Ashe, B., & Smith, C. D. (2004). Transformation of meaning perspectives in clients with rheumatoid arthritis. *American Journal of Occupational Therapy, 58*(4), 398-407.

Dunn, W. (2001). The sensations of everyday life: Empirical, theoretical, and pragmatic considerations. *American Journal of Occupational Therapy, 55*(6), 608-620.

Dunn, W., Brown, C. & McGuigan, A. (1994). The Ecology of human performance: A framework for considering the effect of context. *The American Journal of Occupational Therapy, 48*(7), 595-607.

Dunn, W. W. (1997). The impact of sensory processing abilities on the daily lives of young children and families: A conceptual model. *Infants and Young Children, 9*(4), 23-25.

Dunn, W. W. (2000). Habit: What's the brain got to do with it? *Occupational Therapy Journal of Research, 20*(Suppl), 6-20.

Dunning, H. (1972). Environmental occupational therapy. *American Journal of Occupational Therapy, 26*, 292-298.

Dunton, W. R. (1951). The importance of interest in occupation. *Occupational Therapy and Rehabilitation, 30*, 384-385.

Dutton, R. (Ed.). (1995). *Clinical reasoning in physical disabilities.* Baltimore, MD: Williams & Wilkins.

Dyck, I., & Jongbloed, L. (2000). Women with multiple sclerosis and employment issues: A focus on social and institutional environments. *Canadian Journal of Occupational Therapy, 67*(5), 337-346.

Dyer, G. W. (1963). The fourth dimension of the patient's continuum. *American Journal of Occupational Therapy, 17*, 226-228.

Egan, M., & DeLaat, D. (1994). Considering spirituality in occupational therapy practice. *Canadian Journal of Occupational Therapy, 61*, 95-101.

Eklund, M. (2001). Psychiatric patients' occupational roles: Changes over time and associations with self-rated quality of life. *Scandinavian Journal of Occupational Therapy, 8*(3), 125-130.

Eklund, M., Leufstadius, C., & Bejerholm, U. (2009). Time use among people with psychiatric disabilities: Implications for practice. *Psychiatric Rehabilitation Journal, 32*(3), 177-191.

Elliott, M. S., & Barris, R. (1987). Occupational role performance and life satisfaction in elderly persons. *Occupational Therapy Journal of Research, 7*, 215-224.

Elton, F. G. (1934). Human values: Rehabilitation and conservation. *Occupational Therapy and Rehabilitation, 13*, 367-379.

Emerson, H. (1998). Flow and occupation: A review of the literature. *Canadian Journal of Occupational Therapy, 65*, 37-44.

Engquist, D. E., Short-DeGraff, M., Gliner, J., & Oltjenbruns, K. (1997). Occupational therapists' beliefs and practices with regard to spirituality and therapy. *American Journal of Occupational Therapy, 51*(3), 173-180.

Engström, A., Lexell, J., & Lund, M. L. (2010). Difficulties in using everyday technology after acquired brain injury: A qualitative analysis. *Scandinavian Journal of Occupational Therapy, 17*(3), 233-243.

Erikson, E. H. (1959). *Identity and the Life Cycle.* New York, New York: International Universities Press.

Erlandsson, L. K., Eklund, M., & Persson, D. (2011). Occupational value and relationships to meaning and health: Elaborations of the ValMO-model. *Scandanavian Journal of Occupational Therapy, 18*, 72-80.

Evans, J., & Rodger, S. (2008). Mealtimes and bedtimes: Windows to family routines and rituals. *Journal of Occupational Science, 15*(2), 98-104.

Fasoli, S. E., Trombly, C. A., Tickle-Degnen, L., & Verfaellie, M. H. (2002). Context and goal-directed movement: The effect of materials-based occupation. *Occupational Therapy Journal of Research, 22*, 119-128.

Fearing, V. G., & Clark, J. (2000). *Individuals in context: A practical guide to client-centered practice.* Thorofare, NJ: SLACK Incorporated.

Feuss, C. D. (1959). Occupational therapy in the therapeutic community. *American Journal of Occupational Therapy, 13*, 9-10.

Fine, S. B. (1991). Eleanor Clarke Slagle lecture. Resilience and human adaptability: Who rises above adversity? *American Journal of Occupational Therapy, 45*, 493-503.

Fiorentino, M. R. (1966). The changing dimension of occupational therapy. *American Journal of Occupational Therapy, 20*, 251-252.

Fiorentino, M. R. (1975). Occupational therapy: Realization to activation. *American Journal of Occupational Therapy, 29*, 15-21.

Fitts, P. M., & Posner, M. I. (1967). *Learning and skilled performance in human performance.* Belmont, CA: Brooks/Cole.

Fitzgerald, M., Mullavey-O'Byrne, C., & Clemson, L. (1997). Cultural issues from practice. *Australian Occupational Therapy Journal, 44*, 1-21.

Fleming, J. (2009). Metacognitive occupation-based training in traumatic brain injury. In I. Soderback (Ed.), *International handbook of occupational therapy interventions* (pp. 225-231). New York, NY: Springer.

Fleming, J., & Ownsworth, T. (2006). A review of awareness interventions in brain injury rehabilitation. *Neuropsychological Rehabilitation, 16*(4), 474-500.

Florey, L. L. (1969). Intrinsic motivation: The dynamics of occupational therapy theory. *American Journal of Occupational Therapy, 23*, 319-322.

Florey, L. L. (1970). An approach to play and development. *American Journal of Occupational Therapy, 25*, 275-280.

Forsyth, K., Lai, J., & Kielhofner, G. (1999). The assessment of communication and interaction skills (ACIS): Measurement properties. *British Journal of Occupational Therapy, 62*(2), 69-74.

Franciscus, M. L. (1946). Occupational therapy: Where? How? Why? *Occupational Therapy and Rehabilitation, 25*, 137-140.

Frank, G. (1996). The concept of adaptation as a foundation for occupational science research. In R. Zemke, & F. Clark (Eds.), *Occupational science. The evolving discipline.* Philadelphia, PA: F. A. Davis.

Freud, S (1905). *Three Essays on the Theory of Sexuality* (J. Strachey, 1962, Trans.). New York: Basic Books.

Frieden, L., & Cole, J. A. (1985). Independence: The ultimate goal of rehabilitation for spinal cord-injured persons. *American Journal of Occupational Therapy, 39*, 734-739.

Friedland, J. (2009). *Restoring the spirit: The beginnings of occupational therapy in Canada, 1890-1930.* Kingston, ON: McGill-Queen's University Press.

Gage, M. (1991). The appraisal model of coping: An assessment and intervention model for occupational therapy. *American Journal of Occupational Therapy, 46*, 353-362.

Gage, M., & Polatajko, H. (1994). Enhancing occupational performance through an understanding of perceived self-efficacy. *American Journal of Occupational Therapy, 48*, 452-461.

Galvin, D., Wilding, C., & Whiteford, G. (2011). Utopian visions/ dystopian realities: Exploring practice and taking action to enable human rights and occupational justice in a hospital context. *Australian Occupational Therapy Journal, 58*, 378-385.

Galvin, J., Randall, M., Hewish, S., Rice, J., & MacKay, M. T. (2010). Family-centred outcome measurement following paediatric stroke. *Australian Occupational Therapy Journal, 57*(3), 152-158. doi:http://dx.doi.org/10.1111/j.1440-1630.2010.00853.x

George, L. A., Schkade, J. K., & Ishee, J. H. (2004). Content validity of the relative mastery measurement scale: A measure of occupational adaptation. *OTJR: Occupation, Participation & Health, 24*(3), 92-102.

Gillot, A. J., Holder-Walls, A., Kurtz, J. R., & Varley, N. C. (2003). Perceptions and experiences of two survivors of stroke who participated in constraint-induced movement therapy home programs. *American Journal of Occupational Therapy, 57*(2), 168-176.

Gordon, E. E. (1954). Does occupational therapy meet the demands of total rehabilitation? *American Journal of Occupational Therapy, 8,* 238-240.

Gordon, J. (1987). Assumptions underlying physical therapy intervention: Theoretical and historical perspectives. In J. H. Carr, & R. B. Shepherd (Eds.), *Movement sciences: Foundations for physical therapy in rehabilitation* (pp. 1-30). Rockville, MD: Aspen.

Government of Ontario. (2005). *Accessibility for Ontarians with disabilities act.* Toronto, ON: Government of Ontario.

Grady, A. P. (1995). Building inclusive community: A challenge for occupational therapy. 1994 Eleanor Clarke Slagle Lecture. *American Journal of Occupational Therapy, 49,* 300-310.

Green, A. (2008). Sleep, occupation and the passage of time. *British Journal of Occupational Therapy, 71*(8), 339-347.

Green, N. (1922). Occupational therapy for orthopedic cases. *Archives of Occupational Therapy, 1,* 269-278.

Griffith, J., Caron, C. D., Desrosiers, J., & Thibeault, R. (2007). Defining spirituality and giving meaning to occupation: The perspective of community-dwelling older adults with autonomy loss. *Canadian Journal of Occupational Therapy, 74*(2), 78-90.

Grossman, M. (1946). Coordinating occupational therapy and physical medicine in the Veterans Administration hospitals. *Occupational Therapy and Rehabilitation, 25,* 118-122.

Guay, M., Dubois, M., Desrosiers, J., & Robitaille, J. (2012). Identifying characteristics of 'straightforward cases' for which support personnel could recommend home bathing equipment. *British Journal of Occupational Therapy, 75*(12), 563-569. doi:http://dx.doi.org/10.4276/030802212X13548955545576

Haak, M., Ivanoff, S. D., Fänge, A., Sixsmith, J., & Iwarsson, S. (2007). Home as the locus and origin for participation: Experiences among very old Swedish people. *OTJR: Occupation, Participation & Health, 27*(3), 95-103.

Hachey, R., Boyer, G., & Mercier, C. (2001). Perceived and valued roles of adults with severe mental health problems. *Canadian Journal of Occupational Therapy, 68*(2), 112-120.

Hagedorn, R. (1995). Environment. In R. Hagedorn (Ed.), *Occupational therapy: Perspectives and processes* (pp. 93-101). Edinburgh, Scotland: Churchill Livingstone.

Hahn, H. (1984). Reconceptualizing disability: A political science perspective. *Rehabilitation Literature, 45,* 362-365.

Hall, H. J. (1910). Work-cure: A report of five years' experience at an institution devoted to the therapeutic application of manual work. *Journal of the American Medical Association, 54,* 12-14.

Hall, H. J. (1917). Remunerative occupations for the handicapped. *The Modern Hospital, 8,* 383-386.

Hall, H. J. (1921). Forward steps in occupational therapy during 1920. *The Modern Hospital, 16,* 245-247.

Hammell, K. W. (2001). Intrinsicality: Reconsidering spirituality, meaning(s) and mandates. *Canadian Journal of Occupational Therapy, 68*(3), 186-194.

Hammell, K. W. (2009). Sacred texts: A skeptical exploration of the assumptions underpinning theories of occupation. *Canadian Journal of Occupational Therapy, 76*(1), 6-22.

Hand, C., Law, M., McColl, M., Hanna, S., & Elliott, S. (2012). Neighborhood influences on participation among older adults with chronic health conditions: A scoping review. *OTJR: Occupation, Participation & Health, 32*(3), 95-103.

Hand, C., Wilkins, S., Letts, L., & Law, M. (2013). Renegotiating environments to achieve participation: A metasynthesis of qualitative chronic disease research. *Canadian Journal of Occupational Therapy, 80*(4), 251-262.

Hanna, K., & Rodger, S. (2002). Towards family-centered practice in paediatric occupational therapy: A review of the literature on parent-therapist collaboration. *Australian Occupational Therapy Journal, 49,* 14-24.

Hasselkus, B. R. (2006). 2006 Eleanor Clarke Slagle lecture. The world of everyday occupation: Real people, real lives. *American Journal of Occupational Therapy, 60,* 627-640.

Hasselkus, B. R. (2011). *The meaning of everyday occupation.* Thorofare, NJ: SLACK Incorporated.

Heard, C. (1977). Occupational role acquisition: A perspective on the chronically disabled. *American Journal of Occupational Therapy, 31,* 243-247.

Heaton, T. G. (1937). Occupational therapy for the tuberculous: Motives and methods. *Canadian Journal of Occupational Therapy and Physical Therapy, 4,* 54-61.

Hendrickson, D., Anderson, J., & Gordon, E. E. (1960). A physiological approach to the regulation of activity in the cardiac convalescent. *American Journal of Occupational Therapy, 14,* 292-296.

Hocking, C. (2000). Having and using objects in the western world. *Journal of Occupational Science, 7*(3), 148-157.

Hocking, C. (2009). The challenge of occupation: Describing the things people do. *Journal of Occupational Science, 16*(3), 140.

Hood, M. (1956). Occupational therapy—work tests and assessment. *Canadian Journal of Occupational Therapy, 23,* 57-63.

Hopkins, H. L. (1960). Assistive devices for activities of daily living. *American Journal of Occupational Therapy, 14,* 218-220.

Howard, P. (1956). Motion therapy for the chronically ill. *Canadian Journal of Occupational Therapy, 23,* 19-23.

Howe, M. C., & Briggs, A. K. (1982). Ecological systems model for occupational therapy. *American Journal of Occupational Therapy, 36,* 322-327.

Howell, D., & Pierce, D. (2000). Exploring the forgotten restorative dimension of occupation: Quilting and quilt use. *Journal of Occupational Science, 7*(2), 68-72.

Howie, L., Coulter, M., & Feldman, S. (2004). Crafting the self: Older persons' narratives of occupational identity. *American Journal of Occupational Therapy, 58,* 446-454.

Hughes, J. (2001). Occupational therapy in community mental health teams: A continuing dilemma? Role theory offers an explanation. *British Journal of Occupational Therapy, 64*(1), 34.

Humphreys, E. J. (1937). The value of occupational therapy to the developmentally deficient child. *Occupational Therapy and Rehabilitation, 16,* 1-13.

Hurt, S. (1939). Occupational therapy with traumatic conditions. *Occupational Therapy and Rehabilitation, 18,* 191-194.

Hyde, P. (2001). Support groups for people who have experienced psychosis. *British Journal of Occupational Therapy, 64*(4), 169-173.

Iannone, M. (1987). A cross-cultural investigation of occupational roles. *Occupational Therapy in Health Care, 4*(1), 93-101.

Ikiugu, M. N. (2008). A proposed conceptual model of organizational development for occupational therapists and occupational scientists. *OTJR: Occupation, Participation & Health, 28*(2), 52-63.

Ilg, F. I., & Ames, L. B. (1962). *The Gesell Institute's Child Behavior.* New York: Dell Books.

Isaksson, G., Lexell, J., & Skär, L. (2007). Social support provides motivation and ability to participate in occupation. *OTJR: Occupation, Participation & Health, 27*(1), 23-30.

Iwama, M. K. (2003). Toward culturally relevant epistemologies in occupational therapy. *American Journal of Occupational Therapy, 57*(5), 582-588.

Iwama, M. K. (Ed.). (2006). *The Kawa model: Culturally relevant occupational therapy.* Philadelphia, PA: Elsevier Ltd.

Iwama, M. K., Thomson, N. A., & MacDonald, R. M. (2009). The Kawa model: The power of culturally responsive occupational therapy. *Disability and Rehabilitation, 31*(14), 1125-1135.

Jackson, J., Carlson, M., Mandel, D., Zemke, R., & Clark, F. (1998). Occupation in lifestyle redesign: The well elderly study occupational therapy program. *American Journal of Occupational Therapy, 52*(5), 326-336.

Jackson, J. P., & Schkade, J. K. (2001). Occupational adaptation model versus biomechanical-rehabilitation model in the treatment of patients with hip fractures. *American Journal of Occupational Therapy, 55,* 531-537.

Jakobsen, K. (2001). Employment and the reconstruction of self: A model of space for maintenance of identity by occupation. *Scandinavian Journal of Occupational Therapy, 8*(1), 40-48.

James, W. (1985). Habit. *Occupational Therapy in Mental Health, 5,* 55-67.

Jamieson, M. (1985). The interaction of culture and learning: Implications for occupational therapy. *Canadian Journal of Occupational Therapy, 52,* 5-8.

Jarus, T., Shavit, S., & Ratzon, N. (2000). From hand twister to mind twister: Computer-aided treatment in traumatic wrist fracture. *American Journal of Occupational Therapy, 54*(2), 176-182.

Johnson, D., & Mayers, C. (2005). Spirituality: A review of how occupational therapists acknowledge, assess and meet spiritual needs. *British Journal of Occupational Therapy, 68*(9), 386-392.

Johnson, J., & Smith, M. (1966). Changing concepts of occupational therapy in a community rehabilitation center. *American Journal of Occupational Therapy, 20,* 267-273.

Johnson, J. A. (2006). Describing the phenomenon of homelessness through the theory of occupational adaptation. *Occupational Therapy in Health Care, 20,* 63-80.

Jones, N. A. (1974). Occupational therapy and the aged. *American Journal of Occupational Therapy, 28,* 615-618.

Jongbloed, L., & Crichton, A. (1990). A new definition of disability: Implications for rehabilitation practice and social policy. *Canadian Journal of Occupational Therapy, 57,* 32-37.

Jonsson, H., & Persson, D. (2006). Towards an experiential model of occupational balance: An alternative perspective on flow theory analysis. *Journal of Occupational Science, 13*(1), 62-73.

Kang, C. (2003). A psychosocial integration frame of reference for occupational therapy. Part 1: Conceptual foundations. *Australian Occupational Therapy Journal, 50,* 92-103.

Kantzarksis, S., & Molineaux, M. (2011). The influence of Western society's construction of a healthy daily life on the conceptualization of occupation. *Journal of Occupational Science, 18*(1), 62-80.

Kaponen, R., & Kielhofner, G. (2006). Occupation and meaning in the lives of women with chronic pain. *Scandinavian Journal of Occupational Therapy, 13,* 211-220.

Katz, N. (1985). Occupational therapy domain of concern reconsidered. *American Journal of Occupational Therapy, 39,* 518-524.

Kidner, T. B. (1932). Occupational therapy—its aims and developments. *Occupational Therapy and Rehabilitation, 11,* 233-239.

Kielhofner, G. (1977). Temporal adaptation: A conceptual framework for occupational therapy. *American Journal of Occupational Therapy, 31,* 235-242.

Kielhofner, G. (1978). General systems theory: Implications for theory and action in occupational therapy. *American Journal of Occupational Therapy, 32,* 637.

Kielhofner, G. (1980). A model of human occupation, part 2. Ontogenesis from the perspective of temporal adaptation. *American Journal of Occupational Therapy, 34,* 657-663.

Kielhofner, G. (1992). *Conceptual foundations of occupational therapy.* Philadelphia, PA: F. A. Davis.

Kielhofner, G. (1995). *A model of human occupation: Theory and applications* (2nd ed.). Baltimore, MD: Williams & Wilkins.

Kielhofner, G. (1997). Biomechanical model. In G. Kielhofner (Ed.), *Conceptual foundations of occupational therapy* (2nd ed., pp. 109-125). Philadelphia, PA: F. A. Davis.

Kielhofner, G. (2002). *A model of human occupation: Theory and application* (3rd ed.). Philadelphia, PA: Lippincott, Williams & Wilkins.

Kielhofner, G. (2004). *Conceptual foundations of occupational therapy* (3rd ed.). Philadelphia, PA: F. A. Davis.

Kielhofner, G. (2008). *A model of human occupation: Theory and practice* (4th ed.). Philadelphia, PA: Lippincott, Williams & Wilkins.

Kielhofner, G., Barris, R., & Watts, J. H. (1982). Habits and habit dysfunction: A clinical perspective for psychosocial occupational therapy. *Occupational Therapy in Mental Health, 2,* 1-21.

Kielhofner, G., & Burke, J. P. (1980). A model of human occupation, part 1. Conceptual framework and content. *American Journal of Occupational Therapy, 34*(9), 572-581.

Kiernat, J. (1982). Environment: The hidden modality. *Physical and Occupational Therapy in Geriatrics, 2,* 312.

Kindwall, J. A., & McLean, J. (1941). One hand for the ship. *Occupational Therapy and Rehabilitation, 20,* 223-229.

Klein, J., & Liu, L. (2010). Family-therapist relationships in caring for older adults. *Physical & Occupational Therapy in Geriatrics, 28*(3), 259-270.

Klinger, J. (1965). Activities of daily living: Some comments and recent developments. *American Journal of Occupational Therapy, 19,* 295-299.

Klinger, L. (2005). Occupational adaptation: Perspectives of people with traumatic brain injury. *Journal of Occupational Science, 12*(1), 9-16.

Koenig, K. P., & Rudney, S. G. (2010). Performance challenges for children and adolescents with difficulty processing and integrating sensory information: A systematic review. *American Journal of Occupational Therapy, 64,* 430-442. doi:10.5014/ajot.2010.09073

Kohlberg, L. (1981). *Essays on Moral Development, Vol. I: The Philosophy of Moral Development.* San Francisco, CA: Harper & Row.

Koome, F., Hocking, C., & Sutton, D. (2012). Why routines matter: The nature and meaning of family routines in the context of adolescent mental illness. *Journal of Occupational Science, 19*(4), 312-325. doi:http://dx.doi.org/10.1080/14427591.2012.718245

Kramer, P., Hinojosa, J., & Brasic Royeen, C. (2003). *Perspectives in human occupation: Participation in life.* Philadelphia, PA: Lippincott Williams & Wilkins.

Krefting, L. H., & Krefting, D. V. (1991). Cultural influences on performance. In C. Christiansen, & C. Baum (Eds.), *Occupational Therapy: Overcoming human performance deficits* (pp. 100-122). Thorofare, NJ: SLACK Incorporated.

Krupa, T. (2004). Employment, recovery and schizophrenia: Integrating health and disorder at work. *Psychiatric Rehabilitation Journal, 28,* 8-15.

Krupa, T. M. (2010). Invited commentary…the occupational performance process model in one community mental health setting. *Canadian Journal of Occupational Therapy, 77*(2), 80-81. doi:10.2182/cjot.2010.77.2.3

Krusen, F. H. (1954). Relationships between occupational therapy and physical medicine and rehabilitation. *Canadian Journal of Occupational Therapy, 38,* 522-528.

Kyler, P. L. (2008). Client-centered and family-centered care: Refinement of the concepts. *Occupational Therapy in Mental Health, 24*(2), 100-120.

La Corte, L, F, (2008). New and expanded concepts in neurophysiology, psychology, and sociology complementary to Llorens' developmental theory: Achieving growth and development through occupation for neonatal infants and their families. *Occupational Therapy in Mental Health, 24*(3/4), 201-349.

Larson, E., & von Eye, A. (2010). Beyond flow: Temporality and participations in everyday activities. *American Journal of Occupational Therapy, 64,* 152-163.

Larson, E. A. (2004). Children's work: The less-considered childhood occupation. *American Journal of Occupational Therapy, 58*(4), 369-379.

Larson, E. A., & Zemke, R. (2003). Shaping the temporal patterns of our lives: The social coordination of occupation. *Journal of Occupational Science, 10*(2), 80-89.

Law, M. (1991). 1991 Muriel Driver lecture. The environment: A focus for occupational therapy. *Canadian Journal of Occupational Therapy, 58*(4), 171-180.

Law, M. (2002). Participation in the occupations of everyday life. *American Journal of Occupational Therapy, 56*(6), 640-649.

Law, M., Baptiste, S., Carswell, A., McColl, M. A., Polatajko, H. & Pollock, N. (1991). *The Canadian Occupational Performance Measure and Manual.* Toronto, ON: CAOT.

Law, M., Baptiste, S., McColl, M. A., Polatajko, H., Carswell, A., Pollock, N. (2014). *The Canadian Occupational Performance Measure and Manual* (5th ed.). Ottawa, ON: CAOT.

Law, M., Cooper, B., Strong, S., Stewart, D., Rigby, P., & Letts, L. (1996). The person-environment-occupation model: A transactive approach to occupational performance. *Canadian Journal of Occupational Therapy, 63,* 9-23.

Law, M., & McColl, M. A. (2010). *Interventions, effects and outcomes in occupational therapy: Adults and older adults.* Thorofare, NJ: SLACK Incorporated.

Lee, J. (2010). Achieving best practice: A review of evidence linked to occupation-focused practice models. *Occupational Therapy in Health Care, 24*(3), 206-222. doi:http://dx.doi.org/10.3109/07380577.2010.483270

Lee, J., & Kielhofner, G. (2010). Vocational intervention based on the Model of Human Occupation: A review of the evidence. *Scandinavian Journal of Occupational Therapy, 17,* 177-190.

Lee, M., Madden, V., Mason, K., Rice, S., Wyburd, J., & Hobson, S. (2006). Occupational engagement and adaptation in adults with dementia: A preliminary investigation. *Physical & Occupational Therapy in Geriatrics, 25*(1), 63-81.

Lee, S. W., Taylor R., & Kielhofner, G., (2009). Choice, knowledge and utilization of a practice theory: A national study of occupational therapists who use the model of Human Occupation. *Occupational Therapy in health Care, 23*(1), 60-71.

Lee, S. W., Taylor, R., Kielhofner, G., & Fisher, G. (2008). Theory use in practice: A national survey of therapists who use the model of human occupation. *American Journal of Occupational Therapy, 62*(1), 106-117.

LeVesconte, H. P. (1934). The place of occupational therapy in social work planning. *Canadian Journal of Occupational Therapy, 2,* 13-16.

LeVesconte, H. P. (1935). Expanding the fields of occupational therapy. *Canadian Journal of Occupational Therapy, 3,* 4-12.

Levine, R. (1984). The cultural aspects of home care delivery. *American Journal of Occupational Therapy, 38,* 734-738.

Levit, K. (2008). Optimizing motor behavior using the Bobath approach. In M. Vining Radomski, & C. A. Trombly Latham (Eds.)., *Occupational therapy for physical dysfunction* (6th edition, pp. 643-664). Baltimore, MD: Lippincott Williams & Wilkins.

Lexell, E. M., Iwarsson, S., & Lund, M. L. (2011). Occupational adaptation in people with multiple sclerosis. *OTJR: Occupation, Participation & Health, 31*(3), 127-134.

Licht, S. (1944). Occupational therapy in reconditioning. *Occupational Therapy and Rehabilitation, 23,* 168-173.

Licht, S. (1947). Kinetic analysis of crafts and occupations. *Occupational Therapy and Rehabilitation, 26,* 75-78.

Licht, S., & Reilly, M. (1943). The correlation of physical and occupational therapy. *Occupational Therapy and Rehabilitation, 22,* 171-175.

Lim, S. M., & Rodger, S. (2008). An occupational perspective on the assessment of social competence in children. *British Journal of Occupational Therapy, 71,* 469-481.

Lin, K. C., Wu, C. Y., & Trombly, C. A. (1998). Effects of task goal on movement kinematics and line bisection performance in adults without disabilities. *American Journal of Occupational Therapy, 52,* 179-187.

Llorens, L. (1977). A developmental theory revisited. *American Journal of Occupational Therapy, 31,* 656-657.

Llorens, L. (1984). Theoretical conceptualizations of occupational therapy: 1960-1982. *Occupational Therapy in Mental Health, 4*(2), 1-14.

Llorens, L., Rubin, E., Braun, J., Beck, G., Mottley, N., & Beall, D. (1964). Cognitive perceptual motor functions: A preliminary report on training. *American Journal of Occupational Therapy, 18*, 202-207.

Losada, C. A. (1936). Some values in occupational therapy. *Occupational Therapy and Rehabilitation, 15*, 285-289.

Ludwig, F. M. (1997). How routines facilitate well-being in older women. *Occupational Therapy International, 4*, 213-228.

Lull, G. F. (1926). How occupational therapy promotes recovery. *The Modern Hospital, 26*, 33-37.

Lund, M. L., & Nygård, L. (2004). Occupational life in the home environment: The experiences of people with disabilities. *Canadian Journal of Occupational Therapy, 71*(4), 243-251.

Ma, H., & Trombly, C. A. (2004). Effects of task complexity on reaction time and movement kinematics in elderly people. *American Journal of Occupational Therapy, 58*(2), 150-158.

Marquenie, K., Rodger, S., Mangohig, K., & Cronin, A. (2011). Dinnertime and bedtime routines and rituals in families with a young child with an autism spectrum disorder. *Australian Occupational Therapy Journal, 58*, 145-154.

Mastos, M., Miller, K., Eliasson, A. C., & Imms, C. (2007). Goal-directed training: Linking theories of treatment to clinical practice for improved functional activities in daily life. *Clinical Rehabilitation, 21*, 47-55.

Mathiowetz, V. (1993). Role of physical performance component evaluations in occupational therapy functional assessment. *American Journal of Occupational Therapy, 47*, 225-230.

Matsutsuyu, J. (1971). Occupational behavior: A perspective on work and play. *American Journal of Occupational Therapy, 25*, 291-293.

Matuska, K. M., & Christiansen, C. H. (2008). A proposed model of lifestyle balance. *Journal of Occupational Science, 15*(1), 9-19.

Maurer, P. (1971). Antecedents of work behavior. *American Journal of Occupational Therapy, 25*, 295-297.

McColl, M. A. (2000). Muriel Driver Memorial Lecture: Spirit, occupation and disability. *Canadian Journal of Occupational Therapy, 67*(4), 217-229.

McColl, M. A. (2002). Occupation in stressful times. *American Journal of Occupational Therapy, 56*(3), 350-353.

McColl, M. A. (2011). *Spirituality and occupational therapy* (2nd ed.). Ottawa, ON: CAOT Publications ACE.

McColl, M. A., Carswell, A., Law, M., Pollock, N., Baptiste, S., & Polatajko, H. (2006). *Research on the Canadian Occupational Performance Measure: An annotated resource.* Ottawa, ON: CAOT Publications ACE.

McColl, M. A., & Law, M. (2010). *Interventions, effects, and outcomes in occupational therapy: Adults and older adults.* Thorofare, NJ: SLACK Incorporated.

McColl, M. A., Law, M. C., Doubt, L., Pollock, N., & Stewart, D. (2003). *Theoretical basis of occupational therapy* (2nd ed.). Thorofare, NJ: SLACK Incorporated.

McColl, M. A., Law, M. C., & Stewart, D. (1993). *The theoretical basis of occupational thera*py. Thorofare, NJ: SLACK Incorporated.

McCuaig, M., & Iwama, M. (1989). When daily living becomes a challenge in the workplace. Occupational therapy: The profession that connects. *Canadian Journal of Occupational Therapy, 56*, 161-162.

McGuire, M. (1997). Physical agent modalities: Position paper. *American Journal of Occupational Therapy, 51*(10), 870-871.

McNair, F. E. (1959). Milieu therapy. *Canadian Journal of Occupational Therapy, 26*, 93-98.

McPhee, S. D., Bracciano, A. G., & Rose, B. W., Brayman, S. J., & Commission on Practice. (2003). Physical agent modalities: A position paper. *American Journal of Occupational Therapy, 57*(6), 650-651.

Melton, J., Forsyth, K., & Freeth, D. (2010). A practice development programme to promote the use of the model of human occupation: Contexts, influential mechanisms and levels of engagement amongst occupational therapists. *British Journal of Occupational Therapy, 73*(11), 549-558. doi:http://dx.doi.org/10.4276/030802210X12892992239350

Merritt, M. E. (1938). Occupational therapy modernized. *The Modern Hospital, 51*, 75-77.

Meyer, A. (1918). The mental hygiene movement. *Canadian Medical Association Journal, 8*(7), 632-634.

Meyer, A. (1922). The philosophy of occupational therapy. *Archives of Occupational Therapy, 1*, 1-10.

Meyer, A. (1977). The philosophy of occupational therapy. *American Journal of Occupational Therapy, 31*, 639-642.

Mielicke, C. (1967). The meaning of work and the use of leisure. *Canadian Journal of Occupational Therapy, 34*, 75-81.

Migliore, A. (2004). Improving dyspnea management in three adults with chronic obstructive pulmonary disease. *American Journal of Occupational Therapy, 58*(6), 639-646.

Mirkopolous, C., & Evert, M. M. (1994). Cultural connections: A challenge unmet. *Canadian Journal of Occupational Therapy, 61*, 67-70.

Moher, T. J. (1907). Occupation in treatment of the insane. *Journal of the American Medical Association, 158*, 1664-1666.

Morgan, W. J. (2010). What, exactly, is occupational satisfaction? *Journal of Occupational Science, 17*(4), 216-223.

Mosey, A. C. (1970). *Three frames of reference for mental health.* Thorofare, New Jersey: Charles B. Slack Inc.

Mosey, A. C. (1974). An alternative: The biopsychosocial model. *American Journal of Occupational Therapy, 28*, 137-140.

Mosey, A. C. (1981). Occupational therapy: Configuration of a profession. New York, NY: Raven Press.

Mosey, A. C. (1986). *Psychosocial components of occupational therapy.* New York, NY: Raven Press.

Mosey, A. C. (1997). Partition of occupational science and occupational-therapy. *American Journal of Occupational Therapy, 46*, 851-853.

Murray, H. A. (1938). *Explorations in personality.* New York, NY: Oxford University Press.

Myers, C. T. (2006). The use of infant seating devices in child care centers. *American Journal of Occupational Therapy, 60*(5), 489-493.

Nahemow, L., Lawton, M. P., & Center, P. G. (1973). Toward an ecological theory of adaptation and aging 1.3. *Environmental design research: Selected papers, 1*, 24-32.

Nash, J. B. (1938). The philosophy of busy-ness. *Occupational Therapy and Rehabilitation, 17*, 27-32.

Nayar, S., Hocking, C., & Wilson, J. (2007). An occupational perspective of migrant mental health: Indian women's adjustment to living in New Zealand. *British Journal of Occupational Therapy, 70*(1), 16-23.

Nayar, S., Hocking, C., & Giddings, L. (2012). Using occupation to navigate cultural spaces: Indian immigrant women settling in New Zealand. *Journal of Occupational Science, 19*(1), 62-75.

Neidstadt, M. E. (1990). A critical analysis of occupational therapy approaches for perceptual deficits in adults with brain injury. *American Journal of Occupational Therapy, 44,* 299-303.

Nelson, D. L. (1988). Occupation: Form and performance. *American Journal of Occupational Therapy, 42,* 633-641.

Nelson, D. L., & Peterson, C. Q. (1989). Enhancing therapeutic exercise through purposeful activity: A theoretic analysis. *Topics in Geriatric Rehabilitation, 4*(4), 12-22.

Nelson, D., Peterson, C., Smith, D., Boughton, J., & Whalen, G. (1988). Effects of project versus parallel groups on social interaction and affective responses in senior citizens. *American Journal of Occupational Therapy, 42,* 23-29.

Oakley, F., Kielhofner, G., Barris, R., & Reichler, R. K. (1986). The role checklist: Development and empirical assessment of reliability. *Occupational Therapy Journal of Research, 6*(3), 157–70.

O'Brien, P., Dyck, I., Caron, S., & Mortenson, P. (2002). Environmental analysis: Insights from sociological and geographical perspectives. *Canadian Journal of Occupational Therapy, 69*(4), 229-238.

O'Reilly, J. A. (1954). Occupational therapy in the management of traumatic disabilities. *Canadian Journal of Occupational Therapy, 21,* 75-80.

Olson, L. (2006). One parent-child activity group: A framework and snapshots. *Occupational Therapy in Mental Health, 22*(3/4), 33-47.

Opzoomer, A., & McCordic, L. (1972). The effects of reinforcing working behavior. *American Journal of Occupational Therapy, 26,* 32-35.

Paley, J., Eva, G., & Duncan, E. A. S. (2006). In-order-to analysis: An alternative to classifying different levels of occupational activity. *British Journal of Occupational Therapy, 69*(4), 161-168.

Parham, L. D., & Mailloux, Z. (2010). Sensory Integration. In J. Case-Smith, & J. C. O'Brien (Eds.) *Occupational therapy for children* (6th ed., pp. 325-372). Maryland Heights, MO: Mosby Elsevier.

Patterson, L. M. (1963). Productivity, work study and occupational therapy. *Canadian Journal of Occupational Therapy, 30,* 53-60.

Patterson, W. J. (1939). Opportunity. *Canadian Journal of Occupational Therapy, 6,* 51-56.

Pattison, H. A. (1922). The trend of occupational therapy for the tuberculous. *Archives of Occupational Therapy, 1,* 19-24.

Paul, S. (1995). Culture and its influence on occupational therapy evaluation. *Canadian Journal of Occupational Therapy, 62,* 154-161.

Pedretti, L. W., & Zoltan, B. (1996). *Occupational therapy: Practice skills for physical disability* (4th ed.). St. Louis, MO: C. V. Mosby.

Peloquin, S. (1991). Time as a commodity: Reflections and implications. *American Journal of Occupational Therapy, 45,* 147-154.

Pemberton, S., & Cox, D. (2011). What happened to the time? The relationship of occupational therapy to time. *British Journal of Occupational Therapy, 74*(2), 78-85. doi:http://dx.doi.org/10.4276/030802211X12971689814043

Pendleton, H. M., & Schultz-Krohn, W. (Eds.). (2013). *Pedretti's Occupational Therapy: Practice skills for physical dysfunction* (7th ed.). St. Louis, MO: Mosby.

Pentland, W., & McColl, M. A. (2008). Occupational integrity: Another perspective on "life balance." *Canadian Journal of Occupational Therapy, 75*(3), 135-138.

Persson, D., & Erlandsson, K. L. (2002). Time to reevaluate the machine society: Post-industrial ethics from an occupational perspective. *Journal of Occupational Science, 9*(2), 93-99.

Persson, D., Erlandsson, L. K., Eklund, M., & Iwarsson, S. (2001). Value dimensions, meaning, and complexity in human occupation—a tentative structure for analysis. *Scandinavian Journal of Occupational Therapy, 8,* 7-18.

Phelan, S., & Kinsella, E. A. (2009). Occupational identity: Engaging socio-cultural perspectives. *Journal of Occupational Science, 16*(2), 85-91.

Phillips, P. A., Kelk, N., & Fitzgerald, M. (2007). Object or person: The difference lies in the constructed identity. *Journal of Occupational Science, 14*(3), 162-171.

Piaget, J. (1928). *The Child's Conception of the World.* London: Routledge and Kegan Paul.

Pierce, D. (2001). Untangling occupation and activity. *American Journal of Occupational Therapy, 55*(2), 138-146.

Pierce, D., Atler, K., Baltisberger, J., Fehringer, E., Hunter, E., Malkawi, S., & Parr, T. (2010). Occupational science: A data-based American perspective. *Journal of Occupational Science, 17*(4), 204-215.

Pincus, A. (1968). New findings on learning in old age: Implications for occupational therapy. *American Journal of Occupational Therapy, 22,* 300-303.

Polatajko, H. J., Davis, J. A., Hobson, S. J. G., Landry, J. E., Mandich, A., Street, S. L., … & Yee, S. (2004). Meeting the responsibility that comes with the privilege: Introducing a taxonomic code for understanding occupation. *Canadian Journal of Occupational Therapy, 71*(5), 261-264.

Polatajko, H. J., & Mandich, A. (2005). Cognitive orientation to daily occupational performance. In N. Katz (Ed.), *Cognition and occupation across the lifespan: Models for intervention in occupational therapy* (2nd ed., pp. 237-259). Bethesda, MD: American Occupational Therapy Association.

Pollack, B. (1938). Aims and ideals of occupational therapy in state hospitals. *Occupational Therapy and Rehabilitation, 17,* 291-300.

Pollock, N. (2009). Sensory integration: A review of the current state of the evidence. *Occupational Therapy Now, 11*(5), 6-10.

Preston, G. H. (1942). Relating occupational therapy to reality. *Occupational Therapy and Rehabilitation, 21,* 17-24.

Purves, B., & Suto, M. (2004). In limbo: Creating continuity of identity in a discharge planning unit. *Canadian Journal of Occupational Therapy, 71*(3), 173-181.

Quintana, L. A. (2008). Assessing abilities and capacities: Vision, visual perception, and praxis. In M. Vining Radomski, & C. A. Trombly Latham (Eds.), *Occupational therapy for physical dysfunction* (6th ed., pp. 235-259). Baltimore, MD: Lippincott Williams & Wilkins.

Raber, C., Teitelman, J., Watts, J., & Kielhofner, G. (2010). A phenomenological study of volition in everyday occupations of older people with dementia. *British Journal of Occupational Therapy, 73*(11), 498-506. doi:http://dx.doi.org/10.4276/030802210X12892992239116

Radomski, M. V. (2008). Assessing abilities and capacities: Cognition. In M. Vining Radomski, & C. A. Trombly Latham (Eds.), *Occupational therapy for physical dysfunction* (6th ed., pp. 261-283). Baltimore, MD: Lippincott Williams & Wilkins.

Radomski, M. V., & Davis, E. S. (2008). Optimizing cognitive abilities. In M. Vining Radomski, & C. A. Trombly Latham (Eds.). *Occupational therapy for physical dysfunction* (6th ed., pp. 749-773). Baltimore, MD: Lippincott Williams & Wilkins.

Radomski, M. V., & Trombly, C. A. (2011). *Occupational therapy for physical dysfunction* (7th ed.). Baltimore, MD: Lippincott, Williams & Wilkins.

Rebeiro, K., & Cook, J. (1999). Opportunity, not prescription: An exploratory study of the experience of occupational engagement. *Canadian Journal of Occupational Therapy, 66*(4), 176-187.

Rebeiro, K. L., & Polgar, J. M. (1999). Enabling occupational performance: Optimal experiences in therapy. *Canadian Journal of Occupational Therapy, 66,* 14-22.

Reed, K. D., Hocking, C. S., & Smythe, L. A. (2011). Exploring the meaning of occupation: The case for phenomenology. *Canadian Journal of Occupational Therapy, 78*(5), 303-310. doi:http://dx.doi.org/10.2182/cjot.2011.78.5.5

Reed, K. L., & Sanderson, S. R. (1984). *Concepts of occupational therapy* (2nd ed.). Baltimore, MD: Williams & Wilkins.

Reid, D. (2011). Mindfulness and flow in occupational engagement: Presence in doing. *Canadian Journal of Occupational Therapy, 78,* 50-56.

Reilly, M. (1956). The role of therapist in protective and functional devices. *American Journal of Occupational Therapy, 10,* 118-133.

Reilly, M. (1962). Occupational therapy can be one of the great ideas of 20th century medicine. *American Journal of Occupational Therapy, 16,* 1-9.

Ricksher, C. (1913). Occupation in the treatment of the insane. *Illinois Medical Journal, 23,* 380-385.

Roberts, C. A. (1962). Healing the sick—responsibility or privilege—for the patient or the professional therapist. *Canadian Journal of Occupational Therapy, 29,* 5-14.

Rogers, J. C. (1982). The spirit of independence: The evolution of a philosophy. *American Journal of Occupational Therapy, 36,* 709-715.

Rogers, J. C. (2000). Habits: Do we practice what we preach? *Occupational Therapy Journal of Research, 20,* 119-122.

Rood, M. (1956). Neurophysiological mechanisms utilized in the treatment of neuromuscular dysfunction. *American Journal of Occupational Therapy, 10*(4), 220-225.

Rood, M. (1958). Neurophysiological mechanisms utilized in the treatment of neuromuscular dysfunction. *American Journal of Occupational Therapy, 12,* 326-329.

Ross, L. M., & Nelson, D. L. (2000). Comparing materials-based occupation, imagery-based occupation, and rote movement through kinematic analysis of reach. *Occupational Therapy Journal of Research, 20,* 45-60.

Rowles, G. (1991). Beyond performance: Being in place as a component of occupational therapy. *American Journal of Occupational Therapy, 45,* 265-271.

Rowles, G. (2008). Place in occupational science: A life course perspective on the role of environmental context in the quest for meaning. *Journal of Occupational Science, 15*(3), 127-135.

Rudman, D. L., & Dennhardt, S. (2008). Shaping knowledge regarding occupation: Examining the cultural underpinnings of the evolving concept of occupational identity. *Australian Occupational Therapy Journal, 55*(3), 153-162.

Salvatori, P., Jung, B., Missiuna, C., Stewart, D., Law, M., & Wilkins, S. (2006). *McMaster lens for occupational therapists.* Hamilton, ON: McMaster School of Occupational Therapy.

Sanchez, V. (1964). Relevance of cultural values for occupational therapy programs. *American Journal of Occupational Therapy, 18,* 1-5.

Schaaf, R. C. & Miller, L. J. (2005). Occupational therapy using a sensory integrative approach for children with developmental disabilities. *Mental Retardation and Developmental Disabilities Research Reviews, 11,* 143-148.

Schaber, P. L. (2002). FIRO model: A framework for family-centered care. *Physical & Occupational Therapy in Geriatrics, 20*(3/4), 1-17.

Schimeld, A. (1971). Youth of today and their influences on the practice of occupational therapy. *Canadian Journal of Occupational Therapy, 38*(1), 3-14.

Schkade, J. K., & Schultz, S. (1992). Occupational adaptation: Toward a holistic approach to contemporary practice (part 1). *American Journal of Occupational Therapy, 46,* 829-837.

Schmidt, J., Fleming, J., Ownsworth, T., Lannin, N., & Khan, A. (2012). Feedback interventions for improving self-awareness after brain injury: A protocol for a pragmatic randomized controlled trial. *Australian Occupational Therapy Journal, 59,* 138-146. doi:10.1111/j.1440-1630.2012.00998.x

Schmidt, R. A., & Lee, T. D. (2005). *Motor control and learning: A behavioral emphasis* (4th ed.). Champaign, IL: Human Kinetics.

Schultz-Krohn, W. (2004). The meaning of family routines in a homeless shelter. *American Journal of Occupational Therapy, 58,* 531-542.

Segal, R. (2004). Family routines and rituals: A context for occupational therapy interventions. *American Journal of Occupational Therapy, 58,* 499-508.

Shalinsky, W. (1986). Disabled persons and their environments. *Environments, 17*(1), 1-8.

Shank, K., & Cutchin, M. (2010). Transactional occupations of older women aging-in-place: Negotiating change and meaning. *Journal of Occupational Science, 17*(1), 4-13.

Sharp, N., Dunford, C., & Seddon, L. (2012). A critical appraisal of how occupational therapists can enable participation in adaptive physical activity for children and young people. *British Journal of Occupational Therapy, 75*(11), 486-494. doi:http://dx.doi.org/10.4276/030802212X13522194759815

Shimberg, M. (1936). The rationale of occupational therapy in orthopedic surgery. *Occupational Therapy and Rehabilitation, 15,* 149-161.

Shumway-Cook, A., & Woollacott, M. H. (2012). *Motor control: Translating research into clinical practice* (4th ed.). Baltimore MD, Lippincott Williams & Wilkins.

Slagle, E. C. (1924). A year's development of occupational therapy in New York state hospitals. *The Modern Hospital, 22,* 98-104.

Smith, R. (1995). A client-centered model for equipment prescription. *Occupational Therapy in Health Care, 9*(4), 39-52.

Soeker, M. S. (2011). Occupational adaptation: A return to work perspective of persons with mild to moderate brain injury in South Africa. *Journal of Occupational Science, 18*(1), 81-91. doi:http://dx.doi.org/10.1080/14427591.2011.554155

Spackman, C. S. (1968). A history of the practice of occupational therapy for restoration of physical function: 1917-1967. *American Journal of Occupational Therapy, 22,* 67-71.

Spector, H. I. (1936). In what way does occupational therapy assist in the recovery from tuberculosis? *Occupational Therapy and Rehabilitation, 15,* 41-45.

Stanley, J. (1942). Habit-training. *Occupational Therapy and Rehabilitation, 21,* 82-85.

Sutherland, J. B. (1964). Occupational therapy in the re-establishment of the physically handicapped. *Canadian Journal of Occupational Therapy, 31,* 143-146.

Swaim, L. T. (1921). The relation of occupational therapy to chronic disease. *The Modern Hospital, 17,* 162-168.

Takata, N. (1971). The play milieu: A preliminary appraisal. *American Journal of Occupational Therapy, 25,* 281-284.

Taylor, M. C. (2007). The Casson Memorial Lecture 2007: Diversity amongst occupational therapists—rhetoric or reality? *British Journal of Occupational Therapy, 70*(7), 276-283.

Teitelman, J., Raber, C., & Watts, J. (2010). The power of the social environment in motivating persons with dementia to engage in occupation: Qualitative findings. *Physical & Occupational Therapy in Geriatrics, 28*(4), 321-333.

Thelen, T (1995). Motor development: A new synthesis. *American Psychologist, 50,* 79-95.

Toal-Sullivan, D., & Henderson, P. R. (2004). Client-oriented role evaluation (CORE): The development of a clinical rehabilitation instrument to assess role change associated with disability. *American Journal of Occupational Therapy, 58*(2), 211-220.

Toglia, J. P. (1998). A dynamical interactional model to cognitive rehabilitation. In N. Katz (Ed.), *Cognitive rehabilitation: Models for intervention in occupational therapy,* (pp. 4-50). Bethesda, MD: American Association of Occupational Therapy, Inc.

Toglia, J. P. (2005). A dynamic interactional approach to cognitive rehabilitation. In N. Katz (Ed.), *Cognition and occupation across the lifespan: Models for intervention in occupational therapy* (2nd ed., pp. 29-72). Bethesda, MD: AOTA Press.

Toglia, J. P., & Kirk, U. (2000). Understanding awareness deficits following brain injury. *NeuroRehabilitation, 15,* 57-70.

Townsend, E. A., & Polatajko, H. J. (2007). *Enabling occupation II: Advancing an occupational therapy vision for health, wellbeing, & justice through occupation.* Ottawa, ON: CAOT Publications ACE.

Trombly, C. (1993). Anticipating the future: Assessment of occupational function. *American Journal of Occupational Therapy, 47*(3), 253-257.

Trombly, C. (1995). *Occupational therapy for physical dysfunction* (4th ed.). Baltimore, MD: Williams & Wilkins.

Trombly, C., & Wu, C. Y. (1999). Effect of rehabilitation tasks on organization of movement post stroke. *American Journal of Occupational Therapy, 53,* 333-334.

U.S. Department of Health and Human Services. (1999). *Mental health: A report of the surgeon general.* Rockville, MD: U.S. Department of Health and Human Services, Substance Abuse and Mental Health Services Administration, Center for Mental Health Services, National Institutes of Health, National Institute of Mental Health.

Unruh, A. M., & Elvin, N. (2004). In the eye of the dragon: Women's experience of breast cancer and the occupation of dragon boat racing. *Canadian Journal of Occupational Therapy, 71*(3), 138-149.

Unruh, A. M., Versnel, J., & Kerr, N. (2002). Spirituality unplugged: A review of commonalities and contentions, and a resolution. *Canadian Journal of Occupational Therapy, 69*(1), 5.

Upham, E. G. (1917). Some principles of occupational therapy. *Modern Hospital, 8,* 409.

Urbanowski, R., & Vargo, J. (1994). Spirituality, daily practice, and the occupational performance model. *Canadian Journal of Occupational Therapy, 61,* 88-94.

van Vliet, P., Sheridan, M., Kerwin, D. G., & Fentem, P. (1995). The influence of functional goals on the kinematics of reaching following stroke. *APTA Neurology Report, 19,* 11-15.

Venable, E., Hanson, C., Shechtman, O., & Dasler, P. (2000). The effects of exercise on occupational functioning in the well elderly. *Physical & Occupational Therapy in Geriatrics, 17*(4), 29-42.

Versluys, H. (1980). The remediation of role disorders through focused group work. *American Journal of Occupational Therapy, 34,* 609-614.

Vik, K., Lilja, M., & Nygård, L. (2007). The influence of the environment on participation subsequent to rehabilitation as experienced by elderly people in Norway. *Scandinavian Journal of Occupational Therapy, 14*(2), 86-95.

Vrkljan, B., & Miller-Polgar, J. (2007). Linking occupational participation and occupational identity: An exploratory study of the transition from driving to driving cessation in older adulthood. *Journal of Occupational Science, 14*(1), 30-39.

Wada, M., Backman, C. L., & Forwell, S. J. (2010). Theoretical perspectives of balance and the influence of gender ideologies. *Journal of Occupational Science, 17*(2), 92-103.

Wagman, P., Håkansson, C., & Björklund, A. (2012). Occupational balance as used in occupational therapy: A concept analysis. *Scandinavian Journal of Occupational Therapy, 19,* 322-327.

Wagman, P., Håkansson, C., Jacobsson, C., Falkmer, T., & Björklund, A. (2012). What is considered important for life balance? Similarities and differences among some working adults. *Scandinavian Journal of Occupational Therapy, 19*(4), 377-384

Wagstaff, S. (2005). Supports and barriers for exercise participation for well elders: Implications for occupational therapy. *Physical & Occupational Therapy in Geriatrics, 24*(2), 19-33.

Wahl, H. W. (2001). Environmental influences on aging and behavior. *Handbook of the Psychology of Aging, 5,* 215-237.

Walker, C. (2001). Occupational adaptation in action: Shift workers and their strategies. *Journal of Occupational Science, 8*(1), 3.

Walker, J. (1930). Occupational therapy. *Occupational Therapy and Rehabilitation, 9,* 195-201.

Wallenbert, I., & Jonsson, H. (2005). Waiting to get better: A dilemma regarding habits in daily occupations after stroke. *American Journal of Occupational Therapy, 59,* 218-224.

Walz, N. C., & Baranek, G. T. (2006). Sensory processing patterns in persons with Angelman syndrome. *American Journal of Occupational Therapy, 60,* 472-479.

Whalley-Hammell, K. (2004). Dimensions of meaning in the occupations of daily life. *Canadian Journal of Occupational Therapy, 71,* 296-305.

White, B. P., Mulligan, S., Merrill, K., & Wright, J. (2007). An examination of the relationships between motor and process skills and scores on the Sensory Profile. *American Journal of Occupational Therapy, 61,* 154-160.

Whiteford, G., & Hocking, C. (2012). *Occupational Science: Society, Inclusion, Participation.* Chichester, UK: Wiley-Blackwell.

Whiteford, G., & Wilcock, A. A. (2000). Cultural relativism: Occupation and independence reconsidered. *Canadian Journal of Occupational Therapy, 67,* 324-336.

Whyte, C., Lentin, P., & Farnworth, L. (2013). An investigation into the role and meaning of occupation for people living with on-going health conditions. *Australian Occupational Therapy Journal, 60*(1), 20-29.

Whyte, J., & Hart, T. (2003). It's more than a black box; it's a Russian doll: Defining rehabilitation treatments. *American Journal of Physical Medicine and Rehabilitation, 82*, 639-652.

Wilcock, A. A. (1993). Biological and sociocultural aspects of occupation, health, and health promotion. *British Journal of Occupational Therapy, 56*, 200-203.

Wimpenny, K., Forsyth, K., Jones, C., Matheson, L., & Colley, J. (2010). Implementing the model of human occupation across a mental health occupational therapy service: Communities of practice and a participatory change process. *British Journal of Occupational Therapy, 73*(11), 507-516. doi:http://dx.doi.org/10.4276/030802210X12892992239152

Wiseman, L. M., & Whiteford, G. (2007). Life history as a tool for understanding occupation, identity and context. *Journal of Occupational Science, 14*(2), 108-114.

Wlodkowski, R. (2008). *Enhancing adult motivation to learn: A comprehensive guide for teaching all adults* (3rd ed.). San Francisco, CA: Jossey-Bass.

World Health Organization. (2001). *International Classification of Functioning, Disability, and Health (ICF)*. Geneva, Switzerland: World Health Organization.

Wright-St. Clair, V. A. (2012). The case for multiple research methodologies. In G. Whiteford, & C. Hocking (Eds.), *Occupational science: Society, inclusion, participation* (pp. 137-151). Chichester, UK: Wiley-Blackwell.

Wu, C. Y., Trombly, C. A., & Lin, K. C. (1994). The relationship between occupational form and occupational performance: A kinematic perspective. *American Journal of Occupational Therapy, 48*, 679-687.

Wu, C. Y., Trombly, C. A., Tickle-Degnen, L., & Lin, K. C. (1998). The effects of object affordances on functional reach in adults with and without cerebral vascular accident. *American Journal of Occupational Therapy, 52*, 447-456.

Wu, C. Y., Trombly, C. A., Tickle-Degnen, L., & Lin, K. C. (2000). A kinematic study of contextual effects on reaching performance in persons with and without stroke: Influences of object availability. *Archives of Physical Medicine and Rehabilitation, 81*, 95-101.

Yamada, T., Kawamata, H., Kobayashi, N., Kielhofner, G., & Taylor, R. R. (2010). A randomized clinical trial of a wellness programme for healthy older people. *British Journal of Occupational Therapy, 73*(11), 540-548. doi:http://dx.doi.org/10.4276/030802210X12892992239314

Yerxa, E. J. (1980). Occupational therapy's role in creating a future climate of caring. *American Journal of Occupational Therapy, 34*(8), 529-534.

Yerxa, E. J. (1991) Occupational therapy: an endangered species or an academic discipline in the 21st century? *American Journal of Occupational Therapy, 45*(8), 680-685.

Yerxa, E. J. (1998). Health and the human spirit for occupation. *American Journal of Occupational Therapy, 52*, 412-418.

Zeidner, M., & Endler, N. S. (Eds). (1996). *Handbook of coping: Theory, research and applications*. New York, NY: Wiley and Sons.

Zemke, R. (2004). The 2004 Eleanor Clarke Slagle Lecture: Time, space, and the kaleidoscopes of occupation. *American Journal of Occupational Therapy, 58*, 608-620.

Zemke, R., & Clark, F. (1996). *Occupational science: The evolving discipline*. Philadelphia, PA: F. A. Davis.

Zoltan, B. (2007). *Vision, perception, and cognition: A manual for the evaluation and treatment of the adult with acquired brain injury* (4th ed.). Thorofare, NJ: SLACK Incorporated.

Zwicker, J. G., & Harris, S. R. (2009). A reflection on motor learning theory in pediatric occupational therapy practice. *Canadian Journal of Occupational Therapy, 76*, 29-37.

Appendix

Database of Articles on Occupation From 2012 to 2000

2012

Aguilar, A., Stupans, I., Scutter, S., & King, S. (2012). Exploring professionalism: The professional values of Australian occupational therapists. *Australian Occupational Therapy Journal, 59*(3), 209-217. doi:http://dx.doi.org/10.1111/j.1440-1630.2012.00996.x

Arbesman, M., & Mosley, L. J. (2012). Systematic review of occupation- and activity-based health management and maintenance interventions for community-dwelling older adults. *American Journal of Occupational Therapy, 66*(3), 277-283. doi:http://dx.doi.org/10.5014/ajot.2012.003327

Argentzell, E., Leufstadius, C., & Eklund, M. (2012). Factors influencing subjective perceptions of everyday occupations: Comparing day centre attendees with non-attendees. *Scandinavian Journal of Occupational Therapy, 19*(1), 68-77. doi:http://dx.doi.org/10.3109/11038128.2011.560963

Armstrong, D. (2012). Examining the evidence for interventions with children with developmental coordination disorder. *British Journal of Occupational Therapy, 75*(12), 532-540. doi:http://dx.doi.org/10.4276/030802212X13548955545413

Atasavun Uysal, S., & Düger, T. (2012). Visual perception training on social skills and activity performance in low-vision children. *Scandinavian Journal of Occupational Therapy, 19*(1), 33-41. doi:http://dx.doi.org/10.3109/11038128.2011.582512

Au, E. H., McCluskey, A., & Lannin, N. A. (2012). Inter-rater reliability of three adult handwriting legibility instruments. *Australian Occupational Therapy Journal, 59*(5), 347-354. doi:http://dx.doi.org/10.1111/j.1440-1630.2012.01035.x

Bacon, N., Farnworth, L., & Boyd, R. (2012). The use of Wii Fit in forensic mental health: Exercise for people at risk of obesity. *British Journal of Occupational Therapy, 75*(2), 61-68. doi:http://dx.doi.org/10.4276/030802212X13286281650992

Bagatell, N. (2012). Engaged moments: Mediated action and children with autism in the classroom setting. *OTJR: Occupation, Participation & Health, 32*(1), 258-265.

Bagby, M., S., Dickie, V. A., & Baranek, G. T. (2012). How sensory experiences of children with and without autism affect family occupations. *American Journal of Occupational Therapy, 66*(1), 78-86. doi:http://dx.doi.org/10.5014/ajot.2012.000604

Bannigan, K., & Spring, H. (2012). The evidence base for occupational therapy in mental health: More systematic reviews are needed. *Occupational Therapy in Mental Health, 28*(4), 321-339. doi:http://dx.doi.org/10.1080/0164212X.2012.708573

Basiletti, M., & Townsend, E. (2012). Group decision making in an intersectoral mental health community partnership. *British Journal of Occupational Therapy, 75*(5), 223-229. doi:http://dx.doi.org/10.4276/030802212X13361458480289

Beagan, B. L., De Souza, L., Godbout, C., Hamilton, L., MacLeod, J., Paynter, E., & Tobin, A. (2012). "This is the biggest thing you'll ever do in your life": Exploring the occupations of transgendered people. *Journal of Occupational Science, 19*(3), 226-240. doi:http://dx.doi.org/10.1080/14427591.2012.659169

Beeden, L. (2012). Transformative occupation in practice: Changing media images and lives of people with disabilities. *OTJR: Occupation, Participation & Health, 32*(1), S15-S24.

Bonsall, A. (2012). An examination of the pairing between narrative and occupational science. *Scandinavian Journal of Occupational Therapy, 19*(1), 92-103. doi:http://dx.doi.org/10.3109/11038128.2011.552119

Bowyer, P., Lee, J., Kramer, J., Taylor, R. R., & Kielhofner, G. (2012). Determining the clinical utility of the short child occupational profile (SCOPE). *British Journal of Occupational Therapy, 75*(1), 19-28. doi:http://dx.doi.org/10.4276/030802212X13261082051373

Carman, S. N., & Chapparo, C. J. (2012). Children who experience difficulties with learning: Mother and child perceptions of social competence. *Australian Occupational Therapy Journal, 59*(5), 339-346. doi:http://dx.doi.org/10.1111/j.1440-1630.2012.01034.x

Chippendale, T., & Bear-Lehman, J. (2012). Effect of life review writing on depressive symptoms in older adults: A randomized controlled trial. *American Journal of Occupational Therapy, 66*(4), 438-446. doi:http://dx.doi.org/10.5014/ajot.2012.004291

McColl MA, Law, MC, Stewart D.
Theoretical Basis of Occupational Therapy, Third Edition (pp. 149-177).
© 2015 Taylor & Francis Group.

Colquhoun, H. L., Letts, L. J., Law, M. C., MacDermid, J. C., & Missiuna, C. A. (2012). Administration of the Canadian Occupational Performance Measure: Effect on practice. *Canadian Journal of Occupational Therapy, 79*(2), 120-128. doi:http://dx.doi.org/10.2182/cjot.2012.79.2.7

Corvinelli, A. (2012). Boredom in recovery for adult substance users with HIV/AIDS attending an urban day treatment program. *Occupational Therapy in Mental Health, 28*(3), 201-319. doi:http://dx.doi.org/10.1080/0164212X.2012.708643

de Brito Brandão, M., Gordon, A. M., & Cotta Mancini, M. (2012). Functional impact of constraint therapy and bimanual training in children with cerebral palsy: A randomized controlled trial. *American Journal of Occupational Therapy, 66*(6), 672-681. doi:http://dx.doi.org/10.5014/ajot.2012.004622

Dunn, W., Cox, J., Foster, L., Mische-Lawson, L., & Tanquary, J. (2012). Impact of a contextual intervention on child participation and parent competence among children with autism spectrum disorders: A pretest-posttest repeated-measures design. *American Journal of Occupational Therapy, 66*(5), 520-528. doi:http://dx.doi.org/10.5014/ajot.2012.004119

Eakman, A. M., & Eklund, M. (2012). The relative impact of personality traits, meaningful occupation and occupational value on meaning in life and life satisfaction. *Journal of Occupational Science, 19*(2), 165-177. doi:http://dx.doi.org/10.1080/1442759 1.2012.671762

Eckel, E. (2012). Community dwelling elderly women and meal preparation. *Physical & Occupational Therapy in Geriatrics, 30*(4), 344-360. doi:http://dx.doi.org/10.3109/02703181.201 2.720005

Eklund, M., Hermansson, A., & Håkansson, C. (2012). Meaning in life for people with schizophrenia: Does it include occupation? *Journal of Occupational Science, 19*(2), 93-105. doi:http://dx.doi.org/10.1080/14427591.2011.605833

Enemark Larsen, A., & Carlsson, G. (2012). Utility of the Canadian Occupational Performance Measure as an admission and outcome measure in interdisciplinary community-based geriatric rehabilitation. *Scandinavian Journal of Occupational Therapy, 19*(2), 204-213. doi:http://dx.doi.org/10.3109/11038128.201 1.574151

Estes, J., & Pierce, D. E. (2012). Pediatric therapists' perspectives on occupation-based practice. *Scandinavian Journal of Occupational Therapy, 19*(1), 17-25. doi:http://dx.doi.org/10.3 109/11038128.2010.547598

Fieldhouse, J. (2012). Community participation and recovery for mental health service users: An action research inquiry. *British Journal of Occupational Therapy, 75*(9), 419-428. doi:http://dx.doi.org/10.4276/030802212X13470263980838

Fleming, J., Sampson, J., Cornwell, P., Turner, B., & Griffin, J. (2012). Brain injury rehabilitation: The lived experience of inpatients and their family caregivers. *Scandinavian Journal of Occupational Therapy, 19*(2), 184-193. doi:http://dx.doi.org/10.3109/11038128.2011.611531

Flinn, S. R., Pease, W. S., & Freimer, M. L. (2012). Score reliability and construct validity of the Flinn Performance Screening Tool for adults with symptoms of carpal tunnel syndrome. *American Journal of Occupational Therapy, 66*(3), 330-337. doi:http://dx.doi.org/10.5014/ajot.2012.000935

Forhan, M. A., Law, M. C., Taylor, V. H., & Vrkljan, B. H. (2012). Factors associated with the satisfaction of participation in daily activities for adults with class III obesity. *OTJR: Occupation, Participation & Health, 32*(3), 70-78.

Fox, J., & Quinn, S. (2012). The meaning of social activism to older adults in Ireland. *Journal of Occupational Science, 19*(4), 358-370. doi:http://dx.doi.org/10.1080/14427591.2012.701179

Gitlow, L., Eastman, E., Gefell, A., & Spangenberg, C. (2012). Assessing assistive device needs of community dwelling older adults in Tompkins County. *Physical & Occupational Therapy in Geriatrics, 30*(4), 368-382. doi:http://dx.doi.org/10.3109/02 703181.2012.736125

Guay, M., Dubois, M., Desrosiers, J., & Robitaille, J. (2012). Identifying characteristics of 'straightforward cases' for which support personnel could recommend home bathing equipment. *British Journal of Occupational Therapy, 75*(12), 563-569. doi:http://dx.doi.org/10.4276/030802212X13548955545576

Guptill, C. (2012). Injured professional musicians and the complex relationship between occupation and health. *Journal of Occupational Science, 19*(3), 258-270. doi:http://dx.doi.org/10.1080/14427591.2012.670901

Gustafsson, L., Mitchell, G., Fleming, J., & Price, G. (2012). Clinical utility of the Canadian Occupational Performance Measure in spinal cord injury rehabilitation. *British Journal of Occupational Therapy, 75*(7), 337-342. doi:http://dx.doi.org/1 0.4276/030802212X13418284515910

Hand, C., Law, M. C., McColl, M. A., Hanna, S., & Elliott, S. J. (2012). Neighborhood influences on participation among older adults with chronic health conditions: A scoping review. *OTJR: Occupation, Participation & Health, 32*(3), 95-103.

Holmqvist, K., Kamwendo, K., & Ivarsson, A. (2012). Occupational therapists' practice patterns for clients with cognitive impairment following acquired brain injury: Development of a questionnaire. *Scandinavian Journal of Occupational Therapy, 19*(2), 150-163. doi:http://dx.doi.org/10.3109/11038128.2011 .576428

Honaker, D., Rosello, S., & Candler, C. (2012). Test-retest reliability of family L.I.F.E. (looking into family experiences): An occupation-based assessment. *American Journal of Occupational Therapy, 66*(5), 617-620. doi:http://dx.doi.org/10.5014/ajot.2012.004002

Ikiugu, M. N. (2012). The test-retest reliability and predictive validity of a battery of newly developed occupational performance assessments. *Occupational Therapy in Mental Health, 28*(1), 51-71. doi:http://dx.doi.org/10.1080/0164212X.2012.650985

Ikiugu, M., Pollard, N., Cross, A., Willer, M., Everson, J., & Stockland, J. (2012). Meaning making through occupations and occupational roles: A heuristic study of worker-writer histories. *British Journal of Occupational Therapy, 75*(6), 289-295. doi:http://dx.doi.org/10.4276/030802212X13383757345229

Kadar, M., McDonald, R., & Lentin, P. (2012). Evidence-based practice in occupational therapy services for children with autism spectrum disorders in Victoria, Australia. *Australian Occupational Therapy Journal, 59*(4), 284-293. doi:http://dx.doi.org/10.1111/j.1440-1630.2012.01015.x

Källdalen, A., Marcusson, J., Nägga, K., & Wressle, E. (2012). Occupational performance problems in 85-year-old women and men in Sweden. *OTJR: Occupation, Participation & Health, 32*(2), 30-38.

Kniepmann, K. (2012). Female family carers for survivors of stroke: Occupational loss and quality of life. *British Journal of Occupational Therapy, 75*(5), 208-216. doi:http://dx.doi.org/10.4276/030802212X13361458480207

Koome, F., Hocking, C., & Sutton, D. (2012). Why routines matter: The nature and meaning of family routines in the context of adolescent mental illness. *Journal of Occupational Science, 19*(4), 312-325. doi:http://dx.doi.org/10.1080/144275 91.2012.718245

Kramer-Roy, D. (2012). Supporting ethnic minority families with disabled children: Learning from Pakistani families. *British Journal of Occupational Therapy, 75*(10), 442-448. doi:http:// dx.doi.org/10.4276/030802212X13496921049581

Landa-Gonzalez, B., & Molnar, D. (2012). Occupational therapy intervention: Effects on self-care, performance, satisfaction, self-esteem/self-efficacy, and role functioning of older Hispanic females with arthritis. *Occupational Therapy in Health Care, 26*(2), 109-119. doi:http://dx.doi.org/10.3109/07 380577.2011.644624

Lantz, K., Marcusson, J., & Wressle, E. (2012). Perceived participation and health-related quality of life in 85 year olds in Sweden. *OTJR: Occupation, Participation & Health, 32*(4), 117-125.

Law, M., King, G., Petrenchik, T., Kertoy, M., & Anaby, D. (2012). The assessment of preschool children's participation: Internal consistency and construct validity. *Physical & Occupational Therapy in Pediatrics, 32*(3), 272-287. doi:http://dx.doi.org/10. 3109/01942638.2012.662584

Lindström, M., Hariz, G., & Bernspång, B. (2012). Dealing with real-life challenges: Outcomes of a home-based occupational therapy intervention for people with severe psychiatric disability. *OTJR: Occupation, Participation & Health, 32*(2), 5-13.

Lund, A., Michelet, M., Kjeken, I., Wyller, T. B., & Sveen, U. (2012). Development of a person-centred lifestyle intervention for older adults following a stroke or transient ischaemic attack. *Scandinavian Journal of Occupational Therapy, 19*(2), 140-149. doi:http://dx.doi.org/10.3109/11038128.2011.603353

Lyons, K., Doyle, Hegel, M. T., Hull, J. G., Li, Z., Balan, S., & Bartels, S. (2012). Reliability and validity of the valued activity inventory for adults with cancer. *OTJR: Occupation, Participation & Health, 32*(1), 238-245.

Maclean, F., Carin-Levy, G., Hunter, H., Malcolmson, L., & Locke, E. (2012). The usefulness of the Person-Environment-Occupation model in an acute physical health care setting. *British Journal of Occupational Therapy, 75*(12), 555-562. doi:http://dx.doi.org/10.4276/030802212X13548955545530

Magasi, S. (2012). Negotiating the social service systems: A vital yet frequently invisible occupation. *OTJR: Occupation, Participation & Health, 32*(1), S25-S33.

Mason, J., & Conneeley, L. (2012). The meaning of participation in an allotment project for fathers of preschool children. *British Journal of Occupational Therapy, 75*(5), 230-236. doi:http:// dx.doi.org/10.4276/030802212X13361458480324

Matovu, S. N., La cour, K., & Hemmingsson, H. (2012). Narratives of Ugandan women adhering to HIV/AIDS medication. *Occupational Therapy International, 19*(4), 176-184. doi:http:// dx.doi.org/10.1002/oti.1330

Matuska, K. (2012). Description and development of the life balance inventory. *OTJR: Occupation, Participation & Health, 32*(1), 220-228.

McElroy, T., Muyinda, H., Atim, S., Spittal, P., & Backman, C. (2012). War, displacement and productive occupations in northern Uganda. *Journal of Occupational Science, 19*(3), 198-212. doi:http://dx.doi.org/10.1080/14427591.2011.614681

Mirza, M. (2012). Occupational upheaval during resettlement and migration: Findings of global ethnography with refugees with disabilities. *OTJR: Occupation, Participation & Health, 32*(1), S6-S14.

Morgan, R., & Long, T. (2012). The effectiveness of occupational therapy for children with developmental coordination disorder: A review of the qualitative literature. *British Journal of Occupational Therapy, 75*(1), 10-18. doi:http://dx.doi.org/10.4 276/030802212X13261082051337

Morris, K. F. (2012). Thesis abstracts: Occupational engagement in a regional secure unit [abstract]. *British Journal of Occupational Therapy, 75*(8), 358.

Mulry, C. M. (2012). Transitions to assisted living: A pilot study of residents' occupational perspectives. *Physical & Occupational Therapy in Geriatrics, 30*(4), 328-343. doi:http://dx.doi.org/ 10.3109/02703181.2012.741190

Nayar, S., Hocking, C., & Giddings, L. (2012). Using occupation to navigate cultural spaces: Indian immigrant women settling in New Zealand. *Journal of Occupational Science, 19*(1), 62-75. doi:http://dx.doi.org/10.1080/14427591.2011.602628

Nelson, A., & Wilson, L. (2012). Occupational understandings from the experiences of Holocaust survivors. *Journal of Occupational Science, 19*(2), 178-190. doi:http://dx.doi.org/10 .1080/14427591.2011.595892

Nilsen, D. M., Gillen, G., DiRusso, T., & Gordon, A. M. (2012). Effect of imagery perspective on occupational performance after stroke: A randomized controlled trial. *American Journal of Occupational Therapy, 66*(3), 320-329. doi:http://dx.doi. org/10.5014/ajot.2012.003475

Njelesani, J., Cameron, D., & Polatajko, H. J. (2012). Occupation-for-development: Expanding the boundaries of occupational science into the international development agenda. *Journal of Occupational Science, 19*(1), 36-43. doi:http://dx.doi.org/10.10 80/14427591.2011.639665

Nott, M. T., & Chapparo, C. (2012). Exploring the validity of the perceive, recall, plan and perform system of task analysis: Cognitive strategy use in adults with brain injury. *British Journal of Occupational Therapy, 75*(6), 256-263. doi:http:// dx.doi.org/10.4276/030802212X13383757345067

O'Donoghue, N., & McKay, E. A. (2012). Exploring the impact of sleep apnoea on daily life and occupational engagement. *British Journal of Occupational Therapy, 75*(11), 509-516. doi:http://dx.doi.org/10.4276/030802212X13522194759932

Orellano, E. M., Ito, M., Dorne, R., Irizarry, D., & Dávila, R. (2012). Occupational participation of older adults: Reliability and validity of the activity card sort—Puerto Rican version. *OTJR: Occupation, Participation & Health, 32*(1), 266-272.

Orellano, E., Colón, W. I., & Arbesman, M. (2012). Effect of occupation- and activity-based interventions on instrumental activities of daily living performance among community-dwelling older adults: A systematic review. *American Journal of Occupational Therapy, 66*(3), 292-300. doi:http://dx.doi. org/10.5014/ajot.2012.003053

Parvaneh, S., & Cocks, E. (2012). Framework for describing community integration for people with acquired brain injury. *Australian Occupational Therapy Journal, 59*(2), 131-137. doi:http://dx.doi.org/10.1111/j.1440-1630.2012.01001.x

Peralta-Catipon, T. (2012). Collective occupations among Filipina migrant workers: Bridging disrupted identities. *OTJR: Occupation, Participation & Health, 32*(2), 14-21.

Piernik-Yoder, B., & Beck, A. (2012). The use of standardized assessments in occupational therapy in the United States. *Occupational Therapy in Health Care, 26*(2), 97-108. doi:http://dx.doi.org/10.3109/07380577.2012.695103

Polatajko, H. J., McEwen, S. E., Ryan, J. D., & Baum, C. M. (2012). Pilot randomized controlled trial investigating cognitive strategy use to improve goal performance after stroke. *American Journal of Occupational Therapy, 66*(1), 104-109. doi:http://dx.doi.org/10.5014/ajot.2012.001784

Precin, P., Otto, M., Popalzai, K., & Samuel, M. (2012). The role for occupational therapists in community mobility training for people with autism spectrum disorders. *Occupational Therapy in Mental Health, 28*(2), 129-146. doi:http://dx.doi.org/10.1080/0164212X.2012.679533

Ripat, J., & Becker, P. (2012). Playground usability: What do playground users say? *Occupational Therapy International, 19*(3), 144-153. doi:http://dx.doi.org/10.1002/oti.1331

Robinson, K., Kennedy, N., & Harmon, D. (2012). Happiness: A review of evidence relevant to occupational science. *Journal of Occupational Science, 19*(2), 150-164. doi:http://dx.doi.org/10.1080/14427591.2011.634780

Sakuae, M., & Reid, D. (2012). Making tea in place: Experiences of women engaged in a Japanese tea ceremony. *Journal of Occupational Science, 19*(3), 283-291. doi:http://dx.doi.org/10.1080/14427591.2011.610775

Schulz, C. H., Hersch, G. I., Foust, J. L., Wyatt, A. L., Godwin, K. M., Virani, S., & Ostwald, S. K. (2012). Identifying occupational performance barriers of stroke survivors: Utilization of a home assessment. *Physical & Occupational Therapy in Geriatrics, 30*(2), 109-123. doi:http://dx.doi.org/10.3109/02703181.2012.687441

Scott, P. J., & Brown, V. L. (2012). Resumption of valued activities in the first year post liver transplant. *Occupational Therapy in Health Care, 26*(1), 48-63. doi:http://dx.doi.org/10.3109/07380577.2011.643856

Sharp, N., Dunford, C., & Seddon, L. (2012). A critical appraisal of how occupational therapists can enable participation in adaptive physical activity for children and young people. *British Journal of Occupational Therapy, 75*(11), 486-494. doi:http://dx.doi.org/10.4276/030802212X13522194759815

Skubik-Peplaski, C., Carrico, C., Nichols, L., Chelette, K., & Sawaki, L. (2012). Behavioral, neurophysiological, and descriptive changes after occupation-based intervention. *American Journal of Occupational Therapy, 66*(6), e107-e113. doi:http://dx.doi.org/10.5014/ajot.2012.003590

Skubik-Peplaski, C., Rowles, G. D., & Hunter, E. G. (2012). Toward a physical environmental continuum for occupational intervention in a rehabilitation hospital. *Occupational Therapy in Health Care, 26*(1), 33-47. doi:http://dx.doi.org/10.3109/07380577.2011.621018

Sperens, M., Munkholm, M., & Fisher, A. G. (2012). Gender differences in quality of schoolwork task performance among typically developing students and students at risk of or with mild disabilities. *Scandinavian Journal of Occupational Therapy, 19*(1), 9-16. doi:http://dx.doi.org/10.3109/11038128.2010.533189

Stav, W. B., Hallenen, T., Lane, J., & Arbesman, M. (2012). Systematic review of occupational engagement and health outcomes among community-dwelling older adults. *American Journal of Occupational Therapy, 66*(3), 301-310. doi:http://dx.doi.org/10.5014/ajot.2012.003707

Sutton, D. J., Hocking, C. S., & Smythe, L. A. (2012). A phenomenological study of occupational engagement in recovery from mental illness. *Canadian Journal of Occupational Therapy, 79*(3), 142-150. doi:http://dx.doi.org/10.2182/cjot.2012.79.3.3

Tatzer, V. C., van Nes, F., & Jonsson, H. (2012). Understanding the role of occupation in ageing: Four life stories of older Viennese women. *Journal of Occupational Science, 19*(2), 138-149. doi:http://dx.doi.org/10.1080/14427591.2011.610774

Tomori, K., Uezu, S., Kinjo, S., Ogahara, K., Nagatani, R., & Higashi, T. (2012). Utilization of the iPad application: Aid for decision-making in occupation choice. *Occupational Therapy International, 19*(2), 88-97. doi:http://dx.doi.org/10.1002/oti.325

Turner, K. A., Cohn, E. S., & Koomar, J. (2012). Mothering when mothers and children both have sensory processing challenges. *British Journal of Occupational Therapy, 75*(10), 449-455. doi:http://dx.doi.org/10.4276/030802212X13496921049626

Turpin, M. J., Rodger, S., & Hall, A. R. (2012). Occupational therapy students' perceptions of occupational therapy. *Australian Occupational Therapy Journal, 59*(5), 367-374. doi:http://dx.doi.org/10.1111/j.1440-1630.2011.00988.x

van Nes, F., Jonsson, H., Hirschler, S., Abma, T., & Deeg, D. (2012). Meanings created in co-occupation: Construction of a late-life couple's photo story. *Journal of Occupational Science, 19*(4), 341-357. doi:http://dx.doi.org/10.1080/14427591.2012.679604

Wallen, M. A., & Ziviani, J. M. (2012). Canadian Occupational Performance Measure: Impact of blinded parent-proxy ratings on outcome. *Canadian Journal of Occupational Therapy, 79*(1), 7-14. doi:http://dx.doi.org/10.2182/cjot.2012.79.1.2

Wensley, R., & Slade, A. (2012). Walking as a meaningful leisure occupation: The implications for occupational therapy. *British Journal of Occupational Therapy, 75*(2), 85-92. doi:http://dx.doi.org/10.4276/030802212X13286281651117

Witsø, A. E., Eide, A. H., & Vik, K. (2012). Older homecare service recipients' satisfaction with participation in daily life activities. *Physical & Occupational Therapy in Geriatrics, 30*(2), 85-101. doi:http://dx.doi.org/10.3109/02703181.2012.678970

Wright-St Clair, V. (2012). Being occupied with what matters in advanced age. *Journal of Occupational Science, 19*(1), 44-53. doi:http://dx.doi.org/10.1080/14427591.2011.639135

York, M., & Wiseman, T. (2012). Gardening as an occupation: A critical review. *British Journal of Occupational Therapy, 75*(2), 76-84. doi:http://dx.doi.org/10.4276/030802212X13286281651072

Zachry, A. H., & Mitchell, A. W. (2012). Goal-directed actions and early experience with crawling. *OTJR: Occupation, Participation & Health, 32*(2), 48-55.

2011

Absolom, S., & Roberts, A. (2011). Connecting with others: The meaning of social eating as an everyday occupation for young people. *Journal of Occupational Science, 18*(4), 339-346. doi:http://dx.doi.org/10.1080/14427591.2011.586324

Aiken, F. E., Fourt, A. M., Cheng I. K. S., & Polatajko, H. J. (2011). The meaning gap in occupational therapy: Finding meaning in our own occupation. *Canadian Journal of Occupational Therapy, 78*(5), 294-302. doi:http://dx.doi.org/10.2182/cjot.2011.78.5.4

Aldrich, R. M., & Callanan, Y. (2011). Insights about researching discouraged workers. *Journal of Occupational Science, 18*(2), 153-166. doi:http://dx.doi.org/10.1080/14427591.2011.575756

Amini, D. (2011). Occupational therapy interventions for work-related injuries and conditions of the forearm, wrist, and hand: A systematic review. *American Journal of Occupational Therapy, 65*(1), 29-36. doi:http://dx.doi.org/10.5014/ajot.2011.09186

Anderson, L., Cross, A., Wynthein, D., Schmidt, L., & Grutz, K. (2011). Effects of Dynavision training as a preparatory intervention status postcerebrovascular accident: A case report. *Occupational Therapy in Health Care, 25*(4), 270-282. doi:http://dx.doi.org/10.3109/07380577.2011.589888

Andersson, C., Eklund, M., Sundh, V., Thundal, K., & Spak, F. (2011). Women's patterns of everyday occupations and alcohol consumption. *Scandinavian Journal of Occupational Therapy, 19*(3), 225-238. doi:http://dx.doi.org/10.3109/11038128.2010.527013

Arbesman, M., & Logsdon, D. (2011). Occupational therapy interventions for employment and education for adults with serious mental illness: A systematic review. *American Journal of Occupational Therapy, 65*(3), 238-246. doi:http://dx.doi.org/10.5014/ajot.2011.001289

Asaba, E., & Jackson, J. (2011). Social ideologies embedded in everyday life: A narrative analysis about disability, identities, and occupation. *Journal of Occupational Science, 18*(2), 139-152. doi:http://dx.doi.org/10.1080/14427591.2011.579234

Barclay, L., Callaway, L., McDonald, R., Farnworth, L., Brown, T., & Broom, L. (2011). Time use following spinal cord injury: An examination of the literature. *British Journal of Occupational Therapy, 74*(12), 573-580. doi:http://dx.doi.org/10.4276/030802211X13232584581452

Barstow, B. A., Bennett, D. K., & Vogtle, L. K. (2011). Perspectives on home safety: Do home safety assessments address the concerns of clients with vision loss? *American Journal of Occupational Therapy, 65*(6), 635-642. doi:http://dx.doi.org/10.5014/ajot.2011.001909

Bauerschmidt, B., & Nelson, D. L. (2011). The terms occupation and activity over the history of official occupational therapy publications. *American Journal of Occupational Therapy, 65*(3), 338-345. doi:http://dx.doi.org/10.5014/ajot.2011.000869

Beagan, B. L., & D'Sylva, A. (2011). Occupational meanings of food preparation for Goan Canadian women. *Journal of Occupational Science, 18*(3), 210-222. doi:http://dx.doi.org/10.1080/14427591.2011.586326

Beagan, B. L., & Etowa, J. B. (2011). The meanings and functions of occupations related to spirituality for African Nova Scotian women. *Journal of Occupational Science, 18*(3), 277-290. doi:http://dx.doi.org/10.1080/14427591.2011.594548

Beckelhimer, S. C., Dalton, A. E., Richter, C. A., Hermann, V., & Page, S. J. (2011). Computer-based rhythm and timing training in severe, stroke-induced arm hemiparesis. *American Journal of Occupational Therapy, 65*(1), 96-100. doi:http://dx.doi.org/10.5014/ajot.2011.09158

Bradley, D. M., Hersch, G., Reistetter, T., & Reed, K. (2011). Occupational participation of homeless people. *Occupational Therapy in Mental Health, 27*(1), 26-35. doi:http://dx.doi.org/10.1080/0164212X.2010.518311

Broom, L., Stagnitti, K., & Pepin, G. (2011). Exploring engagement in meaningful occupations following primary brain tumour diagnosis [abstract]. Occupational Therapy Australia 24th National Conference & Exhibition, 29th June-1st July, Gold Coast Convention & Exhibition Centre. *Australian Occupational Therapy Journal, 58*, 89. doi:http://dx.doi.org/10.1111/j.1440-1630.2011.00938.x

Brown, J. A. (2011). Talking about life after early psychosis: The impact on occupational performance. *Canadian Journal of Occupational Therapy, 78*(3), 156-163. doi:http://dx.doi.org/10.2182/cjot.2011.78.3.3

Carson, C., Cummins, A., Bye, R., & Faddy, K. (2011). Occupational engagement of women with post-breast cancer lymphoedema: Using women's perspectives to create an evidence-base [abstract]. Occupational Therapy Australia 24th National Conference & Exhibition, 29th June-1st July, Gold Coast Convention & Exhibition Centre. *Australian Occupational Therapy Journal, 58*, 71-72. doi:http://dx.doi.org/10.1111/j.1440-1630.2011.00938.x

Cheah, S., & Presnell, S. (2011). Older people's experiences of acute hospitalisation: An investigation of how occupations are affected. *Australian Occupational Therapy Journal, 58*(2), 120-128. doi:http://dx.doi.org/10.1111/j.1440-1630.2010.00878.x

Cohn, E., May-Benson, T., & Teasdale, A. (2011). The relationship between behaviors associated with sensory processing and parental sense of competence. *OTJR: Occupation, Participation & Health, 31*(4), 172.

Copley, J. A., Rodger, S. A., Graham, F. P., & Hannay, V. A. (2011). Facilitating student occupational therapists' mastery of occupation-centred approaches for working with children. *Canadian Journal of Occupational Therapy, 78*(1), 37-44. doi:http://dx.doi.org/10.2182/cjot.2011.78.1.5

Crowe, T. K., & Michael, H. J. (2011). Time use of mothers with adolescents: A lasting impact of a child's disability. *OTJR: Occupation, Participation & Health, 31*(3), 118-126.

Dekkers, M. K., & Nielsen, T. L. (2011). Occupational performance, pain, and global quality of life in women with upper extremity fractures. *Scandinavian Journal of Occupational Therapy, 18*(3), 198-209. doi:http://dx.doi.org/10.3109/11038128.2010.510205

Del Fabro Smith, L., Suto, M., Chalmers, A., & Backman, C. L. (2011). Belief in doing and knowledge in being mothers with arthritis. *OTJR: Occupation, Participation & Health, 31*(1), 40-48. doi:http://dx.doi.org/10.3928/15394492-20100222-01

Dickerson, A. E., Reistetter, T., Davis, E. S., & Monahan, M. (2011). Evaluating driving as a valued instrumental activity of daily living. *American Journal of Occupational Therapy, 65*(1), 64-75. doi:http://dx.doi.org/10.5014/ajot.2011.09052

Dickie, V. A. (2011). Experiencing therapy through doing: Making quilts. *OTJR: Occupation, Participation & Health, 31*(4), 209-215.

Du Toit, S. (2011). Dementia care mapping (DCM): Feasible option for improving the quality of formal dementia care in a developing economy [abstract]? Occupational Therapy Australia 24th National Conference & Exhibition, 29th June-1st July, Gold Coast Convention & Exhibition Centre. *Australian Occupational Therapy Journal, 58*, 41. doi:http://dx.doi.org/10.1111/j.1440-1630.2011.00937.x

Dunford, C. (2011). Goal-orientated group intervention for children with developmental coordination disorder. *Physical & Occupational Therapy in Pediatrics, 31*(3), 288-300. doi:http://dx.doi.org/10.3109/01942638.2011.565864

Eakman, A. M. (2011). Convergent validity of the engagement in meaningful activities survey in a college sample. *OTJR: Occupation, Participation & Health, 31*(1), 23-32.

Eakman, A. M., & Eklund, M. (2011). Reliability and structural validity of an assessment of occupational value. *Scandinavian Journal of Occupational Therapy, 18*(3), 231-240. doi:http://dx.doi.org/10.3109/11038128.2010.521948

Ekstam, L., Tham, K., & Borell, L. (2011). Couples' approaches to changes in everyday life during the first year after stroke. *Scandinavian Journal of Occupational Therapy, 18*(1), 49-58. doi:http://dx.doi.org/10.3109/11038120903578791

Eriksson, G. M., Chung, J. C. C., Beng, L. H., Hartman-Maeir, A., Yoo, E., Orellano, E. M., … Baum, C. (2011). Occupations of older adults: A cross cultural description. *OTJR: Occupation, Participation & Health, 31*(4), 182-192. doi:http://dx.doi.org/10.3928/15394492-20110318-01

Erlandsson, L., Eklund, M., & Persson, D. (2011). Occupational value and relationships to meaning and health: Elaborations of the ValMO-model. *Scandinavian Journal of Occupational Therapy, 18*(1), 72-80. doi:http://dx.doi.org/10.3109/11038121003671619

Fallahpour, M., Tham, K., Joghataei, M. T., Eriksson, G., & Jonsson, H. (2011). Occupational gaps in everyday life after stroke and the relation to functioning and perceived life satisfaction. *OTJR: Occupation, Participation & Health, 31*(4), 200-208.

Fitzgerald, M. (2011). An evaluation of the impact of a social inclusion programme on occupational functioning for forensic service users. *British Journal of Occupational Therapy, 74*(10), 465-472. doi:http://dx.doi.org/10.4276/030802211X13182481841903

Forhan, M., Law, M., Vrkljan, B. H., & Taylor, V. H. (2011). Participation profile of adults with class III obesity. *OTJR: Occupation, Participation & Health, 31*(3), 135-142.

Forsyth, K., Parkinson, S., Kielhofner, G., Kramer, J., Mann, L. S., & Duncan, E. (2011). The measurement properties of the model of human occupation screening tool and implications for practice. *New Zealand Journal of Occupational Therapy, 58*(2), 5-13.

Foster, E. R., & Hershey, T. (2011). Everyday executive function is associated with activity participation in Parkinson disease without dementia. *OTJR: Occupation, Participation & Health, 31*(1), S16-S22.

Fuller, K. (2011). The effectiveness of occupational performance outcome measures within mental health practice. *British Journal of Occupational Therapy, 74*(8), 399-405. doi:http://dx.doi.org/10.4276/030802211X13125646371004

Galvin, D., & Wilding, C. (2011). Taking action to enable human rights and occupational justice in an Australian metropolitan hospital [abstract]. Occupational Therapy Australia 24th National Conference & Exhibition, 29th June-1st July, Gold Coast Convention & Exhibition Centre. *Australian Occupational Therapy Journal, 58*, 19. doi:http://dx.doi.org/10.1111/j.1440-1630.2011.00937.x

Gibbs, L. B., & Klinger, L. (2011). Rest is a meaningful occupation for women with hip and knee osteoarthritis. *OTJR: Occupation, Participation & Health, 31*(3), 143-150.

Gibson, R. W., D'Amico, M., Jaffe, L., & Arbesman, M. (2011). Occupational therapy interventions for recovery in the areas of community integration and normative life roles for adults with serious mental illness: A systematic review. *American Journal of Occupational Therapy, 65*(3), 247-256. doi:http://dx.doi.org/10.5014/ajot.2011.001297

Giesbrecht, E. M., Ripat, J. D., Cooper, J. E., & Quanbury, A. O. (2011). Experiences with using a pushrim-activated power-assisted wheelchair for community-based occupations: A qualitative exploration. *Canadian Journal of Occupational Therapy, 78*(2), 127-136. doi:http://dx.doi.org/10.2182/cjot.2011.78.2.8

Graham, F. (2011). Parents' experiences of engaging in occupational performance coaching (OPC) [abstract]. Occupational Therapy Australia 24th National Conference & Exhibition, 29th June-1st July, Gold Coast Convention & Exhibition Centre. *Australian Occupational Therapy Journal, 58*, 43. doi:http://dx.doi.org/10.1111/j.1440-1630.2011.00937.x

Graham, F. (2011). Occupational performance coaching: A contemporary approach for working with parents of children with occupational challenges. *New Zealand Journal of Occupational Therapy, 58*(2), 41-42.

Hahn-Markowitz, J., Manor, I., & Maeir, A. (2011). Effectiveness of cognitive-functional (cog-fun) intervention with children with attention deficit hyperactivity disorder: A pilot study. *American Journal of Occupational Therapy, 65*(4), 384-392. doi:http://dx.doi.org/10.5014/ajot.2011.000901

Håkansson, C., Björkelund, C., & Eklund, M. (2011). Associations between women's subjective perceptions of daily occupations and life satisfaction, and the role of perceived control. *Australian Occupational Therapy Journal, 58*(6), 397-404. doi:http://dx.doi.org/10.1111/j.1440-1630.2011.00976.x

Harris, M., Gladman, B., Hennessy, N., Lloyd, C., Mowry, B., & Waghorn, G. (2011). Reliability and validity of a measure of role functioning among people with psychiatric disabilities. *Australian Occupational Therapy Journal, 58*(3), 203-208. doi:http://dx.doi.org/10.1111/j.1440-1630.2010.00921.x

Heigl, F., Kinéébanian, A., & Josephsson, S. (2011). I think of my family, therefore I am: Perceptions of daily occupations of some Albanians in Switzerland. *Scandinavian Journal of Occupational Therapy, 18*(1), 36-48. doi:http://dx.doi.org/10.3109/11038120903552648

Hocking, C., Murphy, J., & Reed, K. (2011). Strategies older New Zealanders use to participate in day-to-day occupations. *British Journal of Occupational Therapy, 74*(11), 509-516. doi:http://dx.doi.org/10.4276/030802211X13204135680820

Hon, C., Sun, P., Suto, M., & Forwell, S., J. (2011). Moving from China to Canada: Occupational transitions of immigrant mothers of children with special needs. *Journal of Occupational Science, 18*(3), 223-236. doi:http://dx.doi.org/10.1080/14427591.2011.581627

Hooper, B. (2011). The occupation of teaching: Elements of meaning portrayed through educators' teaching diagrams. *Journal of Occupational Science, 18*(2), 167-181. doi:http://dx.doi.org/10.1080/14427591.2011.575757

Ikiugu, M. N., & Smallfield, S. (2011). Ikiugu's eclectic method of combining theoretical conceptual practice models in occupational therapy. *Australian Occupational Therapy Journal, 58*(6), 437-446. doi:http://dx.doi.org/10.1111/j.1440-1630.2011.00968.x

Jacobs, K., Zhu, L., Dawes, M., Franco, J., Huggins, A., Igari, C., ... Umez-Eronini, A. (2011). Wii health: A preliminary study of the health and wellness benefits of Wii Fit on university students. *British Journal of Occupational Therapy, 74*(6), 262-268. doi:http://dx.doi.org/10.4276/030802211X13074383957823

Jensen, L. E., & Padilla, R. (2011). Effectiveness of interventions to prevent falls in people with Alzheimer's disease and related dementias. *American Journal of Occupational Therapy, 65*(5), 532-540. doi:http://dx.doi.org/10.5014/ajot.2011.002626

Johansson, C., & Isaksson, G. (2011). Experiences of participation in occupations of women on long-term sick leave. *Scandinavian Journal of Occupational Therapy, 18*(4), 294-301. doi:http://dx.doi.org/10.3109/11038128.2010.521950

Johansson, M., & Wressle, E. (2011). Validation of the Neurobehavioral Cognitive Status Examination and the Rivermead Behavioural Memory Test in investigations of dementia. *Scandinavian Journal of Occupational Therapy, 19*(3), 282-287. doi:http://dx.doi.org/10.3109/11038128.2010.528789

Jonsson, H. (2011). The first steps into the third age: The retirement process from a Swedish perspective. *Occupational Therapy International, 18*(1), 32-38. doi:http://dx.doi.org/10.1002/oti.311

Keesing, S., & Rosenwax, L. (2011). Is occupation missing from occupational therapy in palliative care? *Australian Occupational Therapy Journal, 58*(5), 329-336. doi:http://dx.doi.org/10.1111/j.1440-1630.2011.00958.x

Kiepek, N., & Magalhães, L. (2011). Addictions and impulse-control disorders as occupation: A selected literature review and synthesis. *Journal of Occupational Science, 18*(3), 254-276. doi:http://dx.doi.org/10.1080/14427591.2011.581628

Lala, A. P., & Kinsella, E. A. (2011). A phenomenological inquiry into the embodied nature of occupation at end of life. *Canadian Journal of Occupational Therapy, 78*(4), 246-254. doi:http://dx.doi.org/10.2182/cjot.2011.78.4.6

LaVesser, P., & Berg, C. (2011). Participation patterns in preschool children with an autism spectrum disorder. *OTJR: Occupation, Participation & Health, 31*(1), 33-39.

Letts, L., Minezes, J., Edwards, M., Berenyi, J., Moros, K., O'Neill, C., & O'Toole, C. (2011). Effectiveness of interventions designed to modify and maintain perceptual abilities in people with Alzheimer's disease and related dementias. *American Journal of Occupational Therapy, 65*(5), 505-513. doi:http://dx.doi.org/10.5014/ajot.2011.002592

Lexell, E. M., Iwarsson, S., & Lund, M. L. (2011). Occupational adaptation in people with multiple sclerosis. *OTJR: Occupation, Participation & Health, 31*(3), 127-134.

Lindstedt, H., Grann, M., & Söderlund, A. (2011). Mentally disordered offenders' daily occupations after one year of forensic care. *Scandinavian Journal of Occupational Therapy, 18*(4), 302-311. doi:http://dx.doi.org/10.3109/11038128.2010.525720

Lipskaya, L., Jarus, T., & Kotler, M. (2011). Influence of cognition and symptoms of schizophrenia on IADL performance. *Scandinavian Journal of Occupational Therapy, 18*(3), 180-187. doi:http://dx.doi.org/10.3109/11038128.2010.490879

Livingston, M. H., Stewart, D., Rosenbaum, P. L., & Russell, D. J. (2011). Exploring issues of participation among adolescents with cerebral palsy: What's important to them? *Physical & Occupational Therapy in Pediatrics, 31*(3), 275-287. doi:http://dx.doi.org/10.3109/01942638.2011.565866

Mailloux, Z., Mulligan, S., Roley, S. S., Blanche, E., Cermak, S., Coleman, G. G., ... Lane, C. J. (2011). Verification and clarification of patterns of sensory integrative dysfunction. *American Journal of Occupational Therapy, 65*(2), 143-151.

Maloney, S. M. (2011). College student high-risk drinking as a maladaptive serious leisure hobby. *Occupational Therapy in Mental Health, 27*(2), 155-177. doi:http://dx.doi.org/10.1080/0164212X.2011.567351

Martin, L. M., Smith, M., Rogers, J., Wallen, T., & Boisvert, R. (2011). Mothers in recovery: An occupational perspective. *Occupational Therapy International, 18*(3), 152-161. doi:http://dx.doi.org/10.1002/oti.318

McCall, M., McEwen, S., Colantonio, A., Streiner, D., & Dawson, D. R. (2011). Modified constraint-induced movement therapy for elderly clients with subacute stroke. *American Journal of Occupational Therapy, 65*(4), 409-418. doi:http://dx.doi.org/10.5014/ajot.2011.002063

McHugh, C. (2011). Wellbeing following stroke: Lost in translation [abstract]. Occupational Therapy Australia 24th National Conference & Exhibition, 29th June-1st July, Gold Coast Convention & Exhibition Centre. *Australian Occupational Therapy Journal, 58*, 42. doi:http://dx.doi.org/10.1111/j.1440-1630.2011.00937.x

Minkoff, Y., & Riley, J. (2011). Perspectives of time-use: Exploring the use of drawings, interviews and rating-scales with children aged 6-7 years. *Journal of Occupational Science, 18*(4), 306-321. doi:http://dx.doi.org/10.1080/14427591.2011.586323

Morgan, D. (2011). Continued living through occupation at end-of-life [abstract]. Occupational Therapy Australia 24th National Conference & Exhibition, 29th June–1st July, Gold Coast Convention & Exhibition Centre. *Australian Occupational Therapy Journal, 58*, 7. doi:http://dx.doi.org/10.1111/j.1440-1630.2011.00937.x

Morgan-Brown, M., Ormerod, M., Newton, R., & Manley, D. (2011). An exploration of occupation in nursing home residents with dementia. *British Journal of Occupational Therapy, 74*(5), 217-225. doi:http://dx.doi.org/10.4276/030802211X13046730116452

Mountain, G. A., & Craig, C. L. (2011). The lived experience of redesigning lifestyle post-retirement in the UK. *Occupational Therapy International, 18*(1), 48-58. doi:http://dx.doi.org/10.1002/oti.309

Müllersdorf, M., & Ivarsson, A. (2011). Occupation as described by academically skilled occupational therapists in Sweden: A Delphi study. *Scandinavian Journal of Occupational Therapy, 18*(2), 85-92. doi:http://dx.doi.org/10.3109/11038128.2010.483689

Njelesani, J., Sedgwick, A., Davis, J. A., & Polatajko, H. J. (2011). The influence of context: A naturalistic study of Ugandan children's doings in outdoor spaces. *Occupational Therapy International, 18*(3), 124-132. doi:http://dx.doi.org/10.1002/oti.310

Öhman, A., Nygård, L., & Kottorp, A. (2011). Occupational performance and awareness of disability in mild cognitive impairment or dementia. *Scandinavian Journal of Occupational Therapy, 18*(2), 133-142. doi:http://dx.doi.org/10.3109/11038121003645993

Pan, A., Fan, C., Chung, L., Chen, T., Kielhofner, G., Wu, M., & Chen, Y. (2011). Examining the validity of the model of human occupation screening tool: Using classical test theory and item response theory. *British Journal of Occupational Therapy, 74*(1), 34-40. doi:http://dx.doi.org/10.4276/030802211X12947686093648

Parkinson, S., Lowe, C., & Vecsey, T. (2011). The therapeutic benefits of horticulture in a mental health service. *British Journal of Occupational Therapy, 74*(11), 525-534. doi:http://dx.doi.org/10.4276/030802211X13204135680901

Pemberton, S., & Cox, D. (2011). What happened to the time? The relationship of occupational therapy to time. *British Journal of Occupational Therapy, 74*(2), 78-85. doi:http://dx.doi.org/10.4276/030802211X12971689814043

Pepin, G., & Deutscher, B. (2011). The lived experience of Australian retirees: 'I'm retired, what do I do now?' *British Journal of Occupational Therapy, 74*(9), 419-426. doi:http://dx.doi.org/10.4276/030802211X13153015305556

Persson, D., Andersson, I., & Eklund, M. (2011). Defying aches and revaluating daily doing: Occupational perspectives on adjusting to chronic pain. *Scandinavian Journal of Occupational Therapy, 18*(3), 188-197. doi:http://dx.doi.org/10.3109/11038128.2010.509810

Pettican, A., & Prior, S. (2011). 'It's a new way of life': An exploration of the occupational transition of retirement. *British Journal of Occupational Therapy, 74*(1), 12-19. doi:http://dx.doi.org/10.4276/030802211X12947686093521

Price, P., Stephenson, S., Krantz, L., & Ward, K. (2011). Beyond my front door: The occupational and social participation of adults with spinal cord injury. *OTJR: Occupation, Participation & Health, 31*(2), 81-88.

Prigg, A., & Froude, E. (2011). Application of the cognitive orientation to occupational performance (co-op) approach to address handwriting goals in a group setting [abstract]. Occupational Therapy Australia 24th National Conference & Exhibition, 29th June-1st July, Gold Coast Convention & Exhibition Centre. *Australian Occupational Therapy Journal, 58*, 57. doi:http://dx.doi.org/10.1111/j.1440-1630.2011.00938.x

Pyatak, E. (2011). Participation in occupation and diabetes self-management in emerging adulthood. *American Journal of Occupational Therapy, 65*(4), 462-469. doi:http://dx.doi.org/10.5014/ajot.2011.001453

Reed, K. D., Hocking, C. S., & Smythe, L. A. (2011). Exploring the meaning of occupation: The case for phenomenology. *Canadian Journal of Occupational Therapy, 78*(5), 303-310. doi:http://dx.doi.org/10.2182/cjot.2011.78.5.5

Riley, J. (2011). Shaping textile-making: Its occupational forms and domain. *Journal of Occupational Science, 18*(4), 322-338. doi:http://dx.doi.org/10.1080/14427591.2011.584518

Rizk, S., Pizur-Barnekow, K., & Darragh, A. R. (2011). Leisure and social participation and health-related quality of life in caregivers of children with autism. *OTJR: Occupation, Participation & Health, 31*(4), 164-171.

Robertson, D., & Carswell, M. A. (2011). Adding a driving task to AMPS: A pilot study. *Canadian Journal of Occupational Therapy, 78*(2), 103-109. doi:http://dx.doi.org/10.2182/cjot.2011.78.2.5

Rotenberg-Shpigelman, S., & Maeir, A. (2011). Participation-centered treatment for elderly with mild cognitive deficits: A 'book club' group case study. *Physical & Occupational Therapy in Geriatrics, 29*(3), 222-232. doi:http://dx.doi.org/10.3109/02703181.2011.604149

Smith, T. M., Drefus, A., & Hersch, G. (2011). Habits, routines, and roles of graduate students: Effects of Hurricane Ike. *Occupational Therapy in Health Care, 25*(4), 283-297. doi:http://dx.doi.org/10.3109/07380577.2011.600426

Smyth, G., Harries, P., & Dorer, G. (2011). Exploring mental health service users' experiences of social inclusion in their community occupations. *British Journal of Occupational Therapy, 74*(7), 323-331. doi:http://dx.doi.org/10.4276/030802211X13099513661072

Soeker, M. S. (2011). Occupational adaptation: A return to work perspective of persons with mild to moderate brain injury in South Africa. *Journal of Occupational Science, 18*(1), 81-91. doi:http://dx.doi.org/10.1080/14427591.2011.554155

Spitzer, J., Tse, T., Baum, C. M., & Carey, L. M. (2011). Mild impairment of cognition impacts on activity participation after stroke in a community-dwelling Australian cohort. *OTJR: Occupation, Participation & Health, 31*(1), S8-S15.

Stanley, M., Jaworski, K., & Rofe, M. (2011). Exploring the shed space: The meaning of the shed for older Australian men [abstract]. Occupational Therapy Australia 24th National Conference & Exhibition, 29th June-1st July, Gold Coast Convention & Exhibition Centre. *Australian Occupational Therapy Journal, 58*, 69-70. doi:http://dx.doi.org/10.1111/j.1440-1630.2011.00938.x

Stein, L. I., Foran, A. C., & Cermak, S. (2011). Occupational patterns of parents of children with autism spectrum disorder: Revisiting Matuska and Christiansen's model of lifestyle balance. *Journal of Occupational Science, 18*(2), 115-130. doi:http://dx.doi.org/10.1080/14427591.2011.575762

Sun Wook, L., Morley, M., Taylor, R. R., Kielhofner, G., Garnham, M., Heasman, D., & Forsyth, K. (2011). The development of care pathways and packages in mental health based on the model of human occupation screening tool. *British Journal of Occupational Therapy, 74*(6), 284-294. doi:http://dx.doi.org/10.4276/030802211X13074383957940

Taylor, R., Lee, S., Wook, Kramer, J., Shirashi, Y., & Kielhofner, G. (2011). Psychometric study of the occupational self assessment with adolescents after infectious mononucleosis. *American Journal of Occupational Therapy, 65*(2), e20-e28. doi:http://dx.doi.org/10.5014/ajot.2011.000778

Thomas, Y., Gray, M., & McGinty, S. (2011). Occupation without occupation: Stories from people experiencing homelessness [abstract]. Occupational Therapy Australia 24th National Conference & Exhibition, 29th June-1st July, Gold Coast Convention & Exhibition Centre. *Australian Occupational Therapy Journal, 58*, 20. doi:http://dx.doi.org/10.1111/j.1440-1630.2011.00937.x

Vaught, E. L., & Prince Wittman, P. (2011). A phenomenological study of the occupational choices of individuals who self identify as adult children of alcoholics. *Journal of Occupational Science, 18*(4), 356-365. doi:http://dx.doi.org/10.1080/14427591.2011.595893

Villagrana Medina D. M., Haltiwanger, E. P., & Funk, K. P. (2011). The experience of chronically ill elderly Mexican-American men with spouses as caregivers. *Physical & Occupational Therapy in Geriatrics, 29*(3), 189-201. doi:http://dx.doi.org/10.3109/02703181.2011.587636

Vrkljan, B. H., Leuty, V., & Law, M. (2011). Aging-in-place: Exploring the transactional relationship between habits and participation in a community context. *OTJR: Occupation, Participation & Health, 31*(3), 151-159.

Wiseman, F., & Urlic, K. (2011). Occupation-based therapy improves functional outcomes for older people participating in rehabilitation [abstract]. Occupational Therapy Australia 24th National Conference & Exhibition, 29th June-1st July, Gold Coast Convention & Exhibition Centre. *Australian Occupational Therapy Journal, 58*, 69. doi:http://dx.doi.org/10.1111/j.1440-1630.2011.00938.x

Wright-St Clair, V. A., Kerse, N., & Smythe, E. (2011). Doing everyday occupations both conceals and reveals the phenomenon of being aged. *Australian Occupational Therapy Journal, 58*(2), 88-94. doi:http://dx.doi.org/10.1111/j.1440-1630.2010.00885.x

Wu, A. J., Radel, J., & Hanna-Pladdy, B. (2011). Improved function after combined physical and mental practice after stroke: A case of hemiparesis and apraxia. *American Journal of Occupational Therapy, 65*(2), 161-168. doi:http://dx.doi.org/10.5014/ajot.2011.000786

Yancosek, K. E., & Howell, D. (2011). Systematic review of interventions to improve or augment handwriting ability in adult clients. *OTJR: Occupation, Participation & Health, 31*(2), 55-63.

Yuen, H. K., Mueller, K., Mayor, E., & Azuero, A. (2011). Impact of participation in a theatre programme on quality of life among older adults with chronic conditions: A pilot study. *Occupational Therapy International, 18*(4), 201-208. doi:http://dx.doi.org/10.1002/oti.327

Zimolag, U. (2011). An evolutionary concept analysis of caring for a pet as an everyday occupation. *Journal of Occupational Science, 18*(3), 237-253. doi:http://dx.doi.org/10.1080/14427591.2011.586325

2010

Aguilar, A., Boerema, C., & Harrison, J. (2010). Meanings attributed by older adults to computer use. *Journal of Occupational Science, 17*(1), 27-33.

Ahmed-Landeryou, M. (2010). 'I have every intention to carry out occupation based therapy sessions, but…' an exploratory study examining neuro occupational therapists' attitudes, intentions and behaviours regarding occupation-based therapy. *British Journal of Occupational Therapy, 73*(7), 333-333.

Alsaker, S., & Josephsson, S. (2010). Occupation and meaning: Narrative in everyday activities of women with chronic rheumatic conditions. *OTJR: Occupation, Participation & Health, 30*(2), 58-67.

Anaby, D. R., Backman, C. L., & Jarus, T. (2010). Measuring occupational balance: A theoretical exploration of two approaches. *Canadian Journal of Occupational Therapy, 77*(5), 280-288. doi:http://dx.doi.org/10.2182/cjot.2010.77.5.4

Anderson, R. L., Doble, S. E., Merritt, B. K., & Kottorp, A. (2010). Assessment of awareness of disability measures among persons with acquired brain injury. *Canadian Journal of Occupational Therapy, 77*(1), 22-29.

Andonian, L. (2010). Community participation of people with mental health issues within an urban environment. *Occupational Therapy in Mental Health, 26*(4), 401-417. doi:http://dx.doi.org/10.1080/0164212X.2010.518435

Arbesman, M., & Lieberman, D. (2010). Methodology for the systematic reviews of occupational therapy for children and adolescents with difficulty processing and integrating sensory information. *American Journal of Occupational Therapy, 64*(3), 368-374. doi:http://dx.doi.org/10.5014/ajot.2010.09068

Ashby, S., & Chandler, B. (2010). An exploratory study of the occupation-focused models included in occupational therapy professional education programmes. *British Journal of Occupational Therapy, 73*(12), 616-624. doi:http://dx.doi.org/10.4276/030802210X12918167234325

Bazyk, S., Glorioso, M., Gordon, R., Haines, J., & Percaciante, M. (2010). Service learning: The process of doing and becoming an occupational therapist. *Occupational Therapy in Health Care, 24*(2), 171-187. doi:http://dx.doi.org/10.3109/07380571003681194

Bigelius, U., Eklund, M., & Erlandsson, L. (2010). The value and meaning of an instrumental occupation performed in a clinical setting. *Scandinavian Journal of Occupational Therapy, 17*(1), 4-9. doi:http://dx.doi.org/10.3109/11038120802714880

Bruni, M., Cameron, D., Dua, S., & Noy, S. (2010). Reported sensory processing of children with Down syndrome. *Physical & Occupational Therapy in Pediatrics, 30*(4), 280-293. doi:http://dx.doi.org/10.3109/01942638.2010.486962

Cahill, M., Connolly, D., & Stapleton, T. (2010). Exploring occupational adaptation through the lives of women with multiple sclerosis. *British Journal of Occupational Therapy, 73*(3), 106-115. doi:http://dx.doi.org/10.4276/030802210X12682330090415

Chantry, J., & Dunford, C. (2010). How do computer assistive technologies enhance participation in childhood occupations for children with multiple and complex disabilities? A review of the current literature. *British Journal of Occupational Therapy, 73*(8), 351-365. doi:http://dx.doi.org/10.4276/030802210X12813483277107

Chapleau, A. (2010). Voices from the street: How structural and individual factors influence homelessness. *Occupational Therapy in Mental Health, 26*(4), 387-400. doi:http://dx.doi.org/10.1080/0164212X.2010.518310

Chilvers, R., Corr, S., & Singlehurst, H. (2010). Investigation into the occupational lives of healthy older people through their use of time. *Australian Occupational Therapy Journal, 57*(1), 24-33. doi:http://dx.doi.org/10.1111/j.1440-1630.2009.00845.x

Colaianni, D., & Provident, I. (2010). The benefits of and challenges to the use of occupation in hand therapy. *Occupational Therapy in Health Care, 24*(2), 130-146. doi:http://dx.doi.org/10.3109/07380570903349378

Cole, F. (2010). Physical activity for its mental health benefits: Conceptualising participation within the Model of Human Occupation. *British Journal of Occupational Therapy, 73*(12), 607-615. doi:http://dx.doi.org/10.4276/030802210X12918167234280

Colquhoun, H., Letts, L., Law, M., MacDermid, J., & Edwards, M. (2010). Feasibility of the Canadian Occupational Performance Measure for routine use. *British Journal of Occupational Therapy, 73*(2), 48-54. doi:http://dx.doi.org/10.4276/030802210X12658062793726

Colquhoun, H., Letts, L., Law, M., MacDermid, J., & Edwards, M. (2010). Routine administration of the Canadian Occupational Performance Measure: Effect on functional outcome. *Australian Occupational Therapy Journal, 57*(2), 111-117. doi:http://dx.doi.org/10.1111/j.1440-1630.2009.00784.x

Copley, J. A., Rodger, S. A., Hannay, V. A., & Graham, F. P. (2010). Occupational therapy students' experiences in learning occupation-centred approaches to working with children. *Canadian Journal of Occupational Therapy, 77*(1), 48-56. doi:http://dx.doi.org/10.2182/cjot.2010.77.1.7

Corvinelli, A. (2010). Boredom in recovery for adult substance users with HIV/AIDS attending an urban day treatment program. *Occupational Therapy in Mental Health, 26*(2), 99-130. doi:http://dx.doi.org/10.1080/01642121003735780

Craik, C., Bryant, W., Ryan, A., Barclay, S., Brooke, N., Mason, A., & Russell, P. (2010). A qualitative study of service user experiences of occupation in forensic mental health. *Australian Occupational Therapy Journal, 57*(5), 339-344.

Crennan, M., & MacRae, A. (2010). Occupational therapy discharge assessment of elderly patients from acute care hospitals. *Physical & Occupational Therapy in Geriatrics, 28*(1), 33-43. doi:http://dx.doi.org/10.3109/02703180903381060

Dhillon, S. K., Wilkins, S., Law, M. C., Stewart, D. A., & Tremblay, M. (2010). Advocacy in occupational therapy: Exploring clinicians' reasons and experiences of advocacy. *Canadian Journal of Occupational Therapy, 77*(4), 241-248.

Doig, E., Fleming, J., Kuipers, P., & Cornwell, P. L. (2010). Clinical utility of the combined use of the Canadian Occupational Performance Measure and goal attainment scaling. *American Journal of Occupational Therapy, 64*(6), 904-914. doi:http://dx.doi.org/10.5014/ajot.2010.08156

Dorer, G. (2010). Focus on research … Community occupations of mental health service users: A quantitative study of engagement and social inclusion. *British Journal of Occupational Therapy, 73*(10), 469-469.

Earley, D., Herlache, E., & Skelton, D. R. (2010). Use of occupations and activities in a modified constraint-induced movement therapy program: A musician's triumphs over chronic hemiparesis from stroke. *American Journal of Occupational Therapy, 64*(5), 735-744. doi:http://dx.doi.org/10.5014/ajot.2010.08073

Egan, M. Y., Kubina, L., Lidstone, R. I., Macdougall, G. H., & Raudoy, A. E. (2010). A critical reflection on occupational therapy within one assertive community treatment team. *Canadian Journal of Occupational Therapy, 77*(2), 70-79.

Eklund, M., Erlandsson, L., & Leufstadius, C. (2010). Time use in relation to valued and satisfying occupations among people with persistent mental illness: Exploring occupational balance. *Journal of Occupational Science, 17*(4), 231-238.

Engström, A., Lexell, J., & Lund, M. L. (2010). Difficulties in using everyday technology after acquired brain injury: A qualitative analysis. *Scandinavian Journal of Occupational Therapy, 17*(3), 233-243. doi:http://dx.doi.org/10.3109/11038120903191806

Falklof, I., & Haglund, L. (2010). Daily occupations and adaptation to daily life described by women suffering from borderline personality disorder. *Occupational Therapy in Mental Health, 26*(4), 354-374. doi:http://dx.doi.org/10.1080/016421 2X.2010.518306

Flinn, N. A., & Stube, J. E. (2010). Post-stroke fatigue: Qualitative study of three focus groups. *Occupational Therapy International, 17*(2), 81-91. doi:http://dx.doi.org/10.1002/oti.286

Forhan, M. (2010). Doing, being, and becoming: A family's journey through perinatal loss. *American Journal of Occupational Therapy, 64*(1), 142-151.

Forhan, M., & Backman, C. (2010). Exploring occupational balance in adults with rheumatoid arthritis. *OTJR: Occupation, Participation & Health, 30*(3), 133-141. doi:http://dx.doi.org/10.3928/15394492-20090625-01

Fox, V., & Dickie, V. (2010). "Breaking in": The politics behind participation in theater. *Journal of Occupational Science, 17*(3), 158-167.

Gal, E., Dyck, M. J., & Passmore, A. (2010). Relationships between stereotyped movements and sensory processing disorders in children with and without developmental or sensory disorders. *American Journal of Occupational Therapy, 64*(3), 453-461. doi:http://dx.doi.org/10.5014/ajot.2010.09075

Galvin, J., Randall, M., Hewish, S., Rice, J., & MacKay, M. T. (2010). Family-centred outcome measurement following paediatric stroke. *Australian Occupational Therapy Journal, 57*(3), 152-158. doi:http://dx.doi.org/10.1111/j.1440-1630.2010.00853.x

Graham, F., Rodger, S., & Ziviani, J. (2010). Enabling occupational performance of children through coaching parents: Three case reports. *Physical & Occupational Therapy in Pediatrics, 30*(1), 4-15. doi:http://dx.doi.org/10.3109/01942630903337536

Gregitis, S., Gelpi, T., Moore, B., & Dees, M. (2010). Self-determination skills of adolescents enrolled in special education: An analysis of four cases. *Occupational Therapy in Mental Health, 26*(1), 67-84. doi:http://dx.doi.org/10.1080/01642120802647683

Haines, C., Smith, T. M., & Baxter, M. F. (2010). Participation in the risk-taking occupation of skateboarding. *Journal of Occupational Science, 17*(4), 239-245.

Hamilton, A., & de Jonge, D. (2010). The impact of becoming a father on other roles: An ethnographic study. *Journal of Occupational Science, 17*(1), 40-46.

Hawes, D., & Houlder, D. (2010). Reflections on using the model of human occupation screening tool in a joint learning disability team. *British Journal of Occupational Therapy, 73*(11), 564-567. doi:http://dx.doi.org/10.4276/030802210X12892992239431

Hayner, K., Gibson, G., & Giles, G. M. (2010). Comparison of constraint-induced movement therapy and bilateral treatment of equal intensity in people with chronic upper-extremity dysfunction after cerebrovascular accident. *American Journal of Occupational Therapy, 64*(4), 528-539. doi:http://dx.doi.org/10.5014/ajot.2010.08027

Hessell, S., Hocking, C., & Davies, S. G. (2010). Participation of boys with developmental coordination disorder in gymnastics. *New Zealand Journal of Occupational Therapy, 57*(1), 14-21.

Hewitt, A., Howie, L., & Feldman, S. (2010). Retirement: What will you do? A narrative inquiry of occupation-based planning for retirement: Implications for practice. *Australian Occupational Therapy Journal, 57*(1), 8-16. doi:http://dx.doi.org/10.1111/j.1440-1630.2009.00820.x

Hillier, S., McIntyre, A., & Plummer, L. (2010). Aquatic physical therapy for children with developmental coordination disorder: A pilot randomized controlled trial. *Physical & Occupational Therapy in Pediatrics, 30*(2), 111-124. doi:http://dx.doi.org/10.3109/01942630903543575

Hoogsteen, L., & Woodgate, R. L. (2010). Can I play? A concept analysis of participation in children with disabilities. *Physical & Occupational Therapy in Pediatrics, 30*(4), 325-339. doi:http://dx.doi.org/10.3109/01942638.2010.481661

Hoppes, S., & Segal, R. (2010). Reconstructing meaning through occupation after the death of a family member: Accommodation, assimilation, and continuing bonds. *American Journal of Occupational Therapy, 64*(1), 133-141.

Horghagen, S., & Josephsson, S. (2010). Theatre as liberation, collaboration and relationship for asylum seekers. *Journal of Occupational Science, 17*(3), 168-176.

Kelly, M., Lamont, S., & Brunero, S. (2010). An occupational perspective of the recovery journey in mental health. *British Journal of Occupational Therapy, 73*(3), 129-135. doi:http://dx.doi.org/10.4276/030802210X12682330090532

Koenig, K. P., & Rudney, S., G. (2010). Performance challenges for children and adolescents with difficulty processing and integrating sensory information: A systematic review. *American Journal of Occupational Therapy, 64*(3), 430-442. doi:http://dx.doi.org/10.5014/ajot.2010.09073

Lee, J. (2010). Achieving best practice: A review of evidence linked to occupation-focused practice models. *Occupational Therapy in Health Care, 24*(3), 206-222. doi:http://dx.doi.org/10.3109/07380577.2010.483270

Lee, J., & Kielhofner, G. (2010). Vocational intervention based on the model of human occupation: A review of evidence. *Scandinavian Journal of Occupational Therapy, 17*(3), 177-190. doi:http://dx.doi.org/10.3109/11038120903082260

Littlechild, R., Bowl, R., & Matka, E. (2010). An independence at home service: The potential and the pitfalls for occupational therapy services. *British Journal of Occupational Therapy, 73*(6), 242-250. doi:http://dx.doi.org/10.4276/03080 2210X12759925468862

Lo, J., Yao, G., & Wang, T. (2010). Development of the Chinese language paediatric daily occupation scale in Taiwan. *Occupational Therapy International, 17*(1), 20-28. doi:http://dx.doi.org/10.1002/oti.281

Lowis, M. J., Knight, J., & Ball, V. (2010). A quantitative analysis of self-related health and occupational aspects of community-dwelling older adults. *Journal of Occupational Science, 17*(1), 20-26.

Magalhaes, L., & Galheigo, S. M. (2010). Enabling international communication among Brazilian occupational therapists: Seeking consensus on occupational terminology. *Occupational Therapy International, 17*(3), 113-124. doi:http://dx.doi.org/10.1002/oti.292

May, M., & Rugg, S. (2010). Electrically powered indoor/outdoor wheelchairs: Recipients' views of their effects on occupational performance and quality of life. *British Journal of Occupational Therapy, 73*(1), 2-12. doi:http://dx.doi.org/10.4276/03080221 0X12629548272583

Melton, J., Forsyth, K., & Freeth, D. (2010). A practice development programme to promote the use of the model of human occupation: Contexts, influential mechanisms and levels of engagement amongst occupational therapists. *British Journal of Occupational Therapy, 73*(11), 549-558. doi:http://dx.doi.org/10.4276/030802210X12892992239350

Mew, M. (2010). Normal movement and functional approaches to rehabilitate lower limb dressing following stroke: A pilot randomised controlled trial. *British Journal of Occupational Therapy, 73*(2), 64-70. doi:http://dx.doi.org/10.4276/0308022 10X12658062793807

Missiuna, C., DeMatteo, C., Hanna, S., Mandich, A., Law, M., Mahoney, W., & Scott, L. (2010). Exploring the use of cognitive intervention for children with acquired brain injury. *Physical & Occupational Therapy in Pediatrics, 30*(3), 205-219. doi:http://dx.doi.org/10.3109/01942631003761554

Moore, K., Merritt, B., & Doble, S. E. (2010). ADL skill profiles across three psychiatric diagnoses. *Scandinavian Journal of Occupational Therapy, 17*(1), 77-85. doi:http://dx.doi.org/10.3109/11038120903165115

Nayar, S. (2010). The theory of navigating cultural spaces [abstract]. *New Zealand Journal of Occupational Therapy, 57*(2), 77.

O'Sullivan, C., & Chard, G. (2010). An exploration of participation in leisure activities post-stroke. *Australian Occupational Therapy Journal, 57*(3), 159-166. doi:http://dx.doi.org/10.1111/j.1440-1630.2009.00833.x

Odawara, E. (2010). Occupations for resolving life crises in old age. *Journal of Occupational Science, 17*(1), 14-19.

Palmadottir, G. (2010). The role of occupational participation and environment among Icelandic women with breast cancer: A qualitative study. *Scandinavian Journal of Occupational Therapy, 17*(4), 299-307. doi:http://dx.doi.org/10.3109/11038120903302874

Parkinson, S., Lowe, C., & Keys, K. (2010). Professional development enhances the occupational therapy work environment. *British Journal of Occupational Therapy, 73*(10), 470-476. doi:http://dx.doi.org/10.4276/030802210X12865330218302

Perruzza, N., & Kinsella, E. A. (2010). Creative arts occupations in therapeutic practice: A review of the literature. *British Journal of Occupational Therapy, 73*(6), 261-268. doi:http://dx.doi.org/10.4276/030802210X12759925468943

Persson, D., & Erlandsson, L. (2010). Evaluating OVal-9, an instrument for detecting experiences of value in daily occupations. *Occupational Therapy in Mental Health, 26*(1), 32-50. doi:http://dx.doi.org/10.1080/01642120903515284

Peterson Bethea, D., Lovett, A., Cooks, K., & Bell, J. (2010). Promoting social participation for adults through arthritis self-management: A pilot study. *Physical & Occupational Therapy in Geriatrics, 28*(3), 297-306. doi:http://dx.doi.org/10.3109/02703181003759528

Pickens, N. D., O'Reilly, K., & Sharp, K. C. (2010). Holding on to normalcy and overshadowed needs: Family caregiving at end of life. *Canadian Journal of Occupational Therapy, 77*(4), 234-240. doi:http://dx.doi.org/10.2182/cjot.2010.77.4.5

Pierce, D., Atler, K., Baltisberger, J., Fehringer, E., Hunter, E., Malkawi, S., & Parr, T. (2010). Occupational science: A data-based American perspective. *Journal of Occupational Science, 17*(4), 204-215.

Pizur-Barnekow, K. (2010). Maternal health after the birth of a medically complex infant: Setting the context for evaluation of co-occupational performance. *American Journal of Occupational Therapy, 64*(4), 642-649. doi:http://dx.doi.org/10.5014/ajot.2010.08160

Raber, C., Teitelman, J., Watts, J., & Kielhofner, G. (2010). A phenomenological study of volition in everyday occupations of older people with dementia. *British Journal of Occupational Therapy, 73*(11), 498-506. doi:http://dx.doi.org/10.4276/030802210X12892992239116

Reed, K., Hocking, C., & Smythe, L. (2010). The interconnected meanings of occupation: The call, being-with, possibilities. *Journal of Occupational Science, 17*(3), 140-149.

Richard, L. F., & Knis-Matthews, L. (2010). Are we really client-centered? Using the Canadian Occupational Performance Measure to see how the client's goals connect with the goals of the occupational therapist. *Occupational Therapy in Mental Health, 26*(1), 51-66. doi:http://dx.doi.org/10.1080/01642120903515292

Rodger, S., & Vishram, A. (2010). Mastering social and organization goals: Strategy use by two children with Asperger syndrome during cognitive orientation to daily occupational performance. *Physical & Occupational Therapy in Pediatrics, 30*(4), 264-276. doi:http://dx.doi.org/10.3109/01942638.2010.500893

Rudman, D. L., Huot, S., Klinger, L., Leipert, B. D., & Spafford, M. M. (2010). Struggling to maintain occupation while dealing with risk: The experiences of older adults with low vision. *OTJR: Occupation, Participation & Health, 30*(2), 87-96.

Sakiyama, M., Josephsson, S., & Asaba, E. (2010). What is participation? A story of mental illness, metaphor, & everyday occupation. *Journal of Occupational Science, 17*(4), 224-230.

Schindler, V. P. (2010). A client-centred, occupation-based occupational therapy programme for adults with psychiatric diagnoses. *Occupational Therapy International, 17*(3), 105-112. doi:http://dx.doi.org/10.1002/oti.291

Shank, K. H., & Cutchin, M. P. (2010). Transactional occupations of older women aging-in-place: Negotiating change and meaning. *Journal of Occupational Science, 17*(1), 4-13.

Simmons, C. D., Griswold, L. A., & Berg, B. (2010). Evaluation of social interaction during occupational engagement. *American Journal of Occupational Therapy, 64*(1), 10-17.

Skjutar Å, Schult, M., Christensson, K., & Müllersdorf, M. (2010). Indicators of need for occupational therapy in patients with chronic pain: Occupational therapists' focus groups. *Occupational Therapy International, 17*(2), 93-103. doi:http://dx.doi.org/10.1002/oti.282

Stark, S. L., Somerville, E. K., & Morris, J. C. (2010). In-home occupational performance evaluation (I-HOPE). *American Journal of Occupational Therapy, 64*(4), 580-589. doi:http://dx.doi.org/10.5014/ajot.2010.08065

Stuber, C. J., & Nelson, D. L. (2010). Convergent validity of three occupational self-assessments. *Physical & Occupational Therapy in Geriatrics, 28*(1), 13-21. doi:http://dx.doi.org/10.3109/02703180903189260

Sutton, D. (2010). Recovery as the re-fabrication of everyday life: Exploring the meaning of doing for people recovering from mental illness. *New Zealand Journal of Occupational Therapy, 57*(1), 41.

Taylor, J. A. (2010). The construction of identities through narratives of occupations. *British Journal of Occupational Therapy, 73*(4), 169.

Taylor, R. R., O'Brien, J., Kielhofner, G., Lee S. W., Katz, B., & Mears, C. (2010). The occupational and quality of life consequences of chronic fatigue syndrome/myalgic encephalomyelitis in young people. *British Journal of Occupational Therapy, 73*(11), 524-530. doi:http://dx.doi.org/10.4276/030802210X12892992239233

Taylor, T. L., Dorer, G., Bradfield, S., & Killaspy, H. (2010). Meeting the needs of women in mental health rehabilitation services. *British Journal of Occupational Therapy, 73*(10), 477-480. doi:http://dx.doi.org/10.4276/030802210X12865330218348

Teitelman, J., Raber, C., & Watts, J. (2010). The power of the social environment in motivating persons with dementia to engage in occupation: Qualitative findings. *Physical & Occupational Therapy in Geriatrics, 28*(4), 321-333. doi:http://dx.doi.org/10.3109/02703181.2010.532582

Toneman, M., Brayshaw, J., Lange, B., & Trimboli, C. (2010). Examination of the change in assessment of motor and process skills performance in patients with acquired brain injury between the hospital and home environment. *Australian Occupational Therapy Journal, 57*(4), 246-252. doi:http://dx.doi.org/10.1111/j.1440-1630.2009.00832.x

Urlic, K., & Lentin, P. (2010). Exploration of the occupations of people with schizophrenia. *Australian Occupational Therapy Journal, 57*(5), 310-317. doi:http://dx.doi.org/10.1111/j.1440-1630.2010.00849.x

Vessby, K., & Kjellberg, A. (2010). Participation in occupational therapy research: A literature review. *British Journal of Occupational Therapy, 73*(7), 319-326. doi:http://dx.doi.org/10.4276/030802210X12759925544380

Vrkljan, B. (2010). Facilitating technology use in older adulthood: The person-environment-occupation model revisited. *British Journal of Occupational Therapy, 73*(9), 396-404. doi:http://dx.doi.org/10.4276/030802210X12839367526011

Vroman, K., Simmons, C. D., & Knight, J. (2010). Service learning can make occupation-based practice a reality: A single case study. *Occupational Therapy in Health Care, 24*(3), 249-265. doi:http://dx.doi.org/10.3109/07380571003706058

Williams, A., Fossey, E., & Harvey, C. (2010). Sustaining employment in a social firm: Use of the work environment impact scale v2.0 to explore views of employees with psychiatric disabilities. *British Journal of Occupational Therapy, 73*(11), 531-539. doi:http://dx.doi.org/10.4276/030802210X12892992239279

Wilson, L. H. (2010). Occupational consequences of weight loss surgery: A personal reflection. *Journal of Occupational Science, 17*(1), 47-54.

Wimpenny, K., Forsyth, K., Jones, C., Matheson, L., & Colley, J. (2010). Implementing the model of human occupation across a mental health occupational therapy service: Communities of practice and a participatory change process. *British Journal of Occupational Therapy, 73*(11), 507-516. doi:http://dx.doi.org/10.4276/030802210X12892992239152

Winston, K. A., Dunbar, S. B., Reed, C. N., & Francis-Connolly, E. (2010). Mothering occupations when parenting children with feeding concerns: A mixed methods study. *Canadian Journal of Occupational Therapy, 77*(3), 181-189.

Yamada, T., Kawamata, H., Kobayashi, N., Kielhofner, G., & Taylor, R. R. (2010). A randomised clinical trial of a wellness programme for healthy older people. *British Journal of Occupational Therapy, 73*(11), 540-548. doi:http://dx.doi.org/10.4276/030802210X12892992239314

Zecevic, A., Magalhaes, L., Madady, M., Halligan, M., & Reeves, A. (2010). Happy and healthy only if occupied? Perceptions of health sciences students on occupation in later life. *Australian Occupational Therapy Journal, 57*(1), 17-23. doi:http://dx.doi.org/10.1111/j.1440-1630.2009.00841.x

Zimolag, U., & Krupa, T. (2010). The occupation of pet ownership as an enabler of community integration in serious mental illness: A single exploratory case study. *Occupational Therapy in Mental Health, 26*(2), 176-196. doi:http://dx.doi.org/10.1080/01642121003736101

2009

Aegler, B., & Satink, T. (2009). Performing occupations under pain: The experience of persons with chronic pain. *Scandinavian Journal of Occupational Therapy, 16*(1), 49-56. doi:http://dx.doi.org/10.1080/11038120802512425

Ásmundsdóttir, E. (2009). Creation of new services: Collaboration between mental health consumers and occupational therapists. *Occupational Therapy in Mental Health, 25*(2), 115-126.

Balaban, T., Hyde, N., & Colantonio, A. (2009). The effects of traumatic brain injury during adolescence on career plans and outcomes. *Physical & Occupational Therapy in Pediatrics, 29*(4), 367-383. doi:http://dx.doi.org/10.3109/01942630903245333

Bar-Shalita, T., Yochman, A., Shapiro-Rihtman, T., Vatine, J., & Parush, S. (2009). The participation in childhood occupations questionnaire (PICO-Q): A pilot study. *Physical & Occupational Therapy in Pediatrics, 29*(3), 295-310.

Bass-Haugen, J. (2009). Health disparities: Examination of evidence relevant for occupational therapy. *American Journal of Occupational Therapy, 63*(1), 24-34.

Bazyk, S., & Bazyk, J. (2009). Meaning of occupation-based groups for low-income urban youths attending after-school care. *American Journal of Occupational Therapy, 63*(1), 69-80.

Beagan, B. L., & Etowa, J. (2009). The impact of everyday racism on the occupations of African Canadian women. *Canadian Journal of Occupational Therapy, 76*(4), 285-293.

Berg, C., Neufeld, P., Harvey, J., Downes, A., & Hayashi, R. J. (2009). Late effects of childhood cancer, participation, and quality of life of adolescents. *OTJR: Occupation, Participation & Health, 29*(3), 116-124.

Blakeney, A. B., & Marshall, A. (2009). Water quality, health, and human occupations. *American Journal of Occupational Therapy, 63*(1), 46-57.

Bundy, A. C., Waugh, K., & Brentnall, J. (2009). Developing assessments that account for the role of the environment: An example using the test of playfulness and test of environmental supportiveness. *OTJR: Occupation, Participation & Health, 29*(3), 135-143.

Chard, G., Faulkner, T., & Chugg, A. (2009). Exploring occupation and its meaning among homeless men. *British Journal of Occupational Therapy, 72*(3), 116-124.

Chard, G., Liu, L., & Mulholland, S. (2009). Verbal cueing and environmental modifications: Strategies to improve engagement in occupations in persons with Alzheimer disease. *Physical & Occupational Therapy in Geriatrics, 27*(3), 197-211.

Cipriani, J., Kreider, M., Sapulak, K., Jacobson, M., Skrypski, M., & Sprau, K. (2009). Understanding object attachment and meaning for nursing home residents: An exploratory study, including implications for occupational therapy. *Physical & Occupational Therapy in Geriatrics, 27*(6), 405-422. doi:http://dx.doi.org/10.3109/02703180903183164

Cook, S., & Chambers, E. (2009). What helps and hinders people with psychotic conditions doing what they want in their daily lives. *British Journal of Occupational Therapy, 72*(6), 238-248.

Cordingley, K., & Ryan, S. (2009). Occupational therapy risk assessment in forensic mental health practice: An exploration. *British Journal of Occupational Therapy, 72*(12), 531-538. doi:http://dx.doi.org/10.4276/030802209X12601857794736

Dawson, D. R., Gaya, A., Hunt, A., Levine, B., Lemsky, C., & Polatajko, H. J. (2009). Using the Cognitive Orientation to Occupational Performance (CO-OP) with adults with executive dysfunction following traumatic brain injury. *Canadian Journal of Occupational Therapy, 76*(2), 115-127.

Dorer, G., Harries, P., & Marston, L. (2009). Measuring social inclusion: A staff survey of mental health service users' participation in community occupations. *British Journal of Occupational Therapy, 72*(12), 520-530. doi:http://dx.doi.org/10.4276/030802209X12601857794691

Ennals, P., & Fossey, E. (2009). Using the OPHI-II to support people with mental illness in their recovery. *Occupational Therapy in Mental Health, 25*(2), 138-150.

Fayed, N., & Kerr, E. N. (2009). Identifying occupational issues among children with intractable epilepsy: Individualized versus norm-referenced approaches. *Canadian Journal of Occupational Therapy, 76*(2), 90-97.

Fingerhut, P. E. (2009). Measuring outcomes of family-centered intervention: Development of the life participation for parents (LPP). *Physical & Occupational Therapy in Pediatrics, 29*(2), 113-128. doi:http://dx.doi.org/10.1080/01942630902784795

Forhan, M., & Law, M. (2009). An evaluation of a workshop about obesity designed for occupational therapists. *Canadian Journal of Occupational Therapy, 76*(5), 351-358.

Giuffrida, C. G., Demery, J. A., Reyes, L. R., Lebowitz, B. K., & Hanlon, R. E. (2009). Functional skill learning in men with traumatic brain injury. *American Journal of Occupational Therapy, 63*(4), 398-407.

Grimm, E. Z., Meus, J. S., Brown, C., Exley, S. M., Hartman, S., Hays, C., & Manner, T. (2009). Meal preparation: Comparing treatment approaches to increase acquisition of skills for adults with schizophrenic disorders. *OTJR: Occupation, Participation & Health, 29*(4), 148-153.

Gunnarsson, A. B., & Eklund, M. (2009). The tree theme method as an intervention in psychosocial occupational therapy: Client acceptability and outcomes. *Australian Occupational Therapy Journal, 56*(3), 167-176. doi:http://dx.doi.org/10.1111/j.1440-1630.2008.00738.x

Hansen, T., Steultjens, E., & Satink, T. (2009). Validation of a Danish translation of an occupational therapy guideline for interventions in apraxia: A pilot study. *Scandinavian Journal of Occupational Therapy, 16*(4), 205-215. doi:http://dx.doi.org/10.3109/11038120802684281

Hitch, D. (2009). Experiences of engagement in occupations and assertive outreach services. *British Journal of Occupational Therapy, 72*(11), 482-490. doi:http://dx.doi.org/10.4276/030802209X12577616538636

Holguin, J. A. (2009). Occupational therapy and the journal citation reports: 10-year performance trajectories. *American Journal of Occupational Therapy, 63*(1), 105-112.

Hudson, M. J., & Aoyama, M. (2009). Hunter-gatherers and the behavioural ecology of human occupation. *Canadian Journal of Occupational Therapy, 76*(1), 48-55.

Ivarsson, A., & Müllersdorf, M. (2009). Occupation as described by occupational therapy students in Sweden: A follow-up study. *Scandinavian Journal of Occupational Therapy, 16*(1), 57-64. doi:http://dx.doi.org/10.1080/11038120802570845

Jacob, C., Guptill, C., & Sumsion, T. (2009). Motivation for continuing involvement in a leisure-based choir: The lived experiences of university choir members. *Journal of Occupational Science, 16*(3), 187-193.

Kåhlin, I., & Haglund, L. (2009). Psychosocial strengths and challenges related to work among persons with intellectual disabilities. *Occupational Therapy in Mental Health, 25*(2), 151-163.

Kielhofner, G., Fogg, L., Braveman, B., Forsyth, K., Kramer, J., & Duncan, E. (2009). A factor analytic study of the model of human occupation screening tool of hypothesized variables. *Occupational Therapy in Mental Health, 25*(2), 127-137.

Kielhofner, G., Forsyth, K., Kramer, J., & Iyenger, A. (2009). Developing the occupational self assessment: The use of Rasch analysis to assure internal validity, sensitivity and reliability. *British Journal of Occupational Therapy, 72*(3), 94-104.

Kinn, L. G., & Aas, R. W. (2009). Occupational therapists' perception of their practice: A phenomenological study. *Australian Occupational Therapy Journal, 56*(2), 112-121. doi:http://dx.doi.org/10.1111/j.1440-1630.2007.00714.x

Kramer, J., Bowyer, P., Kielhofner, G., O'Brien, J., & Maziero-Barbosa, V. (2009). Examining rater behavior on a revised version of the short child occupational profile (SCOPE). *OTJR: Occupation, Participation & Health, 29*(2), 88-96.

Kramer, J., Kielhofner, G., Lee, S. W., Ashpole, E., & Castle, L. (2009). Utility of the model of human occupation screening tool for detecting client change. *Occupational Therapy in Mental Health, 25*(2), 181-191.

Langfield, J., & James, C. (2009). Fishy tales: Experiences of the occupation of keeping fish as pets. *British Journal of Occupational Therapy, 72*(8), 349-356.

Lee, S. W., Taylor, R., & Kielhofner, G. (2009). Choice, knowledge, and utilization of a practice theory: A national study of occupational therapists who use the model of human occupation. *Occupational Therapy in Health Care, 23*(1), 60-71.

Lin, N., Kirsh, B., Polatajko, H., & Seto, M. (2009). The nature and meaning of occupational engagement for forensic clients living in the community. *Journal of Occupational Science, 16*(2), 110-119.

Löfqvist, C., Nygren, C., Brandt Å, & Iwarsson, S. (2009). Very old Swedish women's experiences of mobility devices in everyday occupation: A longitudinal case study. *Scandinavian Journal of Occupational Therapy, 16*(3), 181-192. doi:http://dx.doi.org/10.1080/11038120802613108

Lynch, H. (2009). Patterns of activity of Irish children aged five to eight years: City living in Ireland today. *Journal of Occupational Science, 16*(1), 44-49.

Mahoney, W., & Roberts, E. (2009). Co-occupation in a day program for adults with developmental disabilities. *Journal of Occupational Science, 16*(3), 170-179.

Mason, J., & Reed, K. (2009). Occupation in the environment: A student's perspective. *New Zealand Journal of Occupational Therapy, 56*(2), 21-24.

Mitchell, A. W., & Batorski, R. E. (2009). A study of critical reasoning in online learning: Application of the occupational performance process model. *Occupational Therapy International, 16*(2), 134-153. doi:http://dx.doi.org/10.1002/oti.272

Mynard, L., Howie, L., & Collister, L. (2009). Belonging to a community-based football team: An ethnographic study. *Australian Occupational Therapy Journal, 56*(4), 266-274. doi:http://dx.doi.org/10.1111/j.1440-1630.2008.00741.x

Nott, M. T., Chapparo, C., & Heard, R. (2009). Reliability of the perceive, recall, plan and perform system of task analysis: A criterion-referenced assessment. *Australian Occupational Therapy Journal, 56*(5), 307-314. doi:http://dx.doi.org/10.1111/j.1440-1630.2008.00763.x

Parkinson, S., Forsyth, K., Durose, S., Mason, R., & Harris, D. (2009). The balance of occupation-focused and generic tasks within a mental health and learning disability occupational therapy service. *British Journal of Occupational Therapy, 72*(8), 366-370.

Paul-Ward, A. (2009). Social and occupational justice barriers in the transition from foster care to independent adulthood. *American Journal of Occupational Therapy, 63*(1), 81-88.

Persch, A. C., Pizur-Barnekow, K., Cashin, S., & Pickens, N. D. (2009). Heart rate variability of activity and occupation during solitary and social engagement. *Journal of Occupational Science, 16*(3), 163-169.

Phelan, S., Steinke, L., & Mandich, A. (2009). Exploring a cognitive intervention for children with pervasive developmental disorder. *Canadian Journal of Occupational Therapy, 76*(1), 23-28.

Pizur-Barnekow, K., & Knutson, J. (2009). A comparison of the personality dimensions and behavior changes that occur during solitary and co-occupation. *Journal of Occupational Science, 16*(3), 157-162.

Poole, J. L., Willer, K., & Mendelson, C. (2009). Occupation of motherhood: Challenges for mothers with scleroderma. *American Journal of Occupational Therapy, 63*(2), 214-219.

Price, M. P., & Miner, S. (2009). Mother becoming: Learning to read Mikala's signs. *Scandinavian Journal of Occupational Therapy, 16*(2), 68-77. doi:http://dx.doi.org/10.1080/11038120802409739

Price, P., & Miner, S. (2009). Extraordinarily ordinary moments of co-occupation in a neonatal intensive care unit. *OTJR: Occupation, Participation & Health, 29*(2), 72-78.

Price, P., & Stephenson, S. M. (2009). Learning to promote occupational development through co-occupation. *Journal of Occupational Science, 16*(3), 180-186.

Reed, K. (2009). Resituating the meaning of occupation in the context of living [abstract]. *New Zealand Journal of Occupational Therapy, 56*(1), 46.

Rodger, S., & Brandenburg, J. (2009). Cognitive Orientation to (daily) Occupational Performance (CO-OP) with children with Asperger's syndrome who have motor-based occupational performance goals. *Australian Occupational Therapy Journal, 56*(1), 41-50. doi:http://dx.doi.org/10.1111/j.1440-1630.2008.00739.x

Rodger, S., Pham, C., & Mitchell, S. (2009). Cognitive strategy use by children with Asperger's syndrome during intervention for motor-based goals. *Australian Occupational Therapy Journal, 56*(2), 103-111. doi:http://dx.doi.org/10.1111/j.1440-1630.2007.00719.x

Romero Ayuso, D., & Kramer, J. (2009). Using the Spanish child occupational self-assessment (COSA) with children with ADHD. *Occupational Therapy in Mental Health, 25*(2), 101-114.

Schneider, E. (2009). Longitudinal observations of infants' object play behavior in the home context. *OTJR: Occupation, Participation & Health, 29*(2), 79-87.

Smith, T. M., Ludwig, F., Andersen, L. T., & Copolillo, A. (2009). Engagement in occupation and adaptation to low vision. *Occupational Therapy in Health Care, 23*(2), 119-133.

Stamm, T., Lovelock, L., Stew, G., Nell, V., Smolen, J., Machold, K., ... Sadlo, G. (2009). I have a disease but I am not ill: A narrative study of occupational balance in people with rheumatoid arthritis. *OTJR: Occupation, Participation & Health, 29*(1), 32-39.

Sundsteigen, B., Eklund, K., & Dahlin-Ivanoff, S. (2009). Patients' experience of groups in outpatient mental health services and its significance for daily occupations. *Scandinavian Journal of Occupational Therapy, 16*(3), 172-180. doi:http://dx.doi.org/10.1080/11038120802512433

Taylor, R. R., Kielhofner, G., Smith, C., Butler, S., Cahill, S. M., Ciukaj, M. D., & Gehman, M. (2009). Volitional change in children with autism: A single-case design study of the impact of hippotherapy on motivation. *Occupational Therapy in Mental Health, 25*(2), 192-200.

White, B. P., & Mulligan, S. E. (2009). Application of psychobiological measures in occupational science and occupational therapy research. *OTJR: Occupation, Participation & Health, 29*(4), 163-174.

Zimolag, U., & Krupa, T. (2009). Pet ownership as a meaningful community occupation for people with serious mental illness. *American Journal of Occupational Therapy, 63*(2), 126-137.

Ziviani, J., Poulsen, A., & Hansen, C. (2009). Movement skills proficiency and physical activity: A case for engaging and coaching for health (EACH)-child. *Australian Occupational Therapy Journal, 56*(4), 259-265. doi:http://dx.doi.org/10.1111/j.1440-1630.2008.00758.x

Zlotnik, S., Sachs, D., Rosenblum, S., Shpasser, R., & Josman, N. (2009). Use of the dynamic interactional model in self-care and motor intervention after traumatic brain injury: Explanatory case studies. *American Journal of Occupational Therapy, 63*(5), 549-558.

2008

Agren, K. A., & Kjellberg, A. (2008). Utilization and content validity of the Swedish version of the volitional questionnaire (VQ-S). *Occupational Therapy in Health Care, 22*(2-3), 163-176.

Arnadóttir, G., & Fisher, A. G. (2008). Rasch analysis of the ADL scale of the A-ONE. *American Journal of Occupational Therapy, 62*(1), 51-60.

Asaba, E. (2008). Hashi-ire: Where occupation, chopsticks, and mental health intersect. *Journal of Occupational Science, 15*(2), 74-79.

Asgari, A., & Kramer, J. M. (2008). Construct validity and factor structure of the Persian occupational self-assessment (OSA) with Iranian students. *Occupational Therapy in Health Care, 22*(2-3), 187-200.

Banks, R., Rodger, S., & Polatajko, H. J. (2008). Mastering handwriting: How children with developmental coordination disorder succeed with CO-OP. *OTJR: Occupation, Participation & Health, 28*(3), 100-109.

Bohr, P. C. (2008). Critical review and analysis of the impact of the physical infrastructure on the driving ability, performance, and safety of older adults. *American Journal of Occupational Therapy, 62*(2), 159-172.

Boniface, G., Fedden, T., Hurst, H., Mason, M., Phelps, C., Reagon, C., & Waygood, S. (2008). Using theory to underpin an integrated occupational therapy service through the Canadian Model of Occupational Performance. *British Journal of Occupational Therapy, 71*(12), 531-539.

Bratun, U., & Asaba, E. (2008). From individual to communal experiences of occupation: Drawing upon qi gong practices. *Journal of Occupational Science, 15*(2), 80-86.

Christie, L. (2008). Occupational profile: An interview with Karin Sprague, stone carver. *Journal of Occupational Science, 15*(1), 55-57.

Craig, D. G. (2008). An overview of evidence-based support for the therapeutic use of music in occupational therapy. *Occupational Therapy in Health Care, 22*(1), 73-95.

Creek, J., & Hughes, A. (2008). Occupation and health: A review of selected literature. *British Journal of Occupational Therapy, 71*(11), 456-468.

Di Rezze, B., Wright, V., Curran, C. J., Campbell, K. A., & Macarthur, C. (2008). Individualized outcome measures for evaluating life skill groups for children with disabilities. *Canadian Journal of Occupational Therapy, 75*(5), 282-287.

Dirette, D. K., Plaisier, B. R., & Jones, S. J. (2008). Patterns and antecedents of the development of self-awareness following traumatic brain injury: The importance of occupation. *British Journal of Occupational Therapy, 71*(2), 44-51.

Donica, D. K. (2008). Spirituality and occupational therapy: The application of the psychospiritual integration frame of reference. *Physical & Occupational Therapy in Geriatrics, 27*(2), 107-121.

Downs, M. L. (2008). Leisure routines: Parents and children with disability sharing occupation. *Journal of Occupational Science, 15*(2), 105-110.

Dubouloz, C., Vallerand, J., Laporte, D., Ashe, B., & Hall, M. (2008). Occupational performance modification and personal change among clients receiving rehabilitation services for rheumatoid arthritis. *Australian Occupational Therapy Journal, 55*(1), 30-38.

Eklund, M., & Gunnarsson, A. B. (2008). Content validity, clinical utility, sensitivity to change and discriminant ability of the Swedish satisfaction with daily occupations (SDO) instrument: A screening tool for people with mental disorders. *British Journal of Occupational Therapy, 71*(11), 487-495.

Eklund, M., Ornsberg, L., Ekström, C., Jansson, B., & Kjellin, L. (2008). Outcomes of activity-based assessment (BIA) compared with standard assessment in occupational therapy. *Scandinavian Journal of Occupational Therapy, 15*(4), 196-203.

Evans, J., & Rodger, S. (2008). Mealtimes and bedtimes: Windows to family routines and rituals. *Journal of Occupational Science, 15*(2), 98-104.

Girdler, S., Packer, T. L., & Boldy, D. (2008). The impact of age-related vision loss. *OTJR: Occupation, Participation & Health, 28*(3), 110-120.

Hill-Hermann, V., Strasser, A., Albers, B., Schofield, K., Dunning, K., Levine, P., & Page, S. J. (2008). Task-specific, patient-driven neuroprosthesis training in chronic stroke: Results of a 3-week clinical study. *American Journal of Occupational Therapy, 62*(4), 466-472.

Hocking, C., Pierce, D., Shordike, A., Wright-St. Clair, V., Bunrayong, W., Vittayakorn, S., & Rattakorn, P. (2008). The promise of internationally collaborative research for studying occupation: The example of the older women's food preparation study. *OTJR: Occupation, Participation & Health, 28*(4), 180-190.

Hooper, B. (2008). Stories we teach by: Intersections among faculty biography, student formation, and instructional processes. *American Journal of Occupational Therapy, 62*(2), 228-241.

Hsu, W., Pan, A., & Chen, T. (2008). A psychometric study of the Chinese version of the assessment of communication and interaction skills. *Occupational Therapy in Health Care, 22*(2-3), 177-185.

Hunter, E. G. (2008). Legacy: The occupational transmission of self through actions and artifacts. *Journal of Occupational Science, 15*(1), 48-54.

Ikiugu, M. N. (2008). A proposed conceptual model of organizational development for occupational therapists and occupational scientists. *OTJR: Occupation, Participation & Health, 28*(2), 52-63.

Ivarsson, A., & Müllersdorf, M. (2008). An integrative review combined with a semantic review to explore the meaning of Swedish terms compatible with occupation, activity, doing and task. *Scandinavian Journal of Occupational Therapy, 15*(1), 52-63.

Kang, D. H., Yoo, E. Y., Chung, B. I., Jung, M. Y., Chang, K. Y., & Jeon, H. S. (2008). The application of client-centred occupational therapy for Korean children with developmental disabilities. *Occupational Therapy International, 15*(4), 253-268.

Klein, S., Barlow, I., & Hollis, V. (2008). Evaluating ADL measures from an occupational therapy perspective. *Canadian Journal of Occupational Therapy, 75*(2), 69-81.

Lam, W., Wong, K. W., Fulks, M., & Holsti, L. (2008). Obsessional slowness: A case study. *Canadian Journal of Occupational Therapy, 75*(4), 249-254.

Larsson, Å., Haglund, L., & Hagberg, J. (2008). A review of research with elderly people as respondents reported in occupational therapy journals. *Scandinavian Journal of Occupational Therapy, 15*(2), 116-126.

Lee, S. W., Taylor, R., Kielhofner, G., & Fisher, G. (2008). Theory use in practice: A national survey of therapists who use the model of human occupation. *American Journal of Occupational Therapy, 62*(1), 106-117.

Leufstadius, C., Erlandsson, L., Björkman, T., & Eklund, M. (2008). Meaningfulness in daily occupations among individuals with persistent mental illness. *Journal of Occupational Science, 15*(1), 27-35.

Malekpour, M. (2008). Needs assessment of runaway females in Iran from an occupational therapy perspective. *Occupational Therapy International, 15*(4), 232-252.

Marshall, E., & Mackenzie, L. (2008). Adjustment to residential care: The experience of newly admitted residents to hostel accommodation in Australia. *Australian Occupational Therapy Journal, 55*(2), 123-132.

Martin, A., Burtner, P. A., Poole, J., & Phillips, J. (2008). Case report: ICF-level changes in a preschooler after constraint-induced movement therapy. *American Journal of Occupational Therapy, 62*(3), 282-288.

Martin, L., Miranda, B., & Bean, M. (2008). An exploration of spousal separation and adaptation to long-term disability: Six elderly couples engaged in a horticultural programme. *Occupational Therapy International, 15*(1), 45-55.

Martin, L. M., Bliven, M., & Boisvert, R. (2008). Occupational performance, self-esteem, and quality of life in substance addictions recovery. *OTJR: Occupation, Participation & Health, 28*(2), 81-88.

Matuska, K. M., & Erickson, B. (2008). Lifestyle balance: How it is described and experienced by women with multiple sclerosis. *Journal of Occupational Science, 15*(1), 20-26.

McNulty, M. C., & Beplat, A. L. (2008). The validity of using the Canadian Occupational Performance Measure with older adults with and without depressive symptoms. *Physical & Occupational Therapy in Geriatrics, 27*(1), 1-15.

Mountain, G., Mozley, C., Craig, C., & Ball, L. (2008). Occupational therapy led health promotion for older people: Feasibility of the lifestyle matters programme. *British Journal of Occupational Therapy, 71*(10), 406-413.

Müllersdorf, M., & Ivarsson, A. (2008). Occupation as described by novice occupational therapy students in Sweden: The first step in a theory generative process grounded in empirical data. *Scandinavian Journal of Occupational Therapy, 15*(1), 34-42.

Munkholm, M., & Fisher, A. G. (2008). Differences in schoolwork performance between typically developing students and students with mild disabilities. *OTJR: Occupation, Participation & Health, 28*(3), 121-132.

Nakamura-Thomas, H., & Yamada, T. (2008). Assessing interests in Japanese elders: A descriptive study. *Occupational Therapy in Health Care, 22*(2-3), 151-162.

Norweg, A., Bose, P., Snow, G., & Berkowitz, M. E. (2008). A pilot study of a pulmonary rehabilitation programme evaluated by four adults with chronic obstructive pulmonary disease. *Occupational Therapy International, 15*(2), 114-132.

O'Brien, J., & Sandmire, D. A. (2008). Cardiovascular and electroencephalographic response to purposeful vs. nonpurposeful activity in adults. *Occupational Therapy in Health Care, 22*(4), 19-35.

Parkinson, S., Chester, A., Cratchley, S., & Rowbottom, J. (2008). Application of the model of human occupation screening tool (MOHOST assessment) in an acute psychiatric setting. *Occupational Therapy in Health Care, 22*(2-3), 63-75.

Pépin, G., Guérette, F., Lefebvre, B., & Jacques, P. (2008). Canadian therapists' experiences while implementing the model of human occupation remotivation process. *Occupational Therapy in Health Care, 22*(2-3), 115-124.

Petersen, K., & Bente, H. (2008). A process for translating and validating model of human occupation assessments in the Danish context [corrected] [published erratum appears in Occup Ther Health Care 2009 Jan;23(1):97]. *Occupational Therapy in Health Care, 22*(2-3), 139-149.

Quake-Rapp, C., Miller, B., Ananthan, G., & Chiu, E. (2008). Direct observation as a means of assessing frequency of maladaptive behavior in youths with severe emotional and behavioral disorder. *American Journal of Occupational Therapy, 62*(2), 206-211.

Rayner, L. (2008). How satisfied are intermediate care patients with their perceived change in performance in the occupational performance areas of self-care, productivity and leisure as described by the Canadian model of occupational therapy (CMOP) (CAOT 1997). *British Journal of Occupational Therapy, 71*(5), 195.

Riley, J. (2008). Weaving an enhanced sense of self and a collective sense of self through creative textile-making. *Journal of Occupational Science, 15*(2), 63-73.

Rochman, D. L., Ray, S. A., Kulich, R. J., Mehta, N. R., & Driscoll, S. (2008). Validity and utility of the Canadian Occupational Performance Measure as an outcome measure in a craniofacial pain center. *OTJR: Occupation, Participation & Health, 28*(1), 4-11.

Rodger, S., Ireland, S., & Vun, M. (2008). Can cognitive orientation to daily occupational performance (CO-OP) help children with Asperger's syndrome to master social and organisational goals? *British Journal of Occupational Therapy, 71*(1), 23-32.

Rodger, S., & Liu, S. (2008). Cognitive orientation to (daily) occupational performance: Changes in strategy and session time use over the course of intervention. *OTJR: Occupation, Participation & Health, 28*(4), 168-179.

Rosenstein, L., Ridgel, A. L., Thota, A., Samame, B., & Alberts, J. L. (2008). Effects of combined robotic therapy and repetitive-task practice on upper-extremity function in a patient with chronic stroke. *American Journal of Occupational Therapy, 62*(1), 28-35.

Sandmire, D. A., O'Brien, J., Lemieux, S. M., Meyer, S. A., & Moutinho, S. D. (2008). Cardiovascular and electroencephalographic responses to purposeful versus nonpurposeful activities in children. *Occupational Therapy in Health Care, 22*(4), 1-18.

Schnell, G. (2008). Monitoring the progress of young people's occupational performance in an inpatient mental health setting. *New Zealand Journal of Occupational Therapy, 55*(2), 4-10.

Stav, W. B. (2008). Review of the evidence related to older adult community mobility and driver licensure policies. *American Journal of Occupational Therapy, 62*(2), 149-158.

Stav, W. B., Arbesman, M., & Lieberman, D. (2008). Background and methodology of the older driver evidence-based systematic literature review. *American Journal of Occupational Therapy, 62*(2), 130-135.

Steindl, C., Winding, K., & Runge, U. (2008). Occupation and participation in everyday life: Women's experiences of an Austrian refugee camp. *Journal of Occupational Science, 15*(1), 36-42.

Stoffel, A., & Berg, C. (2008). Spanish translation and validation of the preschool activity card sort. *Physical & Occupational Therapy in Pediatrics, 28*(2), 171-189.

Taylor, J. (2008). An autoethnographic exploration of an occupation: Doing a PhD. *British Journal of Occupational Therapy, 71*(5), 176-184.

Timmons, A., & MacDonald, E. (2008). 'Alchemy and magic': The experience of using clay for people with chronic illness and disability. *British Journal of Occupational Therapy, 71*(3), 86-94.

Todorova, L. (2008). Assessing employment needs of Bulgarian youths with intellectual impairments. *Occupational Therapy in Health Care, 22*(2-3), 77-84.

Tonneijck, H., Kinébanian, A., & Josephsson, S. (2008). An exploration of choir singing: Achieving wholeness through challenge. *Journal of Occupational Science, 15*(3), 173-180.

Turner, N., & Lydon, C. (2008). Psychosocial programming in Ireland based on the model of human occupation: A program evaluation study. *Occupational Therapy in Health Care, 22*(2-3), 105-114.

Vik, K., Nygård, L., Borell, L., & Josephsson, S. (2008). Agency and engagement: Older adults' experiences of participation in occupation during home-based rehabilitation. *Canadian Journal of Occupational Therapy, 75*(5), 262-271.

Wilding, C., & Whiteford, G. (2008). Language, identity and representation: Occupation and occupational therapy in acute settings. *Australian Occupational Therapy Journal, 55*(3), 180-187.

Williams, B. J. (2008). An exploratory study of older adults' perspectives of spirituality. *Occupational Therapy in Health Care, 22*(1), 3-19.

Yazdani, F., Jibril, M., & Kielhofner, G. (2008). A study of the relationship between variables from the model of human occupation and subjective well-being among university students in Jordan. *Occupational Therapy in Health Care, 22*(2-3), 125-138.

Ziviani, J., Lim, C., Jendra-Smith, D., & Nolan, D. (2008). Variability in daily time use: Methodological considerations in the use of time diaries for children. *Journal of Occupational Science, 15*(2), 111-116.

2007

Beagan, B. L. (2007). Experiences of social class: Learning from occupational therapy students. *Canadian Journal of Occupational Therapy, 74*(2), 125-133.

Bejerholm, U., & Eklund, M. (2007). Occupational engagement in persons with schizophrenia: Relationships to self-related variables, psychopathology, and quality of life. *American Journal of Occupational Therapy, 61*(1), 21-32.

Blanche, E. I. (2007). The expression of creativity through occupation. *Journal of Occupational Science, 14*(1), 21-29.

Bowyer, P. L., Kramer, J., Kielhofner, G., Maziero-Barbosa, V., & Girolami, G. (2007). Measurement properties of the short child occupational profile (SCOPE). *Physical & Occupational Therapy in Pediatrics, 27*(4), 67-85.

Brooke, K. E., Desmarais, C. D., & Forwell, S. J. (2007). Types and categories of personal projects: A revelatory means of understanding human occupation. *Occupational Therapy International, 14*(4), 281-296.

Brott, T., Hocking, C., & Paddy, A. (2007). Occupational disruption: Living with motor neurone disease. *British Journal of Occupational Therapy, 70*(1), 24-31.

Brown, G. T., Rodger, S., Brown, A., & Roever, C. (2007). A profile of Canadian pediatric occupational therapy practice. *Occupational Therapy in Health Care, 21*(4), 39-69.

Carmody, S., Nolan, R., Chonchuir, N. N., Curry, M., Halligan, C., & Robinson, K. (2007). The guiding nature of the Kawa (river) model in Ireland: Creating both opportunities and challenges for occupational therapists. *Occupational Therapy International, 14*(4), 221-236.

Cordeiro, J. R., Camelier, A., Oakley, F., & Jardim, J. R. (2007). Cross-cultural reproducibility of the Brazilian Portuguese version of the role checklist for persons with chronic obstructive pulmonary disease. *American Journal of Occupational Therapy, 61*(1), 33-40.

Corvinelli, A. (2007). An emerging theory of boredom in recovery for adult substance users with HIV/AIDS attending an urban day treatment program. *Occupational Therapy in Mental Health, 23*(2), 27-50.

Cruz, E. D. (2007). Habits in place: The lives of elders in assisted living. *OTJR: Occupation, Participation & Health, 27*, 80S-82S.

Devine, R., & Nolan, C. (2007). Sexual identity & human occupation: A qualitative exploration. *Journal of Occupational Science, 14*(3), 154-161.

Edwards, M., Baptiste, S., Stratford, P. W., & Law, M. (2007). Recovery after hip fracture: What can we learn from the Canadian Occupational Performance Measure? *American Journal of Occupational Therapy, 61*(3), 335-344.

Eklund, M. (2007). Perceived control: How is it related to daily occupation in patients with mental illness living in the community? *American Journal of Occupational Therapy, 61*(5), 535-542.

Eklund, M., & Bejerholm, U. (2007). Temperament, character, and self-esteem in relation to occupational performance in individuals with schizophrenia. *OTJR: Occupation, Participation & Health, 27*(2), 52-58.

Eklund, M., & Gunnarsson, A. B. (2007). Satisfaction with daily occupations: Construct validity and test-retest reliability of a screening tool for people with mental health disorders. *Australian Occupational Therapy Journal, 54*(1), 59-65.

Eklund, M., & Leufstadius, C. (2007). Relationships between occupational factors and health and well-being in individuals with persistent mental illness living in the community. *Canadian Journal of Occupational Therapy, 74*(4), 303-313.

Ekstam, L., Uppgard, B., Kottorp, A., & Tham, K. (2007). Relationship between awareness of disability and occupational performance during the first year after a stroke. *American Journal of Occupational Therapy, 61*(5), 503-511.

Ennals, P., & Fossey, E. (2007). The occupational performance history interview in community mental health case management: Consumer and occupational therapist perspectives. *Australian Occupational Therapy Journal, 54*(1), 11-21.

Erikson, A., Karlsson, G., Borell, L., & Tham, K. (2007). The lived experience of memory impairment in daily occupation after acquired brain injury. *OTJR: Occupation, Participation & Health, 27*(3), 84-94.

Fenger, K., & Kramer, J. M. (2007). Worker role interview: Testing the psychometric properties of the Icelandic version. *Scandinavian Journal of Occupational Therapy, 14*(3), 160-172.

Fisher, G. S., Emerson, L., Firpo, C., Ptak, J., Wonn, J., & Bartolacci, G. (2007). Chronic pain and occupation: An exploration of the lived experience. *American Journal of Occupational Therapy, 61*(3), 290-302.

Friedland, J., & Davids-Brumer, N. (2007). From education to occupation: The story of Thomas Bessell Kidner. *Canadian Journal of Occupational Therapy, 74*(1), 27-37.

Griffith, J., Caron, C. D., Desrosiers, J., & Thibeault, R. (2007). Defining spirituality and giving meaning to occupation: The perspective of community-dwelling older adults with autonomy loss. *Canadian Journal of Occupational Therapy, 74*(2), 78-90.

Haak, M., Ivanoff, S. D., Fänge, A., Sixsmith, J., & Iwarsson, S. (2007). Home as the locus and origin for participation: Experiences among very old Swedish people. *OTJR: Occupation, Participation & Health, 27*(3), 95-103.

Häggblom-Kronlöf, G., Hultberg, J., Eriksson, B. G., & Sonn, U. (2007). Experiences of daily occupations at 99 years of age. *Scandinavian Journal of Occupational Therapy, 14*(3), 192-200.

Harmer, B. J. (2007). Focus on research…What is meaningful activity? A study to examine and compare the perceptions of older people with dementia living in care homes with those of staff and family carers. *British Journal of Occupational Therapy, 70*(8), 348.

Hasselkus, B. R., & Murray, B. J. (2007). Everyday occupation, well-being, and identity: The experience of caregivers in families with dementia. *American Journal of Occupational Therapy, 61*(1), 9-20.

Holthe, T., Thorsen, K., & Josephsson, S. (2007). Occupational patterns of people with dementia in residential care: An ethnographic study. *Scandinavian Journal of Occupational Therapy, 14*(2), 96-107.

Hovbrandt, P., Fridlund, B., & Carlsson, G. (2007). Very old people's experience of occupational performance outside the home: Possibilities and limitations. *Scandinavian Journal of Occupational Therapy, 14*(2), 77-85.

Howell, D. M., & Cleary, K. K. (2007). Rural seniors' perceptions of quality of life. *Physical & Occupational Therapy in Geriatrics, 25*(4), 55-71.

Iannelli, S., & Wilding, C. (2007). Health-enhancing effects of engaging in productive occupation: Experiences of young people with mental illness. *Australian Occupational Therapy Journal, 54*(4), 285-293.

Isaksson, G., Lexell, J., & Skär, L. (2007). Social support provides motivation and ability to participate in occupation. *OTJR: Occupation, Participation & Health, 27*(1), 23-30.

Knight, J., Ball, V., Corr, S., Turner, A., Lowis, M., & Ekberg, M. (2007). An empirical study to identify older adults' engagement in productivity occupations. *Journal of Occupational Science, 14*(3), 145-153.

Kramer, J. M. (2007). Using a participatory action approach to identify habits and routines to support self-advocacy. *OTJR: Occupation, Participation & Health, 27*, 84S-85S.

Levin, M., Kielhofner, G., Braveman, B., & Fogg, L. (2007). Narrative slope as a predictor of work and other occupational participation. *Scandinavian Journal of Occupational Therapy, 14*(4), 258-264.

Ludwig, F. M., Hattjar, B., Russell, R. L., & Winston, K. (2007). How caregiving for grandchildren affects grandmothers' meaningful occupations. *Journal of Occupational Science, 14*(1), 40-51.

MacLachlan, J., Rudman, D. L., & Klinger, L. (2007). Low vision: A preliminary exploration of its impact on the daily lives of older women and perceived constraints to service use. *Physical & Occupational Therapy in Geriatrics, 26*(2), 43-62.

Martins, V., & Reid, D. (2007). New-immigrant women in urban Canada: Insights into occupation and sociocultural context. *Occupational Therapy International, 14*(4), 203-220.

McKenna, K., Broome, K., & Liddle, J. (2007). What older people do: Time use and exploring the link between role participation and life satisfaction in people aged 65 years and over. *Australian Occupational Therapy Journal, 54*(4), 273-284.

McNamara, P., & Humphry, R. (2007). Now this is what you do: Developing structured routines. *OTJR: Occupation, Participation & Health, 27*, 88S-89S.

Moats, G. (2007). Discharge decision-making, enabling occupations, and client-centred practice. *Canadian Journal of Occupational Therapy, 74*(2), 91-101.

Molineux, M. (2007). The occupational careers of men living with HIV infection in the United Kingdom: Insights into engaging in and orchestrating occupations. *Australian Occupational Therapy Journal, 54*(1), 85-85.

Murray, J. B., Klinger, L., & McKinnon, C. C. (2007). The deaf: An exploration of their participation in community life. *OTJR: Occupation, Participation & Health, 27*(3), 113-120.

Nayar, S., Hocking, C., & Wilson, J. (2007). An occupational perspective of migrant mental health: Indian women's adjustment to living in New Zealand. *British Journal of Occupational Therapy, 70*(1), 16-23.

Nilsson, I., Bernspång, B., Fisher, A. G., Gustafson, Y., & Löfgren, B. (2007). Occupational engagement and life satisfaction in the oldest-old: The Umeå 85+ study. *OTJR: Occupation, Participation & Health, 27*(4), 131-139.

Odawara, E. (2007). Reconstruction of habitual occupations in an old Japanese woman. *OTJR: Occupation, Participation & Health, 27*, 90S.

Petersson, I., Fisher, A. G., Hemmingsson, H., & Lilja, M. (2007). The client-clinician assessment protocol (C-CAP): Evaluation of its psychometric properties for use with people aging with disabilities in need of home modifications. *OTJR: Occupation, Participation & Health, 27*(4), 140-148.

Phipps, S., & Richardson, P. (2007). Occupational therapy outcomes for clients with traumatic brain injury and stroke using the Canadian Occupational Performance Measure. *American Journal of Occupational Therapy, 61*(3), 328-334.

Price, P., & Miner, S. (2007). Occupation emerges in the process of therapy. *American Journal of Occupational Therapy, 61*(4), 441-450.

Roberts, J. E., King-Thomas, L., & Boccia, M. L. (2007). Behavioral indexes of the efficacy of sensory integration therapy. *American Journal of Occupational Therapy, 61*(5), 555-562.

Rodger, S., Springfield, E., & Polatajko, H. J. (2007). Cognitive orientation for daily occupational performance approach for children with Asperger's syndrome: A case report. *Physical & Occupational Therapy in Pediatrics, 27*(4), 7-22.

Schaaf, R. C., & Nightlinger, K. M. (2007). Occupational therapy using a sensory integrative approach: A case study of effectiveness. *American Journal of Occupational Therapy, 61*(2), 239-246.

Schaber, P. (2007). Beyond participation: Selecting quality of life outcomes for an adult day service program. *OTJR: Occupation, Participation & Health, 27*, 91S-92S.

Singlehurst, H., Corr, S., Griffiths, S., & Beaulieu, K. (2007). The impact of binge eating disorder on occupation: A pilot study. *British Journal of Occupational Therapy, 70*(11), 493-501.

Stamm, T. A. (2007). Focus on research…Occupational balance in people with rheumatoid arthritis. *British Journal of Occupational Therapy, 70*(10), 425-425.

Stevenson, T., & Thalman, L. (2007). A modified constraint-induced movement therapy regimen for individuals with upper extremity hemiplegia. *Canadian Journal of Occupational Therapy, 74*(2), 115-124.

Stewart, P., & Craik, C. (2007). Occupation, mental illness and medium security: Exploring time-use in forensic regional secure units. *British Journal of Occupational Therapy, 70*(10), 416-425.

Taylor, S., Fayed, N., & Mandich, A. (2007). CO-OP intervention for young children with developmental coordination disorder. *OTJR: Occupation, Participation & Health, 27*(4), 124-130.

Thompson, K. (2007). Occupational therapy and substance use disorders: Are practitioners addressing these disorders in practice? *Occupational Therapy in Health Care, 21*(3), 61-77.

Turner, N., Jackson, D., Renwick, L., Sutton, M., Foley, S., McWilliams, S., ... O'Callaghan, E. (2007). What influences purpose in life in first-episode psychosis? *British Journal of Occupational Therapy, 70*(9), 401-406.

Tzanidaki, D. (2007). Focus on research...Women from Crete after retirement: Exploring their engagement in art making as a meaningful occupation that contributes to wellbeing. *British Journal of Occupational Therapy, 70*(5), 198-198.

van Huet, H., & Williams, D. (2007). Self-beliefs about pain and occupational performance: A comparison of two measures used in a pain management program. *OTJR: Occupation, Participation & Health, 27*(1), 4-12.

Vik, K., Lilja, M., & Nygård, L. (2007). The influence of the environment on participation subsequent to rehabilitation as experienced by elderly people in Norway. *Scandinavian Journal of Occupational Therapy, 14*(2), 86-95.

Vik, K., Nygård, L., & Lilja, M. (2007). Perceived environmental influence on participation among older adults after home-based rehabilitation. *Physical & Occupational Therapy in Geriatrics, 25*(4), 1-20.

Vrkljan, B. H. (2007). Collaborative participation: An occupational analysis of the older driver-copilot relationship. *OTJR: Occupation, Participation & Health, 27*, 96S.

Ward, K., Mitchell, J., & Price, P. (2007). Occupation-based practice and its relationship to social and occupational participation in adults with spinal cord injury. *OTJR: Occupation, Participation & Health, 27*(4), 149-156.

White, B. P., Mulligan, S., Merrill, K., & Wright, J. (2007). An examination of the relationships between motor and process skills and scores on the sensory profile. *American Journal of Occupational Therapy, 61*(2), 154-160.

Wilding, C., & Whiteford, G. (2007). Occupation and occupational therapy: Knowledge paradigms and everyday practice. *Australian Occupational Therapy Journal, 54*(3), 185-193.

Wiseman, L. M., & Whiteford, G. (2007). Life history as a tool for understanding occupation, identity and context. *Journal of Occupational Science, 14*(2), 108-114.

Wright, J. J., Sadlo, G., & Stew, G. (2007). Further explorations into the conundrum of flow process. *Journal of Occupational Science, 14*(3), 136-144.

2006

Alsaker, S., Jakobsen, K., Magnus, E., Bendixen, H. J., Kroksmark, U., & Nordell, K. (2006). Everyday occupations of occupational therapy and physiotherapy students in Scandinavia. *Journal of Occupational Science, 13*(1), 17-26.

Bergan-Gander, R., & von Kürthy, H. (2006). Sexual orientation and occupation: Gay men and women's lived experiences of occupational participation. *British Journal of Occupational Therapy, 69*(9), 402-408.

Borell, L., Asaba, E., Rosenberg, L., Schult, M., & Townsend, E. (2006). Exploring experiences of "participation" among individuals living with chronic pain. *Scandinavian Journal of Occupational Therapy, 13*(2), 76-85.

Bowman, J. (2006). Challenges to measuring outcomes in occupational therapy: A qualitative focus group study. *British Journal of Occupational Therapy, 69*(10), 464-472.

Chan, V., Chung, J., & Packer, T. L. (2006). Validity and reliability of the activity card sort—Hong Kong version. *OTJR: Occupation, Participation & Health, 26*(4), 152-158.

Coutinho, F., Hersch, G., & Davidson, H. (2006). The impact of informal caregiving on occupational therapy: Practice review and analysis. *Physical & Occupational Therapy in Geriatrics, 25*(1), 47-61.

Craik, C., & Pieris, Y. (2006). Without leisure...'it wouldn't be much of life': The meaning of leisure for people with mental health problems. *British Journal of Occupational Therapy, 69*(5), 209-216.

Cruz, E. D. (2006). Elders' and family caregivers' experience of place at an assisted living center. *OTJR: Occupation, Participation & Health, 26*(3), 97-107.

Diamantis, A. D. (2006). Use of standardised tests in paediatrics: The practice of private occupational therapists working in the United Kingdom. *British Journal of Occupational Therapy, 69*(6), 281-287.

Dunbar, S. B., & Roberts, E. (2006). An exploration of mothers' perceptions regarding mothering occupations and experiences. *Occupational Therapy in Health Care, 20*(2), 51-73.

Egan, M., Hobson, S., & Fearing, V. G. (2006). Dementia and occupation: A review of the literature. *Canadian Journal of Occupational Therapy, 73*(3), 132-140.

Eklund, K., & Ivanoff, S. D. (2006). Health education for people with macular degeneration: Learning experiences and the effect on daily occupations. *Canadian Journal of Occupational Therapy, 73*(5), 272-280.

Eklund, M. (2006). Occupational factors and characteristics of the social network in people with persistent mental illness. *American Journal of Occupational Therapy, 60*(5), 587-594.

Eklund, M., & Bäckström, M. (2006). The role of perceived control for the perception of health by patients with persistent mental illness. *Scandinavian Journal of Occupational Therapy, 13*(4), 249-256.

Erlandsson, L., & Eklund, M. (2006). Levels of complexity in patterns of daily occupations: Relationship to women's well-being. *Journal of Occupational Science, 13*(1), 27-36.

Falkdal, A. H., Edlund, C., & Dahlgren, L. (2006). Experiences within the process of sick leave. *Scandinavian Journal of Occupational Therapy, 13*(3), 170-182.

Fleming, J. M., Lucas, S. E., & Lightbody, S. (2006). Using occupation to facilitate self-awareness in people who have acquired brain injury: A pilot study. *Canadian Journal of Occupational Therapy, 73*(1), 44-55.

Fossey, E., Harvey, C., Plant, G., & Pantelis, C. (2006). Occupational performance of people diagnosed with schizophrenia in supported housing and outreach programmes in Australia. *British Journal of Occupational Therapy, 69*(9), 409-419.

Gevir, D., Goldstand, S., Weintraub, N., & Parush, S. (2006). A comparison of time use between mothers of children with and without disabilities. *OTJR: Occupation, Participation & Health, 26*(3), 117-127.

Häggblom-Kronlöf, G., & Sonn, U. (2006). Interests that occupy 86-year-old persons living at home: Associations with functional ability, self-rated health and sociodemographic characteristics. *Australian Occupational Therapy Journal, 53*(3), 196-204.

Håkansson, C., Dahlin-Ivanoff, S., & Sonn, U. (2006). Achieving balance in everyday life. *Journal of Occupational Science, 13*(1), 74-82.

Harper, K., Stalker, C. A., & Templeton, G. (2006). The use and validity of the Canadian Occupational Performance Measure in a posttraumatic stress program. *OTJR: Occupation, Participation & Health, 26*(2), 45-55.

Helfrich, C. A., Aviles, A. M., Badiani, C., Walens, D., & Sabol, P. (2006). Life skill interventions with homeless youth, domestic violence victims and adults with mental illness. *Occupational Therapy in Health Care, 20*(3-4), 189-207.

Helfrich, C. A., & Rivera, Y. (2006). Employment skills and domestic violence survivors: A shelter-based intervention. *Occupational Therapy in Mental Health, 22*(1), 33-48.

Heward, K., Molineux, M., & Gough, B. (2006). A grounded theory analysis of the occupational impact of caring for a partner who has multiple sclerosis. *Journal of Occupational Science, 13*(3), 188-197.

Holubar, M. N., & Rice, M. S. (2006). The effects of contextual relevance and ownership on a reaching and placing task. *Australian Occupational Therapy Journal, 53*(1), 35-42.

Hooper, B. (2006). Beyond active learning: A case study of teaching practices in an occupation-centered curriculum. *American Journal of Occupational Therapy, 60*(5), 551-562.

Huebner, R. A., Custer, M. G., Freudenberger, L., & Nichols, L. (2006). The occupational therapy practice checklist for adult physical rehabilitation. *American Journal of Occupational Therapy, 60*(4), 388-396.

Johnson, C. R., Koenig, K. P., Piersol, C. V., Santalucia, S. E., & Wachter-Schutz, W. (2006). Level I fieldwork today: A study of contexts and perceptions. *American Journal of Occupational Therapy, 60*(3), 275-287.

Jonsson, H., & Persson, D. (2006). Towards an experiential model of occupational balance: An alternative perspective on flow theory analysis. *Journal of Occupational Science, 13*(1), 62-73.

Karlsson, B., Berglin, E., & Wållberg-Jonsson, S. (2006). Life satisfaction in early rheumatoid arthritis: A prospective study. *Scandinavian Journal of Occupational Therapy, 13*(3), 193-199.

Keponen, R., & Kielhofner, G. (2006). Occupation and meaning in the lives of women with chronic pain. *Scandinavian Journal of Occupational Therapy, 13*(4), 211-220.

Kuipers, K., McKenna, K., & Carlson, G. (2006). Factors influencing occupational therapists' clinical decision making for clients with upper limb performance dysfunction following brain injury. *British Journal of Occupational Therapy, 69*(3), 106-114.

Lee, K., & Kirsh, B. (2006). An occupational journey: Narratives of two women who divorced a spouse with alcoholism. *Journal of Occupational Science, 13*(2), 134-144.

Lee, M., Madden, V., Mason, K., Rice, S., Wyburd, J., & Hobson, S. (2006). Occupational engagement and adaptation in adults with dementia: A preliminary investigation. *Physical & Occupational Therapy in Geriatrics, 25*(1), 63-81.

Leufstadius, C., Erlandsson, L., & Eklund, M. (2006). Time use and daily activities in people with persistent mental illness. *Occupational Therapy International, 13*(3), 123-141.

Lexell, E. M., Iwarsson, S., & Lexell, J. (2006). The complexity of daily occupations in multiple sclerosis. *Scandinavian Journal of Occupational Therapy, 13*(4), 241-248.

Lindstedt, H. (2006). Focus on research…Daily occupations in mentally disordered offenders in Sweden: Exploring occupational performance and social participating. *British Journal of Occupational Therapy, 69*(11), 524.

McDonald, A. E. (2006). The after-school occupations of homeless youth: Three narrative accounts. *Occupational Therapy in Health Care, 20*(3-4), 115-133.

Missiuna, C., Moll, S., Law, M., King, S., & King, G. (2006). Mysteries and mazes: Parents' experiences of children with developmental coordination disorder. *Canadian Journal of Occupational Therapy, 73*(1), 7-17.

Mortenson, P. A., & Harris, S. R. (2006). Playfulness in children with traumatic brain injury: A preliminary study. *Physical & Occupational Therapy in Pediatrics, 26*(1), 181-198.

Muñoz, J., Garcia, T., Lisak, J., & Reichenbach, D. (2006). Assessing the occupational performance priorities of people who are homeless. *Occupational Therapy in Health Care, 20*(3-4), 135-148.

Niva, B., & Skär, L. (2006). A pilot study of the activity patterns of five elderly persons after a housing adaptation. *Occupational Therapy International, 13*(1), 21-34.

Olson, L. (2006). Closing thoughts about promoting parent-child co-occupation through parent-child activity intervention. *Occupational Therapy in Mental Health, 22*(3-4), 153-156.

Olson, L. (2006). Engaging psychiatrically hospitalized teens with their parents through a parent-adolescent activity group. *Occupational Therapy in Mental Health, 22*(3-4), 121-133.

Parker, D. M., & Sykes, C. H. (2006). A systematic review of the Canadian Occupational Performance Measure: A clinical practice perspective. *British Journal of Occupational Therapy, 69*(4), 150-160.

Reid, D., Chiu, T., Sinclair, G., Wehrmann, S., & Naseer, Z. (2006). Outcomes of an occupational therapy school-based consultation service for students with fine motor difficulties. *Canadian Journal of Occupational Therapy, 73*(4), 215-224.

Reynolds, F., & Prior, S. (2006). Creative adventures and flow in art-making: A qualitative study of women living with cancer. *British Journal of Occupational Therapy, 69*(6), 255-262.

Rodger, S., Brown, G. T., Brown, A., & Roever, C. (2006). A comparison of paediatric occupational therapy university program curricula in New Zealand, Australia, and Canada. *Physical & Occupational Therapy in Pediatrics, 26*(1), 153-180.

Rudman, D. L., Hebert, D., & Reid, D. (2006). Living in a restricted occupational world: The occupational experiences of stroke survivors who are wheelchair users and their caregivers. *Canadian Journal of Occupational Therapy, 73*(3), 141-152.

Sakellariou, D., & Algado, S. S. (2006). Sexuality and disability: A case of occupational injustice. *British Journal of Occupational Therapy, 69*(2), 69-76.

Schultz-Krohn, W., Drnek, S., & Powell, K. (2006). Occupational therapy intervention to foster goal setting skills for homeless mothers. *Occupational Therapy in Health Care, 20*(3-4), 149-166.

Segal, R., & Hinojosa, J. (2006). The activity setting of homework: An analysis of three cases and implications for occupational therapy. *American Journal of Occupational Therapy, 60*(1), 50-59.

Tariah, H. A., Hersch, G., & Ostwald, S. K. (2006). Factors associated with quality of life: Perspectives of stroke survivors. *Physical & Occupational Therapy in Geriatrics, 25*(2), 33-50.

Thompson, B. E., & MacNeil, C. (2006). A phenomenological study exploring the meaning of a seminar on spirituality for occupational therapy students. *American Journal of Occupational Therapy, 60*(5), 531-539.

VanLeit, B., Starrett, R., & Crowe, T. K. (2006). Occupational concerns of women who are homeless and have children: An occupational justice critique. *Occupational Therapy in Health Care, 20*(3-4), 47-62.

Walz, N. C., & Baranek, G. T. (2006). Sensory processing patterns in persons with Angelman syndrome. *American Journal of Occupational Therapy, 60*(4), 472-479.

Wehrmann, S., Chiu, T., Reid, D., & Sinclair, G. (2006). Evaluation of occupational therapy school-based consultation service for students with fine motor difficulties. *Canadian Journal of Occupational Therapy, 73*(4), 225-235.

Wicks, A., & Whiteford, G. (2006). Conceptual and practical issues in qualitative research: Reflections on a life-history study. *Scandinavian Journal of Occupational Therapy, 13*(2), 94-100.

Wright, J. J., Sadlo, G., & Stew, G. (2006). Challenge-skills and mindfulness: An exploration of the conundrum of flow process. *OTJR: Occupation, Participation & Health, 26*(1), 25-32.

Yang, S., Shek, M. P., Tsunaka, M., & Lim, H. B. (2006). Cultural influences on occupational therapy practice in Singapore: A pilot study. *Occupational Therapy International, 13*(3), 176-192.

Yeager, J. (2006). Theater engagement and self-concept in college undergraduates. *Journal of Occupational Science, 13*(3), 198-208.

2005

Aldehag, A. S., Jonsson, H., & Ansved, T. (2005). Effects of a hand training programme in five patients with myotonic dystrophy type 1. *Occupational Therapy International, 12*(1), 14-27.

Andersen, S., Kielhofner, G., & Lai, J. (2005). An examination of the measurement properties of the pediatric volitional questionnaire. *Physical & Occupational Therapy in Pediatrics, 25*(1), 39-57.

Apte, A., Kielhofner, G., Paul-Ward, A., & Braveman, B. (2005). Therapists' and clients' perceptions of the occupational performance history interview. *Occupational Therapy in Health Care, 19*(1), 173-192.

Bailey, D., & Jackson, J. (2005). The occupation of household financial management among lesbian couples. *Journal of Occupational Science, 12*(2), 57-68.

Barbosa, V. M., Campbell, S. K., Smith, E., & Berbaum, M. (2005). Comparison of test of infant motor performance (TIMP) item responses among children with cerebral palsy, developmental delay, and typical development. *American Journal of Occupational Therapy, 59*(4), 446-456.

Beagan, B., & Saunders, S. (2005). Occupations of masculinity: Producing gender through what men do and don't do. *Journal of Occupational Science, 12*(3), 161-169.

Birch, M. (2005). Cultivating wildness: Three conservation volunteers' experiences of participation in the green gym scheme. *British Journal of Occupational Therapy, 68*(6), 244-252.

Birken, M. (2005). Exploring the relationship between mental health and occupation in a community development project. *British Journal of Occupational Therapy, 68*(9), 417.

Chapparo, C. J., & Hooper, E. (2005). Self-care at school: Perceptions of 6-year-old children. *American Journal of Occupational Therapy, 59*(1), 67-77.

Crist, P., Fairman, A., Muñoz, J., Hansen, A., Sciulli, J., & Eggers, M. (2005). Education and practice collaborations: A pilot case study between a university faculty and county jail practitioners. *Occupational Therapy in Health Care, 19*(1), 193-210.

Cutajar, R., & Roberts, A. (2005). The relationship between engagement in occupations and pressure sore development in Saudi men with paraplegia. *British Journal of Occupational Therapy, 68*(7), 307-314.

Daunhauer, L. A., Bolton, A., & Cermak, S. A. (2005). Time-use patterns of young children institutionalized in Eastern Europe. *OTJR: Occupation, Participation & Health, 25*(1), 33-40.

Donovan, J. M., VanLeit, B. J., Crowe, T. K., & Keefe, E. B. (2005). Occupational goals of mothers of children with disabilities: Influence of temporal, social, and emotional contexts. *American Journal of Occupational Therapy, 59*(3), 249-261.

Eschenfelder, V. G. (2005). Shaping the goal setting process in OT: The role of meaningful occupation. *Physical & Occupational Therapy in Geriatrics, 23*(4), 67-81.

Eyres, L., & Unsworth, C. A. (2005). Occupational therapy in acute hospitals: The effectiveness of a pilot program to maintain occupational performance in older clients. *Australian Occupational Therapy Journal, 52*(3), 218-224.

Fisher, S. (2005). The Canadian Occupational Performance Measure: Does it address the cultural occupations of ethnic minorities? *British Journal of Occupational Therapy, 68*(5), 224-234.

Flinn, N. A., Schamburg, S., Fetrow, J. M., & Flanigan, J. (2005). The effect of constraint-induced movement treatment on occupational performance and satisfaction in stroke survivors. *OTJR: Occupation, Participation & Health, 25*(3), 119-127.

Gould, A., DeSouza, S., & Rebeiro-Gruhl, K. (2005). And then I lost that life: A shared narrative of four young men with schizophrenia. *British Journal of Occupational Therapy, 68*(10), 467-473.

Guptill, C., Zaza, C., & Paul, S. (2005). Treatment preferences of injured college student musicians. *OTJR: Occupation, Participation & Health, 25*(1), 4-8.

Hoppes, S. (2005). Meanings and purposes of caring for a family member: An autoethnography. *American Journal of Occupational Therapy, 59*(3), 262-272.

Hoppes, S. (2005). When a child dies the world should stop spinning: An autoethnography exploring the impact of family loss on occupation. *American Journal of Occupational Therapy, 59*(1), 78-87.

Hull Garci, T., & Mandich, A. (2005). Going for gold: Understanding occupational engagement in elite-level wheelchair basketball athletes. *Journal of Occupational Science, 12*(3), 170-175.

Ikiugu, M. N., & Rosso, H. M. (2005). Understanding the occupational human being as a complex, dynamical, adaptive system. *Occupational Therapy in Health Care, 19*(4), 43-65.

Kjorstad, M., O'Hare, S., Soseman, K., Spellman, C., & Thomas, P. (2005). The effects of post-traumatic stress disorder on children's social skills and occupation of play. *Occupational Therapy in Mental Health, 21*(1), 39-56.

Klinger, L. (2005). Occupational adaptation: Perspectives of people with traumatic brain injury. *Journal of Occupational Science, 12*(1), 9-16.

Knis-Matthews, L., Richard, L., Marquez, L., & Mevawala, N. (2005). Implementation of occupational therapy services for an adolescent residence program. *Occupational Therapy in Mental Health, 21*(1), 57-72.

Law, M., Majnemer, A., McColl, M. A., Bosch, J., Hanna, S., Wilkins, S.,…Stewart, D. (2005). Home and community occupational therapy for children and youth: A before and after study. *Canadian Journal of Occupational Therapy, 72*(5), 289-297.

Legarth, K. H., Ryan, S., & Avlund, K. (2005). The most important activity and the reasons for that experience reported by a Danish population at age 75 years. *British Journal of Occupational Therapy, 68*(11), 501-508.

Lyons, K. D., & Tickle-Degnen, L. (2005). Reliability and validity of a videotape method to describe expressive behavior in persons with Parkinson's disease. *American Journal of Occupational Therapy, 59*(1), 41-49.

Lysaght, R., & Wright, J. (2005). Professional strategies in work-related practice: An exploration of occupational and physical therapy roles and approaches. *American Journal of Occupational Therapy, 59*(2), 209-217.

Miller, K. S., Bunch-Harrison, S., Brumbaugh, B., Kutty, R. S., & FitzGerald, K. (2005). The meaning of computers to a group of men who are homeless. *American Journal of Occupational Therapy, 59*(2), 191-197.

Mortenson, W. B., Miller, W. C., Boily, J., Steele, B., Odell, L., Crawford, E. M., & Desharnais, G. (2005). Perceptions of power mobility use and safety within residential facilities. *Canadian Journal of Occupational Therapy, 72*(3), 142-152.

Odawara, E. (2005). Cultural competency in occupational therapy: Beyond a cross-cultural view of practice. *American Journal of Occupational Therapy, 59*(3), 325-334.

Öhman, A., & Nygård, L. (2005). Meanings and motives for engagement in self-chosen daily life occupations among individuals with Alzheimer's disease. *OTJR: Occupation, Participation & Health, 25*(3), 89-97.

Rexroth, P., Fisher, A. G., Merritt, B. K., & Gliner, J. (2005). ADL differences in individuals with unilateral hemispheric stroke. *Canadian Journal of Occupational Therapy, 72*(4), 212-221.

Roche, R., & Taylor, R. R. (2005). Coping and occupational participation in chronic fatigue syndrome. *OTJR: Occupation, Participation & Health, 25*(2), 75-83.

Rodger, S., Brown, G. T., & Brown, A. (2005). Profile of paediatric occupational therapy practice in Australia. *Australian Occupational Therapy Journal, 52*(4), 311-325.

Rudman, D. L. (2005). Understanding political influences on occupational possibilities: An analysis of newspaper constructions of retirement. *Journal of Occupational Science, 12*(3), 149-160.

Sandqvist, G., Åkesson, A., & Eklund, M. (2005). Daily occupations and well-being in women with limited cutaneous systemic sclerosis. *American Journal of Occupational Therapy, 59*(4), 390-397.

Sangster, C. A., Beninger, C., Polatajko, H. J., & Mandich, A. (2005). Cognitive strategy generation in children with developmental coordination disorder. *Canadian Journal of Occupational Therapy, 72*(2), 67-77.

Segal, R. (2005). Occupations and identity in the life of a primary caregiving father. *Journal of Occupational Science, 12*(2), 82-90.

Shordike, A., & Pierce, D. (2005). Cooking up Christmas in Kentucky: Occupation and tradition in the stream of time. *Journal of Occupational Science, 12*(3), 140-148.

Stone, S. D. (2005). Being as doing: Occupational perspectives of women survivors of hemorrhagic stroke. *Journal of Occupational Science, 12*(1), 17-25.

Tam, C., Archer, J., Mays, J., & Skidmore, G. (2005). Measuring the outcomes of word cueing technology. *Canadian Journal of Occupational Therapy, 72*(5), 301-308.

Vikström, S., Borell, L., Stigsdotter-Neely, A., & Josephsson, S. (2005). Caregivers' self-initiated support toward their partners with dementia when performing an everyday occupation together at home. *OTJR: Occupation, Participation & Health, 25*(4), 149-159.

Wagstaff, S. (2005). Supports and barriers for exercise participation for well elders: Implications for occupational therapy. *Physical & Occupational Therapy in Geriatrics, 24*(2), 19-33.

Watts, J. H., & Teitelman, J. (2005). Achieving a restorative mental break for family caregivers of persons with Alzheimer's disease. *Australian Occupational Therapy Journal, 52*(4), 282-292.

Wicks, A. (2005). Thesis abstract. Understanding occupational potential across the life course: Life stories of older women. *Australian Occupational Therapy Journal, 52*(2), 175.

Wicks, A. (2005). Understanding occupational potential. *Journal of Occupational Science, 12*(3), 130-139.

Wilding, C., May, E., & Muir-Cochrane, E. (2005). Experience of spirituality, mental illness and occupation: A life-sustaining phenomenon. *Australian Occupational Therapy Journal, 52*(1), 2-9.

Wilson, L., & Wilcock, A. (2005). Occupational balance: What tips the scales for new students? *British Journal of Occupational Therapy, 68*(7), 319-323.

Wilson, L. H. (2005). Thesis abstract. Role differentiation in a professionalising occupation: The case of occupational therapy, New Zealand. *New Zealand Journal of Occupational Therapy, 52*(2), 39.

Winkler, D., Unsworth, C., & Sloan, S. (2005). Time use following a severe traumatic brain injury. *Journal of Occupational Science, 12*(2), 69-81.

Wiseman, J. O., Davis, J. A., & Polatajko, H. J. (2005). Occupational development: Towards an understanding of children's doing. *Journal of Occupational Science, 12*(1), 26-35.

2004

Bejerholm, U., & Eklund, M. (2004). Time use and occupational performance among persons with schizophrenia. *Occupational Therapy in Mental Health, 20*(1), 27-47.

Belcham, C. (2004). Spirituality in occupational therapy: Theory in practice? *British Journal of Occupational Therapy, 67*(1), 39-46.

Birnboim, S. (2004). Strategy application test: Discriminate validity studies. *Canadian Journal of Occupational Therapy, 71*(1), 47-55.

Black, W., & Living, R. (2004). Volunteerism as an occupation and its relationship to health and wellbeing. *British Journal of Occupational Therapy, 67*(12), 526-532.

Bontje, P., Kinébanian, A., Josephsson, S., & Tamura, Y. (2004). Occupational adaptation: The experiences of older persons with physical disabilities. *American Journal of Occupational Therapy, 58*(2), 140-149.

Bryant, W., Craik, C., & McKay, E. A. (2004). Living in a glasshouse: Exploring occupational alienation. *Canadian Journal of Occupational Therapy, 71*(5), 282-289.

Carlsson, G. (2004). Travelling by urban public transport: Exploration of usability problems in a travel chain perspective. *Scandinavian Journal of Occupational Therapy, 11*(2), 78-89.

Carswell, A., McColl, M. A., Baptiste, S., Law, M., Polatajko, H., & Pollock, N. (2004). The Canadian Occupational Performance Measure: A research and clinical literature review. *Canadian Journal of Occupational Therapy, 71*(4), 210-222.

Chaffey, L., & Fossey, E. (2004). Caring and daily life: Occupational experiences of women living with sons diagnosed with schizophrenia. *Australian Occupational Therapy Journal, 51*(4), 199-207.

Chan, J., & Spencer, J. (2004). Adaptation to hand injury: An evolving experience. *American Journal of Occupational Therapy, 58*(2), 128-139.

Chan, S. (2004). Chronic obstructive pulmonary disease and engagement in occupation. *American Journal of Occupational Therapy, 58*(4), 408-415.

Coates, G., & Crist, P. A. (2004). Brief or new: Professional development of fieldwork students: Occupational adaptation, clinical reasoning, and client-centeredness. *Occupational Therapy in Health Care, 18*(1), 39-47.

DeGrace, B. W. (2004). The everyday occupation of families with children with autism. *American Journal of Occupational Therapy, 58*(5), 543-550.

Dirette, D., & Kolak, L. (2004). Brief report. Occupational performance needs of adolescents in alternative education programs. *American Journal of Occupational Therapy, 58*(3), 337-341.

Dubouloz, C., Laporte, D., Hall, M., Ashe, B., & Smith, C. D. (2004). Transformation of meaning perspectives in clients with rheumatoid arthritis. *American Journal of Occupational Therapy, 58*(4), 398-407.

Eklund, M. (2004). Satisfaction with daily occupations: A tool for client evaluation in mental health care. *Scandinavian Journal of Occupational Therapy, 11*(3), 136-142.

Erlandsson, L., Rognvaldsson, T., & Eklund, M. (2004). Recognition of similarities: A methodological approach to analysing and characterising patterns of daily occupations. *Journal of Occupational Science, 11*(1), 3-13.

Farnworth, L., Nikitin, L., & Fossey, E. (2004). Being in a secure forensic psychiatric unit: Every day is the same, killing time or making the most of it. *British Journal of Occupational Therapy, 67*(10), 430-438.

Freeman, A. R., MacKinnon, J. R., & Miller, L. T. (2004). Assistive technology and handwriting problems: What do occupational therapists recommend? *Canadian Journal of Occupational Therapy, 71*(3), 150-160.

George, L. A., Schkade, J. K., & Ishee, J. H. (2004). Content validity of the relative mastery measurement scale: A measure of occupational adaptation. *OTJR: Occupation, Participation & Health, 24*(3), 92-102.

Haley, L., & McKay, E. A. (2004). 'Baking gives you confidence': Users' views of engaging in the occupation of baking. *British Journal of Occupational Therapy, 67*(3), 125-128.

Hardy, P. (2004). Powered wheelchair mobility: An occupational performance evaluation perspective. *Australian Occupational Therapy Journal, 51*(1), 34-42.

Ivarsson, A., Carlsson, M., & Sidenvall, B. (2004). Performance of occupations in daily life among individuals with severe mental disorders. *Occupational Therapy in Mental Health, 20*(2), 33-50.

Jacques, N. D., & Hasselkus, B. R. (2004). The nature of occupation surrounding dying and death. *OTJR: Occupation, Participation & Health, 24*(2), 44-53.

James, S., & Corr, S. (2004). The Morriston occupational therapy outcome measure (MOTOM): Measuring what matters. *British Journal of Occupational Therapy, 67*(5), 210-216.

Kennedy, B. L., & Vecitis, R. N. (2004). Contexts of the flow experience of women with HIV/AIDS. *OTJR: Occupation, Participation & Health, 24*(3), 83-91.

Larson, E. A. (2004). Children's work: The less-considered childhood occupation. *American Journal of Occupational Therapy, 58*(4), 369-379.

Levin, M., & Helfrich, C. (2004). Mothering role identity and competence among parenting and pregnant homeless adolescents. *Journal of Occupational Science, 11*(3), 95-104.

Lindstedt, H., Söderlund, A., Stålenheim, G., & Sjödén, P. (2004). Mentally disordered offenders' abilities in occupational performance and social participation. *Scandinavian Journal of Occupational Therapy, 11*(3), 118-127.

Lund, M. L., & Nygård, L. (2004). Occupational life in the home environment: The experiences of people with disabilities. *Canadian Journal of Occupational Therapy, 71*(4), 243-251.

Ma, H., & Trombly, C. A. (2004). Effects of task complexity on reaction time and movement kinematics in elderly people. *American Journal of Occupational Therapy, 58*(2), 150-158.

McGuire, B. K., Crowe, T. K., Law, M., & VanLeit, B. (2004). Mothers of children with disabilities: Occupational concerns and solutions. *OTJR: Occupation, Participation & Health, 24*(2), 54-63.

McPherson, J. (2004). Thesis abstract. Partner or carer: Role perceptions in the presence of spinal cord injury. *Australian Occupational Therapy Journal, 51*(4), 216-217.

Mee, J., Sumsion, T., & Craik, C. (2004). Mental health clients confirm the value of occupation in building competence and self-identity. *British Journal of Occupational Therapy, 67*(5), 225-233.

Miller, B. K., & Nelson, D. (2004). Constructing a program development proposal for community-based practice: A valuable learning experience for occupational therapy students. *Occupational Therapy in Health Care, 18*(1), 137-150.

Minato, M., & Zemke, R. (2004). Occupational choices of persons with schizophrenia living in the community. *Journal of Occupational Science, 11*(1), 31-39.

Molke, D. K., Laliberte-Rudman, D., & Polatajko, H. J. (2004). The promise of occupational science: A developmental assessment of an emerging academic discipline. *Canadian Journal of Occupational Therapy, 71*(5), 269-281.

Niemeyer, L. O., Aronow, H. U., & Kasman, G. S. (2004). A pilot study to investigate shoulder muscle fatigue during a sustained isometric wheelchair-propulsion effort using surface EMG. *American Journal of Occupational Therapy, 58*(5), 587-593.

Nygård, L. (2004). Responses of persons with dementia to challenges in daily activities: A synthesis of findings from empirical studies. *American Journal of Occupational Therapy, 58*(4), 435-445.

Passmore, A. (2004). A measure of perceptions of generalized self-efficacy adapted for adolescents. *OTJR: Occupation, Participation & Health, 24*(2), 64-71.

Preminger, F., Weiss, P. L., & Weintraub, N. (2004). Predicting occupational performance: Handwriting versus keyboarding. *American Journal of Occupational Therapy, 58*(2), 193-201.

Purves, B., & Suto, M. (2004). In limbo: Creating continuity of identity in a discharge planning unit. *Canadian Journal of Occupational Therapy, 71*(3), 173-181.

Reynolds, F. (2004). Textile art promoting well-being in long-term illness: Some general and specific influences. *Journal of Occupational Science, 11*(2), 58-67.

Satink, T., Winding, K., & Jonsson, H. (2004). Daily occupations with or without pain: Dilemmas in occupational performance. *OTJR: Occupation, Participation & Health, 24*(4), 144-150.

Scheerer, C. R., Cahill, L. G., Kirby, K., & Lane, J. (2004). Cake decorating as occupation: Meaning and motivation. *Journal of Occupational Science, 11*(2), 68-74.

Siporin, S., & Lysack, C. (2004). Quality of life and supported employment: A case study of three women with developmental disabilities. *American Journal of Occupational Therapy, 58*(4), 455-465.

Stagnitti, K., & Unsworth, C. (2004). The test-retest reliability of the child-initiated pretend play assessment. *American Journal of Occupational Therapy, 58*(1), 93-99.

Stark, S. (2004). Removing environmental barriers in the homes of older adults with disabilities improves occupational performance. *OTJR: Occupation, Participation & Health, 24*(1), 32-39.

Stevens-Ratchford, R., & Cebulak, B. J. (2004). Living well with arthritis: A study of engagement in social occupations and successful aging. *Physical & Occupational Therapy in Geriatrics, 22*(4), 31-52.

Tebben, A. B., & Thomas, J. J. (2004). Trowels labeled ergonomic versus standard design: Preferences and effects on wrist range of motion during a gardening occupation. *American Journal of Occupational Therapy, 58*(3), 317-323.

Toal-Sullivan, D., & Henderson, P. R. (2004). Client-oriented role evaluation (CORE): The development of a clinical rehabilitation instrument to assess role change associated with disability. *American Journal of Occupational Therapy, 58*(2), 211-220.

Unruh, A. M., & Elvin, N. (2004). In the eye of the dragon: Women's experience of breast cancer and the occupation of dragon boat racing. *Canadian Journal of Occupational Therapy, 71*(3), 138-149.

Ward, A., & Rodger, S. (2004). The application of cognitive orientation to daily occupational performance (CO-OP) with children 5-7 years with developmental coordination disorder. *British Journal of Occupational Therapy, 67*(6), 256-264.

Whitcher, K., & Tse, S. (2004). Counselling skills in occupational therapy: A grounded theory approach to explain their use within mental health in New Zealand. *British Journal of Occupational Therapy, 67*(8), 361-368.

Wright-St. Clair, V., Bunrayong, W., Vittayakorn, S., Rattakorn, P., & Hocking, C. (2004). Offerings: Food traditions of older Thai women at Songkran. *Journal of Occupational Science, 11*(3), 115-124.

2003

Ahlström, S., & Bernspång, B. (2003). Occupational performance of persons who have suffered a stroke: A follow-up study. *Scandinavian Journal of Occupational Therapy, 10*(2), 88-94.

Alsaker, S., & Josephsson, S. (2003). Negotiating occupational identities while living with chronic rheumatic disease. *Scandinavian Journal of Occupational Therapy, 10*(4), 167-176.

Atwal, A., Owen, S., & Davies, R. (2003). Struggling for occupational satisfaction: Older people in care homes. *British Journal of Occupational Therapy, 66*(3), 118-124.

Baker, N. A., Jacobs, K., & Tickle-Degnen, L. (2003). A methodology for developing evidence about meaning in occupation: Exploring the meaning of working. *OTJR: Occupation, Participation & Health, 23*(2), 57-66.

Bazyk, S., Stalnaker, D., Llerena, M., Ekelman, B., & Bazyk, J. (2003). Play in Mayan children. *American Journal of Occupational Therapy, 57*(3), 273-283.

Björklund, A., & Henriksson, M. (2003). On the context of elderly persons' occupational performance. *Physical & Occupational Therapy in Geriatrics, 21*(3), 49-58.

Candler, C. (2003). Sensory integration and therapeutic riding at summer camp: Occupational performance outcomes. *Physical & Occupational Therapy in Pediatrics, 23*(3), 51-64.

Case-Smith, J. (2003). Outcomes in hand rehabilitation using occupation therapy services. *American Journal of Occupational Therapy, 57*(5), 499-506.

Cederfeldt, M., Lundgren, P. B., & Sadlo, G. (2003). Occupational status as documented in records for stroke inpatients in Sweden. *Scandinavian Journal of Occupational Therapy, 10*(2), 81-87.

Corr, S., & Wilmer, S. (2003). Returning to work after a stroke: An important but neglected area. *British Journal of Occupational Therapy, 66*(5), 186-192.

Craik, J., & Rappolt, S. (2003). Theory of research utilization enhancement: A model for occupational therapy. *Canadian Journal of Occupational Therapy, 70*(5), 266-275.

Deane, K., Ellis-Hill, C., Dekker, K., Davies, P., & Clarke, C. E. (2003). A survey of current occupational therapy practice for Parkinson's disease in the United Kingdom. *British Journal of Occupational Therapy, 66*(5), 193-200.

Denshire, S., & Mullavey-O'Byrne, C. (2003). 'Named in the lexicon': Meanings ascribed to occupation in personal and professional life spaces. *British Journal of Occupational Therapy, 66*(11), 519-527.

Dickie, V. A. (2003). Establishing worker identity: A study of people in craft work. *American Journal of Occupational Therapy, 57*(3), 250-261.

Dickie, V. A. (2003). The role of learning in quilt making. *Journal of Occupational Science, 10*(3), 120-129.

Donati, S. (2003). Focus on research … Ordinary lives: Occupational perspectives of people with severe learning disabilities. *British Journal of Occupational Therapy, 66*(3), 100.

Dychawy-Rosner, I., & Eklund, M. (2003). Content validity and clinical applicability of the Irena daily activity assessment measuring occupational performance in adults with developmental disability. *Occupational Therapy International, 10*(2), 127-149.

Ekelman, B. A., Bazyk, S. S., & Dal Bello-Haas, V. (2003). An occupational perspective of the well-being of Maya women in southern Belize. *OTJR: Occupation, Participation & Health, 23*(4), 130-142.

Eklund, M., Erlandsson, L., & Persson, D. (2003). Occupational value among individuals with long-term mental illness. *Canadian Journal of Occupational Therapy, 70*(5), 276-284.

Erlandsson, L., & Eklund, M. (2003). Women's experiences of hassles and uplifts in their everyday patterns of occupations. *Occupational Therapy International, 10*(2), 95-114.

Fieldhouse, J. (2003). The impact of an allotment group on mental health clients' health, wellbeing and social networking. *British Journal of Occupational Therapy, 66*(7), 286-296.

Graff, M., Vernooij-Dassen, M., Hoefnagels, W., Dekker, J., & de Witte, L. (2003). Occupational therapy at home for older individuals with mild to moderate cognitive impairments and their primary caregivers: A pilot study. *OTJR: Occupation, Participation & Health, 23*(4), 155-164.

Gray, M. I., & Fossey, E. M. (2003). Illness experience and occupations of people with chronic fatigue syndrome. *Australian Occupational Therapy Journal, 50*(3), 127-136.

Hackett, J. (2003). Perceptions of play and leisure in junior school aged children with juvenile idiopathic arthritis: What are the implications for occupational therapy? *British Journal of Occupational Therapy, 66*(7), 303-310.

Helbig, K., & McKay, E. (2003). An exploration of addictive behaviours from an occupational perspective. *Journal of Occupational Science, 10*(3), 140-145.

Henare, D., Hocking, C., & Smythe, L. (2003). Chronic pain: Gaining understanding through the use of art. *British Journal of Occupational Therapy, 66*(11), 511-518.

Hogan, V. M., Lisy, E. D., Savannah, R. L., Henry, L., Kuo, F., & Fisher, G. S. (2003). Role change experienced by family caregivers of adults with Alzheimer's disease: Implications for occupational therapy [corrected] [published erratum appears in Phys Occup Ther Geriatr 2003;22(2):80]. *Physical & Occupational Therapy in Geriatrics, 22*(1), 21-43.

Howie, L. (2003). Ritualising in book clubs: Implications for evolving occupational identities. *Journal of Occupational Science, 10*(3), 130.

Hvalsøe, B., & Josephsson, S. (2003). Characteristics of meaningful occupations from the perspective of mentally ill people. *Scandinavian Journal of Occupational Therapy, 10*(2), 61-71.

Katz, N., Karpin, H., Lak, A., Furman, T., & Hartman-Maeir, A. (2003). Participation in occupational performance: Reliability and validity of the activity card sort. *OTJR: Occupation, Participation & Health, 23*(1), 10-17.

Klos, R. (2003). Gainful occupation (paid employment) is the only valid vocational outcome. *New Zealand Journal of Occupational Therapy, 50*(2), 34-36.

Krupa, T., McLean, H., Eastabrook, S., Bonham, A., & Baksh, L. (2003). Daily time use as a measure of community adjustment for persons served by assertive community treatment teams. *American Journal of Occupational Therapy, 57*(5), 558-565.

Lammi, B. M., & Law, M. (2003). The effects of family-centred functional therapy on the occupational performance of children with cerebral palsy. *Canadian Journal of Occupational Therapy, 70*(5), 285-297.

Lampinen, J., & Tham, K. (2003). Interaction with the physical environment in everyday occupation after stroke: A phenomenological study of persons with visuospatial agnosia. *Scandinavian Journal of Occupational Therapy, 10*(4), 147-156.

Lawlor, M. C. (2003). The significance of being occupied: The social construction of childhood occupations. *American Journal of Occupational Therapy, 57*(4), 424-434.

Lee, C. J., Skarakis-Doyle, E., & Dempsey, L. (2003). The contributions of activity and occupation to young children's comprehension of picture books. *Journal of Occupational Science, 10*(3), 146-149.

Lyons, K. D., & Tickle-Degnen, L. (2003). Dramaturgical challenges of Parkinson's disease. *OTJR: Occupation, Participation & Health, 23*(1), 27-34.

MacKinnon, J. R., & Miller, W. C. (2003). Rheumatoid arthritis and self esteem: The impact of quality occupation. *Journal of Occupational Science, 10*(2), 90-98.

Maitra, K. K., Curry, D., Gamble, C., Martin, M., Phelps, J., Santisteban, M. E., ... Telage, K. M. (2003). Using speech sounds to enhance occupational performance in young and older adults. *OTJR: Occupation, Participation & Health, 23*(1), 35-44.

Molyneaux-Smith, L., Townsend, E., & Guernsey, J. R. (2003). Occupation disrupted: Impacts, challenges, and coping strategies for farmers with disabilities. *Journal of Occupational Science, 10*(1), 14-20.

Nurit, W., & Michal, A. (2003). Rest: A qualitative exploration of the phenomenon. *Occupational Therapy International, 10*(4), 227-238.

Padilla, R. (2003). Clara: A phenomenology of disability. *American Journal of Occupational Therapy, 57*(4), 413-423.

Palmadottir, G. (2003). Client perspectives on occupational therapy in rehabilitation services. *Scandinavian Journal of Occupational Therapy, 10*(4), 157-166.

Pan, A., Chung, L., & Hsin-Hwei, G. (2003). Reliability and validity of the Canadian Occupational Performance Measure for clients with psychiatric disorders in Taiwan. *Occupational Therapy International, 10*(4), 269-277.

Passmore, A. (2003). The occupation of leisure: Three typologies and their influence on mental health in adolescence. *OTJR: Occupation, Participation & Health, 23*(2), 76-83.

Randles, N., Randolph, E., Schell, B., & Grant, S. (2003). The impact of occupational therapy intervention on adults with osteoporosis: A pilot study. *Physical & Occupational Therapy in Geriatrics, 22*(2), 43-56.

Reich, J. W., & Williams, J. (2003). Exploring the properties of habits and routines in daily life. *OTJR: Occupation, Participation & Health, 23*(2), 48-56.

Reynolds, F. (2003). Reclaiming a positive identity in chronic illness through artistic occupation. *OTJR: Occupation, Participation & Health, 23*(3), 118-127.

Sachs, D., & Josman, N. (2003). The activity card sort: A factor analysis. *OTJR: Occupation, Participation & Health, 23*(4), 165-174.

Shimitras, L., Fossey, E., & Harvey, C. (2003). Time use of people living with schizophrenia in a north London catchment area. *British Journal of Occupational Therapy, 66*(2), 46-54.

Taylor, J. (2003). Women's leisure activities, their social stereotypes and some implications for identity. *British Journal of Occupational Therapy, 66*(4), 151-158.

Wright, C. V., & Rebeiro, K. L. (2003). Exploration of a single case in a consumer-governed mental health organization. *Occupational Therapy in Mental Health, 19*(2), 19-32.

Yuen, M., & Fossey, E. M. (2003). Working in a community recreation program: A study of consumer-staff perspectives. *Australian Occupational Therapy Journal, 50*(2), 54-63.

2002

Andree, M. E., & Maitra, K. K. (2002). Intermanual transfer of a new writing occupation in young adults without disability. *Occupational Therapy International, 9*(1), 41-56.

Andresen, M., & Runge, U. (2002). Co-housing for seniors experienced as an occupational generative environment. *Scandinavian Journal of Occupational Therapy, 9*(4), 156-166.

Baranek, G. T., Chin, Y. H., Hess, L., Yankee, J. G., Hatton, D. D., & Hooper, S. R. (2002). Sensory processing correlates of occupational performance in children with fragile X syndrome: Preliminary findings. *American Journal of Occupational Therapy, 56*(5), 538-546.

Burtner, P. A., Ortega, S. G., Morris, C. G., Scott, K., & Qualls, C. (2002). Discriminative validity of the motor-free visual perceptual test revised in children with and without learning disabilities. *OTJR: Occupation, Participation & Health, 22*(4), 161-163.

Cena, L., McGruder, J., & Tomlin, G. (2002). Representations of race, ethnicity, and social class in case examples in the American journal of occupational therapy. *American Journal of Occupational Therapy, 56*(2), 130-139.

Chen, Y., Rodger, S., & Polatajko, H. (2002). Experiences with the COPM and client-centred practice in adult neurorehabilitation in Taiwan. *Occupational Therapy International, 9*(3), 167-184.

Chesworth, C., Duffy, R., Hodnett, J., & Knight, A. (2002). Measuring clinical effectiveness in mental health: Is the Canadian occupational performance an appropriate measure? *British Journal of Occupational Therapy, 65*(1), 30-34.

Chugg, A., & Craik, C. (2002). Some factors influencing occupational engagement for people with schizophrenia living in the community. *British Journal of Occupational Therapy, 65*(2), 67-74.

Daniëls, R., Winding, K., & Borell, L. (2002). Experiences of occupational therapists in stroke rehabilitation: Dilemmas of some occupational therapists in inpatient stroke rehabilitation. *Scandinavian Journal of Occupational Therapy, 9*(4), 167-175.

Eriksson, M., & Dahlin-Ivanoff, S. (2002). How adults with acquired brain damage perceive computer training as a rehabilitation tool: A focus-group study. *Scandinavian Journal of Occupational Therapy, 9*(3), 119-129.

Fasoli, S. E., Trombly, C. A., Tickle-Degnen, L., & Verfaellie, M. H. (2002). Context and goal-directed movement: The effect of materials-based occupation. *OTJR: Occupation, Participation & Health, 22*(3), 119-128.

Finlayson, M., Baker, M., Rodman, L., & Herzberg, G. (2002). The process and outcomes of a multimethod needs assessment at a homeless shelter. *American Journal of Occupational Therapy, 56*(3), 313-321.

French, G. (2002). Occupational disfranchisement in the dependency culture of a nursing home. *Journal of Occupational Science, 9*(1), 28-37.

Hocking, C., Wright-St. Clair, V., & Bunrayong, W. (2002). The meaning of cooking and recipe work for older Thai and New Zealand women. *Journal of Occupational Science, 9*(3), 117-127.

Ivanoff, S. D. (2002). Focus group discussions as a tool for developing a health education programme for elderly persons with visual impairment. *Scandinavian Journal of Occupational Therapy, 9*(1), 3-9.

Ivanoff, S. D., Sonn, U., & Svensson, E. (2002). A health education program for elderly persons with visual impairments and perceived security in the performance of daily occupations: A randomized study. *American Journal of Occupational Therapy, 56*(3), 322-330.

Ivarsson, A., & Carlsson, M. (2002). Development of the experiences of occupational performance questionnaire: Validity and reliability in a sample of individuals with severe mental disorders. *Scandinavian Journal of Occupational Therapy, 9*(4), 184-191.

Kizony, R., & Katz, N. (2002). Relationships between cognitive abilities and the process scale and skills of the assessment of motor and process skills (AMPS) in patients with stroke. *OTJR: Occupation, Participation & Health, 22*(2), 82-92.

Larivière, N., Gélinas, I., Mazer, B., Tallant, B., & Paquette, I. (2002). Discharging older adults with a severe and chronic mental illness in the community. *Canadian Journal of Occupational Therapy, 69*(2), 71-83.

Lentin, P. (2002). The human spirit and occupation: Surviving and creating a life. *Journal of Occupational Science, 9*(3), 143-152.

Lyons, M., Orozovic, N., Davis, J., & Newman, J. (2002). Doing-being-becoming: Occupational experiences of persons with life-threatening illnesses. *American Journal of Occupational Therapy, 56*(3), 285-295.

Lysack, C. L., & Seipke, H. L. (2002). Communicating the occupational self: A qualitative study of oldest-old American women. *Scandinavian Journal of Occupational Therapy, 9*(3), 130-139.

McCarron, K. A., & D'Amico, F. (2002). The impact of problem-based learning on clinical reasoning in occupational therapy education. *Occupational Therapy in Health Care, 16*(1), 1-13.

McIntyre, G., & Howie, L. (2002). Adapting to widowhood through meaningful occupations: A case study. *Scandinavian Journal of Occupational Therapy, 9*(2), 54-62.

Nagle, S., Cook, J. V., & Polatajko, H. J. (2002). I'm doing as much as I can: Occupational choices of persons with a severe and persistent mental illness. *Journal of Occupational Science, 9*(2), 72-81.

Nygård, L., & Öhman, A. (2002). Managing changes in everyday occupations: The experience of persons with Alzheimer's disease. *OTJR: Occupation, Participation & Health, 22*(2), 70-81.

Ratcliff, E., Farnworth, L., & Lentin, P. (2002). Journey to wholeness: The experience of engaging in physical occupation for women survivors of childhood abuse. *Journal of Occupational Science, 9*(2), 65-71.

Sanford, J. A., Pynoos, J., Tejral, A., & Browne, A. (2002). Development of a comprehensive assessment for delivery of home modifications. *Physical & Occupational Therapy in Geriatrics, 20*(2), 43-55.

Schisler, A., & Polatajko, H. J. (2002). The individual as mediator of the person-occupation-environment interaction: Learning from the experience of refugees. *Journal of Occupational Science, 9*(2), 82-92.

Tam, C., Reid, D., Naumann, S., & O'Keefe, B. (2002). Perceived benefits of word prediction intervention on written productivity in children with spina bifida and hydrocephalus. *Occupational Therapy International, 9*(3), 237-255.

Taylor, L., Poland, F., & Stephenson, R. (2002). Are occupational therapists losing sight of hemianopia? *British Journal of Occupational Therapy, 65*(11), 495-501.

Thomas, J. J., & Rice, M. S. (2002). Perceived risk and its effects on quality of movement in occupational performance of well-elderly individuals. *OTJR: Occupation, Participation & Health, 22*(3), 104-110.

Trombly, C. A., Radomski, M. V., Trexel, C., & Burnett-Smith, S. (2002). Occupational therapy and achievement of self-identified goals by adults with acquired brain injury: Phase II. *American Journal of Occupational Therapy, 56*(5), 489-498.

VanLeit, B., & Crowe, T. K. (2002). Outcomes of occupational therapy program for mothers of children with disabilities: Impact on satisfaction with time use and occupational performance. *American Journal of Occupational Therapy, 56*(4), 402-410.

Van't Leven, N., & Jonsson, H. (2002). Doing and being in the atmosphere of the doing: Environmental influences on occupational performance in a nursing home. *Scandinavian Journal of Occupational Therapy, 9*(4), 148-155.

Veneri, A. (2002). Focus on research ... Occupational performance: Perceptions of children with developmental coordination disorder. *British Journal of Occupational Therapy, 65*(8), 380-380.

Warren, A. (2002). An evaluation of the Canadian Model of Occupational Performance and the Canadian Occupational Performance Measure in mental health practice. *British Journal of Occupational Therapy, 65*(11), 515-521.

Wilson, L. H. (2002). A review of the journals of the New Zealand Association of Occupation Therapists, 1949-2002. *New Zealand Journal of Occupational Therapy, 49*(2), 5-13.

Wressle, E., Marcusson, J., & Henriksson, C. (2002). Clinical utility of the Canadian Occupational Performance Measure—Swedish version. *Canadian Journal of Occupational Therapy, 69*(1), 40-48.

2001

Bickes, M. B., DeLoache, S. N., Dicer, J. R., & Miller, S. C. (2001). Effectiveness of experiential and verbal occupational therapy groups in a community mental health setting. *Occupational Therapy in Mental Health, 17*(1), 51-72.

Bonder, B. R. (2001). Culture and occupation: A comparison of weaving in two traditions. *Canadian Journal of Occupational Therapy, 68*(5), 310-319.

Borell, L., Lilja, M., Svidén, G., & Sadlo, G. (2001). Occupations and signs of reduced hope: An explorative study of older adults with functional impairments. *American Journal of Occupational Therapy, 55*(3), 311-316.

Braveman, B., & Helfrich, C. A. (2001). Occupational identity: Exploring the narratives of three men living with AIDS. *Journal of Occupational Science, 8*(2), 25-31.

Brock, M. J. (2001). Focus on research ... The qualities of meaningful occupation. *British Journal of Occupational Therapy, 64*(2), 99.

Brown, F., Shiels, M., & Hall, C. (2001). A pilot community living skills group: An evaluation. *British Journal of Occupational Therapy, 64*(3), 144-150.

Buning, M. E., Angelo, J. A., & Schmeler, M. R. (2001). Occupational performance and the transition to powered mobility: A pilot study. *American Journal of Occupational Therapy, 55*(3), 339-344.

Burke, J. P. (2001). How therapists' conceptual perspectives influence early intervention evaluations. *Scandinavian Journal of Occupational Therapy, 8*(1), 49-61.

Cameron, D., Leslie, M., Teplicky, R., Pollock, N., Stewart, D., Toal, C., & Gaik, S. (2001). The clinical utility of the test of playfulness. *Canadian Journal of Occupational Therapy, 68*(2), 104-111.

Carpenter, L., Baker, G. A., & Tyldesley, B. (2001). The use of the Canadian Occupational Performance Measure as an outcome of a pain management program. *Canadian Journal of Occupational Therapy, 68*(1), 16-22.

Denshire, S. (2001). Thesis abstract. Imagination, occupation, reflection: Ways of coming to understand practice. *Australian Occupational Therapy Journal, 48*(4), 200.

Drew, J., & Rugg, S. (2001). Activity use in occupational therapy: Occupational therapy students' fieldwork experience. *British Journal of Occupational Therapy, 64*(10), 478-486.

Dubouloz, C., Chevrier, J., & Savoie-Zajc, L. (2001). Transformation learning among persons with cardiac problems to achieve a balance of occupation. *Canadian Journal of Occupational Therapy, 68*(3), 171-185.

Eklund, M. (2001). Psychiatric patients' occupational roles: Changes over time and associations with self-rated quality of life. *Scandinavian Journal of Occupational Therapy, 8*(3), 125-130.

Erlandsson, L., & Eklund, M. (2001). Describing patterns of daily occupations—a methodological study comparing data from four different methods. *Scandinavian Journal of Occupational Therapy, 8*(1), 31-39.

Ferguson, M. C., & Rice, M. S. (2001). The effect of contextual relevance on motor skill transfer. *American Journal of Occupational Therapy, 55*(5), 558-565.

Frank, G., Fishman, M., Crowley, C., Blair, B., Murphy, S. T., Montoya, J. A., ... Bensimon, E. M. (2001). The new stories/new cultures after-school enrichment program: A direct cultural intervention. *American Journal of Occupational Therapy, 55*(5), 501-508.

George, S., Wilcock, A. A., & Stanley, M. (2001). Depression and lability: The effects on occupation following stroke. *British Journal of Occupational Therapy, 64*(9), 455-461.

Hanson, C. S., Nabavi, D., & Yuen, H. K. (2001). The effect of sports on level of community integration as reported by persons with spinal cord injury. *American Journal of Occupational Therapy, 55*(3), 332-338.

Jakobsen, K. (2001). Employment and the reconstruction of self. A model of space for maintenance of identity by occupation. *Scandinavian Journal of Occupational Therapy, 8*(1), 40-48.

Jonsson, H., Josephsson, S., & Kielhofner, G. (2001). Narratives and experience in an occupational transition: A longitudinal study of the retirement process. *American Journal of Occupational Therapy, 55*(4), 424-432.

Josman, N., & Birnboim, S. (2001). Measuring kitchen performance: What assessment should we choose? *Scandinavian Journal of Occupational Therapy, 8*(4), 193-202.

Kielhofner, G., & Forsyth, K. (2001). Measurement properties of a client self-report for treatment planning and documenting therapy outcomes. *Scandinavian Journal of Occupational Therapy, 8*(3), 131-139.

Kielhofner, G., Mallinson, T., Forsyth, K., & Lai, J. (2001). Psychometric properties of the second version of the occupational performance history interview (OPHI-II). *American Journal of Occupational Therapy, 55*(3), 260-267.

Legault, E., & Rebeiro, K. L. (2001). Case report. Occupation as means to mental health: A single-case study. *American Journal of Occupational Therapy, 55*(1), 90-96.

Lilja, M., & Borell, L. (2001). Occupational therapy practice patterns with older Swedish persons at home. *Canadian Journal of Occupational Therapy, 68*(1), 51-59.

Magnus, E. (2001). Everyday occupations and the process of redefinition: A study of how meaning in occupation influences redefinition of identity in women with a disability. *Scandinavian Journal of Occupational Therapy, 8*(3), 115-124.

Mee, J., & Sumsion, T. (2001). Mental health clients confirm the motivating power of occupation. *British Journal of Occupational Therapy, 64*(3), 121-128.

Meltzer, P. J. (2001). Using the self-discovery tapestry to explore occupational careers. *Journal of Occupational Science, 8*(2), 16-24.

Miller, L. T., Missiuna, C. A., Macnab, J. J., Malloy-Miller, T., & Polatajko, H. J. (2001). Clinical description of children with developmental coordination disorder. *Canadian Journal of Occupational Therapy, 68*(1), 5-15.

Murphy, S., & Tickle-Degnen, L. (2001). Participation in daily living tasks among older adults with fear of falling. *American Journal of Occupational Therapy, 55*(5), 538-544.

Oxer, S. S., & Miller, B. K. (2001). Effects of choice in an art occupation with adolescents living in residential treatment facilities. *Occupational Therapy in Mental Health, 17*(1), 39-49.

Pierre, B. L. (2001). Occupational therapy as documented in patients' records—part III. Valued but not documented. Underground practice in the context of professional written communication. *Scandinavian Journal of Occupational Therapy, 8*(4), 174-183.

Ralston, L. S., Bell, S. L., Mote, J. K., Rainey, T. B., Brayman, S., & Shotwell, M. (2001). Giving up the car keys: Perceptions of well elders and families. *Physical & Occupational Therapy in Geriatrics, 19*(4), 59-70.

Rebeiro, K. L. (2001). Enabling occupation: The importance of an affirming environment. *Canadian Journal of Occupational Therapy, 68*(2), 80-89.

Rebeiro, K. L., Day, D. G., Semeniuk, B., O'Brien, M., & Wilson, B. (2001). Northern initiative for social action: An occupation-based mental health program. *American Journal of Occupational Therapy, 55*(5), 493-500.

Reid, D. T., Hebert, D., & Rudman, D. (2001). Occupational performance in older stroke wheelchair users living at home. *Occupational Therapy International, 8*(4), 273-286.

Ripat, J., Etcheverry, E., Cooper, J., & Tate, R. (2001). A comparison of the Canadian Occupational Performance Measure and the health assessment questionnaire. *Canadian Journal of Occupational Therapy, 68*(4), 247-253.

Royeen, C. B., Zardetto-Smith, A., Duncan, M., & Mu, K. (2001). What do young school-age children know about occupational therapy? An evaluation study. *Occupational Therapy International, 8*(4), 263-272.

Sewell, L., & Singh, S. J. (2001). The Canadian Occupational Performance Measure: Is it a reliable measure in clients with chronic obstructive pulmonary disease? *British Journal of Occupational Therapy, 64*(6), 305-310.

Southon, K. A. (2001). Focus on research ... A study of the occupational performance goals of elderly patients when in hospital and at home, and the implications for the provision of occupational therapy. *British Journal of Occupational Therapy, 64*(7), 356-356.

Stenbeck, B., Eklund, M., & Hallberg, R. (2001). The domain of concern of Swedish occupational therapists working in psychiatric care. *Scandinavian Journal of Occupational Therapy, 8*(4), 184-192.

Vrkljan, B., & Miller-Polgar, J. (2001). Meaning of occupational engagement in life-threatening illness: A qualitative pilot project. *Canadian Journal of Occupational Therapy, 68*(4), 237-246.

Walker, C. (2001). Occupational adaptation in action: Shift workers and their strategies. *Journal of Occupational Science, 8*(1), 3.

Wikström, I., Isacsson, Å., & Jacobsson, T. H. (2001). Leisure activities in rheumatoid arthritis: Change after disease onset and associated factors. *British Journal of Occupational Therapy, 64*(2), 87-92.

Ziviani, J., Boyle, M., & Rodger, S. (2001). An introduction to play and the preschool child with autistic spectrum disorder. *British Journal of Occupational Therapy, 64*(1), 17-22.

2000

Allen, J. M., Kellegrew, D. H., & Jaffe, D. (2000). The experience of pet ownership as a meaningful occupation. *Canadian Journal of Occupational Therapy, 67*(4), 271-278.

Björklund, A., & Svensson, T. (2000). Health, the body and occupational therapy. *Scandinavian Journal of Occupational Therapy, 7*(1), 26-32.

Boyer, G., Hachey, R., & Mercier, C. (2000). Perceptions of occupational performance and subjective quality of life in persons with severe mental illness. *Occupational Therapy in Mental Health, 15*(2), 1-15.

Breeden, L. E., Fultz, R. L., Gersbacher, C. A., Murrell, J. L., Pedersen, K. D., Thomas, K. E., & Hanna-Stewart, J. (2000). The relationship among demographic variables, professionalism, and level of involvement in a state occupational therapy association. *Occupational Therapy in Health Care, 12*(2), 53-72.

Crist, P. H., Davis, C. G., & Coffin, P. S. (2000). The effects of employment and mental health status on the balance of work, play/leisure, self-care, and rest. *Occupational Therapy in Mental Health, 15*(1), 27-42.

Davis, S. F., & Bannigan, K. (2000). Priorities in mental health research: The results of a live research project. *British Journal of Occupational Therapy, 63*(3), 98-104.

Dennis, D. M., & Rebeiro, K. L. (2000). Occupational therapy in pediatric mental health: Do we practice what we preach? *Occupational Therapy in Mental Health, 16*(2), 5-25.

Dyck, I., & Jongbloed, L. (2000). Women with multiple sclerosis and employment issues: A focus on social and institutional environments. *Canadian Journal of Occupational Therapy, 67*(5), 337-346.

Evans, R. (2000). The effect of electrically powered indoor/outdoor wheelchairs on occupation: A study of users' views. *British Journal of Occupational Therapy, 63*(11), 547-553.

Farber, R. S. (2000). Mothers with disabilities: In their own voice. *American Journal of Occupational Therapy, 54*(3), 260-268.

Francis-Connolly, E. (2000). Toward an understanding of mothering: A comparison of two motherhood stages. *American Journal of Occupational Therapy, 54*(3), 281-289.

Gilbertson, L., & Langhorne, P. (2000). Home-based occupational therapy: Stroke patients' satisfaction with occupational performance and service provision. *British Journal of Occupational Therapy, 63*(10), 464-468.

Green, S., & Cooper, B. A. (2000). Occupation as a quality of life constituent: A nursing home perspective. *British Journal of Occupational Therapy, 63*(1), 17-24.

Haglund, L., Ekbladh, E., Thorell, L., & Hallberg, I. R. (2000). Practice models in Swedish psychiatric occupational therapy. *Scandinavian Journal of Occupational Therapy, 7*(3), 107-113.

Hartman, B. A., Miller, B. K., & Nelson, D. L. (2000). The effects of hands-on occupation versus demonstration on children's recall memory. *American Journal of Occupational Therapy, 54*(5), 477-483.

Ivarsson, A., Söderback, I., & Stein, F. (2000). Goal, intervention and outcome of occupational therapy in individuals with psychoses. Content analysis through a chart review. *Occupational Therapy International, 7*(1), 21-41.

Josephsson, S., Bäckman, L., Nygård, L., & Borell, L. (2000). Non-professional caregivers' experience of occupational performance on the part of relatives with dementia: Implications for caregiver program in occupational therapy. *Scandinavian Journal of Occupational Therapy, 7*(2), 61-66.

Kao, C., & Kellegrew, D. H. (2000). Self-concept, achievement and occupation in gifted Taiwanese adolescents. *Occupational Therapy International, 7*(2), 121-133.

Kingsley, P., & Molineux, M. (2000). True to our philosophy? Sexual orientation and occupation. *British Journal of Occupational Therapy, 63*(5), 205-210.

Laliberte-Rudman, D., Yu, B., Scott, E., & Pajouhandeh, P. (2000). Exploration of the perspectives of persons with schizophrenia regarding quality of life. *American Journal of Occupational Therapy, 54*(2), 137-147.

Larson, E. A. (2000). The orchestration of occupation: The dance of mothers. *American Journal of Occupational Therapy, 54*(3), 269-280.

Liu, K., Chan, C., & Hui-Chan, C. (2000). Clinical reasoning and the occupational therapy curriculum. *Occupational Therapy International, 7*(3), 173-183.

Lo, J., & Huang, S. (2000). Affective experiences during daily occupations: Measurement and results. *Occupational Therapy International, 7*(2), 134-144.

Mandich, A. D., Polatajko, H. J., Missiuna, C., & Miller, L. T. (2000). Cognitive strategies and motor performance in children with developmental coordination disorder. *Physical & Occupational Therapy in Pediatrics, 20*(2), 125-143.

McColl, M. A., Paterson, M., Davies, D., Doubt, L., & Law, M. (2000). Validity and community utility of the Canadian Occupational Performance Measure. *Canadian Journal of Occupational Therapy, 67*(1), 22-30.

McGrath, W. L., Meuller, M. M., Brown, C., Teitelman, J., & Watts, J. (2000). Caregivers of persons with Alzheimer's disease: An exploratory study of occupational performance and respite. *Physical & Occupational Therapy in Geriatrics, 18*(2), 51-69.

McKinnon, A. L. (2000). Client values and satisfaction with occupational therapy. *Scandinavian Journal of Occupational Therapy, 7*(3), 99-106.

Mee, J. D. (2000). Focus on research … The value of occupation for people with enduring mental health problems. *British Journal of Occupational Therapy, 63*(5), 224.

Packer, T. L., Paterson, M., Krupa, T., Avtchoukhova, L., Tchebotareva, L., & Krasnova, L. (2000). Client outcomes after student community fieldwork in Russia. *Occupational Therapy International, 7*(3), 191-197.

Peachey-Hill, C., & Law, M. (2000). Impact of environmental sensitivity on occupational performance. *Canadian Journal of Occupational Therapy, 67*(5), 304-313.

Pierce, D. (2000). Maternal management of the home as a developmental play space for infants and toddlers. *American Journal of Occupational Therapy, 54*(3), 290-299.

Primeau, L. (2000). Divisions of household work, routines, and child care occupations in families. *Journal of Occupational Science, 7*(1), 19-28.

Rebeiro, K. L. (2000). Client perspectives on occupational therapy practice: Are we truly client-centred? *Canadian Journal of Occupational Therapy, 67*(1), 7-14.

Rice, M. S., & Thomas, J. J. (2000). Perceived risk as a constraint on occupational performance during hot and cold water pouring. *American Journal of Occupational Therapy, 54*(5), 525-532.

Segal, R. (2000). Adaptive strategies of mothers with children with attention deficit hyperactivity disorder: Enfolding and unfolding occupations. *American Journal of Occupational Therapy, 54*(3), 300-306.

Simmons, D. C., Crepeau, E. B., & White, B. P. (2000). The predictive power of narrative data in occupational therapy evaluation. *American Journal of Occupational Therapy, 54*(5), 471-476.

Stagnitti, K., Unsworth, C., & Rodger, S. (2000). Development of an assessment to identify play behaviours that discriminate between the play of typical preschoolers and preschoolers with pre-academic problems. *Canadian Journal of Occupational Therapy, 67*(5), 291-303.

Stewart, S., & Neyerlin-Beale, J. (2000). The impact of community paediatric occupational therapy on children with disabilities and their carers. *British Journal of Occupational Therapy, 63*(8), 373-379.

Turner, H., Chapman, S., McSherry, A., Krishnagiri, S., & Watts, J. (2000). Leisure assessment in occupational therapy: An exploratory study. *Occupational Therapy in Health Care, 12*(2), 73-85.

Unruh, A. M., Smith, N., & Scammel, C. (2000). The occupation of gardening in life-threatening illness: A qualitative pilot project. *Canadian Journal of Occupational Therapy, 67*(1), 70-77.

Van Deusen, J. (2000). The body image for four women recovered from alcohol abuse. *Occupational Therapy in Mental Health, 16*(2), 27-44.

Venable, E., Hanson, C., Shechtman, O., & Dasler, P. (2000). The effects of exercise on occupational functioning in the well elderly. *Physical & Occupational Therapy in Geriatrics, 17*(4), 29-42.

Whiteford, G. E., & Wilcock, A. A. (2000). Cultural relativism: Occupation and independence reconsidered. *Canadian Journal of Occupational Therapy, 67*(5), 324-336.

Financial Disclosures

Dr. Briano Di Rezze has no financial or proprietary interest in the materials presented herein.

Dr. Terry Krupa has no financial or proprietary interest in the materials presented herein.

Dr. Mary Law has no financial or proprietary interest in the materials presented herein.

Dr. Mary Ann McColl has no financial or proprietary interest in the materials presented herein.

Nancy Pollock has no financial or proprietary interest in the materials presented herein.

Debra Stewart has no financial or proprietary interest in the materials presented herein.

Dr. Michelle Villeneuve has no financial or proprietary interest in the materials presented herein.

Index